Brain drug targeting
The future of brain drug development

Innovation in the therapeutics of brain disorders depends critically on the delivery of drugs to the appropriate region of the central nervous system, across the blood–brain barrier. The thesis of this innovative and challenging book is that brain drug development has been restricted by the failure of adequate brain drug targeting, and that this is an increasingly urgent problem as developments in genomics lead to new generations of therapeutic macromolecules.

The author, a world leader in the study of the blood–brain barrier and its clinical implications, reviews the field of neurotherapeutics from the point of view of drug targeting. He surveys the scientific and clinical basis of drug delivery across biological membranes, including topics such as carrier-mediated transport, receptor-mediated transcytosis, genetically engineered Trojan horses for drug targeting, antisense neurotherapeutics, and gene therapy of brain disorders.

At a time when there are few significant new drug treatments in prospect for Alzheimer's disease, Parkinson's disease, stroke, brain cancer, or brain injury, this authoritative review will encourage a wide range of clinicians and neuroscientists to reexamine the development and use of drugs in treating disorders of the central nervous system.

William M. Pardridge is Professor of Medicine at UCLA School of Medicine and an authority on the blood–brain barrier. Among his many publications in this field, he is the editor of *Introduction to the Blood–Brain Barrier: Methodology, Biology and Pathology* (Cambridge University Press, 1998).

Brain drug targeting

The future of brain drug development

WILLIAM M. PARDRIDGE

Professor of Medicine
UCLA School of Medicine
Los Angeles

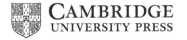
CAMBRIDGE
UNIVERSITY PRESS

CAMBRIDGE UNIVERSITY PRESS
Cambridge, New York, Melbourne, Madrid, Cape Town, Singapore,
São Paulo, Delhi, Dubai, Tokyo, Mexico City

Cambridge University Press
The Edinburgh Building, Cambridge CB2 8RU, UK

Published in the United States of America by Cambridge University Press, New York

www.cambridge.org
Information on this title: www.cambridge.org/9780521154468

First published 2001
First paperback printing 2010

A catalogue record for this publication is available from the British Library

ISBN 978-0-521-80077-8 Hardback
ISBN 978-0-521-15446-8 Paperback

Additional resources for this publication at www.cambridge.org/9780521154468

To Rhonda

Contents

Plates between pages 174 and 175
*These plates are available for download in colour from
www.cambridge.org/9780521154468

Preface

The theme of this book is that brain drug development in the twenty-first century will be limited by the innovation in brain drug-targeting science. In the twentieth century, drug development for the brain, and other organs, was a chemistry-driven science that created small molecule pharmaceuticals. These drugs are lipid soluble and have molecular weights under a threshold of approximately 500 Da. In the twenty-first century, central nervous system (CNS) drug development will be biology-driven and will create large molecule pharmaceuticals, such as recombinant proteins, monoclonal antibodies, antisense drugs, and gene medicines.

The singular driving force behind the future development of large molecule pharmaceuticals is the new science of genomics and the availability of the complete sequence of the human genome. The use of gene microarray technologies will enable the discovery of thousands of disease-specific genes, and thousands of secreted proteins and their cognate receptors. However, in the absence of a functional platform for CNS drug-targeting science, the large molecule pharmaceuticals cannot be delivered to brain and, accordingly, the therapeutic potential of these molecules will not be realized. When brain drug-targeting science develops, and the remarkable pharmacologic actions of large molecule pharmaceuticals in the brain are documented (because these molecules were actually delivered to brain cells), the development of large molecule neuropharmaceuticals will continue to expand in the twenty-first century. In this scenario, the separation of the "cart" and the "horse" is clear. Brain drug-targeting science is the "horse" and large molecule pharmaceuticals are the "cart." If brain drug-targeting science is not developed, then the large molecules will not be developed as neuropharmaceuticals.

Finally, if small molecule drugs are so effective, why should one even consider the need to develop large molecule pharmaceuticals, and thus the need to develop brain drug-targeting science? The answer to this question is found in another question. Can you name a single chronic disease of the brain that is cured by a small molecule drug? Indeed, can you name a single chronic disease of the body that is cured by small molecules? Are patients with brain cancer being cured? Are patients with solid cancers of the body being systematically cured? Small molecules do not cure solid cancer or chronic disease because small molecules are essentially pallia-tive medicines. Conversely, large molecule pharmaceuticals have the potential to be curative medicines. Cures for brain cancer and chronic diseases that are brought about by the development of large molecule pharmaceuticals in the twenty-first century must all pass through the blood–brain barrier. This can only happen with the development of brain drug-targeting science. The "magic bullets" of the twenty-first century will need their "magic gun."

William M. Pardridge
Los Angeles, June 2000

Abbreviations

%ID/g   percentage of injected dose per gram brain
3-NPA   3-nitropropionic acid
AA   amino acid
AAAD   aromatic amino acid decarboxylase
AAG α_1-acid glycoprotein
AAV   adeno-associated virus
ABC   ATP-binding cassette
Ac   acetyl
ACTH   adrenocorticotropic hormone
AD   Alzheimer's disease
AET   active efflux transport
AIDS   acquired immune deficiency syndrome
ALS   amyotrophic lateral sclerosis
AMP   adenosine monophosphate
ANP   atrial natriuretic peptide
APP   amyloid peptide precursor
ATP   adenosine triphosphate
AUC   area under the plasma concentration curve
AV   avidin
AZT   azidothymidine
BBB   blood–brain barrier
BCM   brain cell membrane
BCNU   1,3-*bis*(2-chloroethyl)-1-nitrosourea
BDNF   brain-derived neurotrophic factor
BEP   brain capillary-enriched protein
bFGF   basic fibroblast growth factor
bio   biotin
BMV   brain microvessels
BSA   bovine serum albumin

BSAT	BBB-specific anion transporter
BSP	brain capillary-specific protein
BTB	blood–tumor barrier
BT-CGAP	Brain Tumor Cancer Genome Anatomy Project
BUI	brain uptake index
CBF	cerebral blood flow
CCK	cholecystokinin
CDF	cholinergic neuron differentiation factor
CDR	complementary determining region
CHO	Chinese hamster ovary
cHSA	cationized human serum albumin
cHSA-AV	conjugate of cationized human serum albumin and avidin
cIgG	cationized IgG
Cl	clearance
CMT	carrier-mediated transport
CNS	central nervous system
CNTF	ciliary neurotrophic factor
Cpase E	carboxypeptidase E
CSF	cerebral spinal fluid
CTZ	chemical triggering zone
CVO	circumventricular organ
D_2R	dopamine-2 receptor
DAGO	Tyr-d-Ala-Gly-Phe(N-methyl)-Gly-ol
DDAB	didodecyldimethyl ammonium bromide
DDC	dideoxycytidine
DHA	docosahexanenoic acid
DHP	dihydropyridine
DIG	digoxigenin
DIG-II-UTP	digoxigenin-II-uridine triphosphate
dl-NAM	dl-2-amino-7-bis[(2-chloroethyl)amino]-1,2,3,4,tetrahydro-2-naphthoic acid
DMSO	dimethylsulfoxide
DPDPE	[d-penicallimine[2,5]] enkephalin
DRP	dystrophin-related protein
DSPE	distearoylphosphatidyl ethanolamine
DSS	disuccinimidylsuberate
DTPA	diethylenetriaminepentaacetic acid
DTT	dithiothreitol
EBNA	Epstein–Barr nuclear antigen
ECS	extracellular space

EDAC	*N*-methyl-*n*'-3' (dimethylaminopropyl) carbodiimide hydrochloride
EEG	electroencephalogram
EGF	epidermal growth factor
EGFR	epidermal growth factor receptor
ELISA	enzyme-linked immunosorbent assay
ENT	equilibrative nucleoside transporter
EPO	erythropoietin
EST	expressed sequence tag
EVAC	poly(ethylenecovinyl acetate)
FAB	fast atom bombardment
FDA	Food and Drug Administration
FDG	2-fluoro-2-deoxyglucose
FDG	fluorodeoxyglucose
Fe	iron
FGCV	$[^{18}F]$ganciclovir
FGF	fibroblast growth factor
FIAU	$[^{124}I]$-2'-fluoro-1-β-D-arabinfuranosyluracil
flt-1	vascular endothelial growth factor receptor
FPLC	fast protein liquid chromatography
FR	folate receptor
FR	framework region
G3PDH	glyceraldehyde 3-phosphate dehydrogenase
GABA	γ-aminobutyric acid
GAPDH	glyceraldehyde phosphate dehydrogenase
GASB	β-glucuronidase
GBM	glioblastoma multiforme
GDNF	glial-derived neurotrophic factor
GFAP	glial fibrillary acidic protein
GLUT	glucose transporter
GMP	guanosine monophosphate
GTPase	guanosine triphosphatase
HA-2	hemagglutinin
HBNF	heparin-binding growth factor
HD	Huntington's disease
HGF	hepatocyte growth factor
hHDL	human high density lipoprotein
HIR	human insulin receptor
HIV	human immunodeficiency virus
hLDL	human low density lipoprotein

HPLC	high performance liquid chromatography
HRP	horseradish peroxidase
HSA	human serum albumin
HSV	herpes simplex virus
HSV-tk	HSV-thymidine kinase
HTP	high-throughput
HTS	high-throughput screening
hVLDL	human very low density lipoprotein
Hz	hydrazide
ICAP	internal carotid artery perfusion
ICV	intracerebroventricular
ID	injected dose
IEF	isoelectric focusing
IGF	insulin-like growth factor
IgG	immunoglobulin G
IL-1ra	interleukin-1 receptor antagonist
IL-2	interleukin-2
IMAC	immobilized metal affinity chromatography
IR	insulin receptor
ISF	interstitial fluid
ISH	in situ hybridization
IV	intravenous
K7DA	$[Lys^7]$ dermorphin analog
K_D	binding dissociation constant in vitro
K_d	constant of nonsaturable transport
$K_D{}^a$	apparent dissociation constant in vivo
K_m	half saturation constant
KRC	Kety–Renkin–Crone
LAT	large neutral amino acid transporter
LDL	low density lipoprotein
LIF	leukemia-inhibitory factor
LRP	LDL-related protein
luc	luciferase
M6G	morphine-6-glucuronide
M6P	mannose-6-phosphate
MAb	monoclonal antibody
MABP	mean arterial blood pressure
MAL	maleimide
MALDI	matrix-assisted laser desorption ionization
MARCKS	myristoylated alanine-rich C kinase substrate

MBP	myelin basic protein
MBS	*m*-maleimidobenzoyl *N*-hydroxysuccinimide ester
MCAO	middle cerebral artery occlusion
MCT	monocarboxylic acid transporter
MDR	multidrug resistance
MHC	multiple histocompatibility complex
MLV	multivesicular liposomes
MMP	matrix metalloproteinases
MRgs5	mouse regulator of G protein signaling
MS	multiple sclerosis
MTFA	methyltetrahydrofolic acid
MW	molecular weight
nBSA	native bovine serum albumin
NBTI	*S*-4-nitrobenzyl-(6-thioinosine)
NGF	nerve growth factor
NHS	*N*-hydroxysuccinimide
NIMH	National Institute of Mental Health
NLA	neutral light avidin
Nle	norleucine
N-MDA	*N*-methyl D-aspartic acid
NO	nitric oxide
NOS	nitrous oxide synthase
NPC	nuclear pore complex
nRSA	native rat serum albumin
NSE	neuron-specific enolase
NSP	*N*-succinimidyl propionate
NT	neurotrophin
NTP	nucleotide triphosphates
oatp2	organic anion transporting polypeptide type 2
OB	leptin
OBR	leptin receptor
ODN	oligodeoxynucleotide
OPT	oligopeptide transporter
OR	opioid peptide receptor
orf	open reading frame
OVLT	organum vasculosum of the lamina terminalis
OX26	monoclonal antibody to rat transferrin receptor
OX26-NLA	conjugate of OX26 monoclonal antibody and neutral light avidin
OX26-SA	conjugate of OX26 monoclonal antibody and streptavidin
P	1-octanol/saline lipid partition coefficient

PAG	periaqueductal gray
PAGE	polyacrylamide gel electrophoresis
PAH	*para*-aminohippuric acid
PAS	periarterial spaces
PCR	polymerase chain reaction
PDI	protein disulfide isomerase
PE	phosphatidyl ethanolamine
PEG	polyethylene glycol
PET	positron emission tomography
PNA	peptide nucleic acid
PO	phosphodiester
PO-ODN	phosphodiester oligodeoxynucleotide
POPC	1-palmitoyl-2-oleoyl-sn-glycero-3-phosphocholine
PS	permeability–surface area
PS	phosphorothioate
PS-ODN	phosphorothioate oligodeoxynucleotide
PTH	parathyroid hormone
PTS	peptide transport systems
QAR	quantitative autoradiography
QSAR	quantitative SAR
QSTR	quantitative STR
RB	retinoblastoma
RES	reticuloendothelial system
RFC	reduced folate carrier
RGS	regulator of G protein signaling
RLU	relative light units
RMT	receptor-mediated transcytosis
RPA	RNAse protection assay
RRA	radioreceptor assay
RSA	rat serum albumin
S	thioether
SA	streptavidin
SAR	structure–activity relationship
SAS	subarachnoid space
SBF	salivary gland blood flow
ScFv	single chain Fv antibody
SCO	subcommissural organ
SDGF	Schwannoma-derived growth factor
SDS	sodium dodecylsulfate
SDS-PAGE	sodium dodecylsulfate polyacrylamide gel electrophoresis

SFO	subfornical organ
SH	sulfhydryl
SOD	superoxide dismutase
SPECT	single photon emission computed tomography
SR	scavenger receptors
SS	disulfide
SSH	suppressive subtractive hybridization
STR	structure–transport relationship
SUV	small unilamellar vesicles
STZ	streptozotocin
suc	succinylated
T_3	triiodothyronine
T_4	thyroxine
TCA	trichloroacetic acid
TCM	tumor cell membrane
Tf	transferrin
TFI	transient forebrain ischemia
TfR	transferrin receptor
TGF	transforming growth factor
TGN	trans-Golgi network
tk	thymidine kinase
TNF	tumor necrosis factor
TNFR	tumor necrosis factor receptor
tPA	tissue plasminogen activator
trkB	BDNF receptor
TTC	triphenyltetrazolium chloride
UTP	uridine triphosphate
UTR	untranslated region
V_D	organ volume of distribution
VEGF	vascular endothelial growth factor
VH	variable region of the heavy chain
VIP	vasoactive intestinal peptide
VIPa	VIP analog
VL	variable region of the light chain
V_{max}	maximal transport capacity
V_O	plasma volume of distribution
WGA	wheat germ agglutinin
XX	*bis*-aminohexanoyl
ZO	zonula occludin

Drug targeting, drug discovery, and brain drug development

The brain of all vertebrates is protected from substances in the blood by the blood–brain barrier (BBB). Owing to the presence of the BBB, >98% of new drugs discovered for the central nervous system (CNS) do not enter the brain following systemic administration. Twentieth-century CNS drug development, like drug development in general, relied almost exclusively on small molecule pharmaceuticals, as it was generally believed that small molecules cross the BBB. In fact, most small molecules do not cross the BBB, as reviewed in Chapter 3. The few small molecules that did cross the BBB enabled twentieth-century CNS drug development to focus on small molecule drug discovery without a parallel program in CNS drug targeting. The sole reliance on small molecules will change in the twenty-first century as large molecule pharmaceuticals are developed. Large molecule drugs are peptides, recombinant proteins, monoclonal antibodies, antisense drugs, and gene medicines. Since these large molecule drugs do not cross the BBB, it will not be possible to develop large molecules as CNS pharmaceuticals unless there is a parallel development of BBB drug-targeting technology. The future of brain drug development will, therefore, be limited by progress in brain drug targeting.

The driving force in the discovery and development of large molecule drugs is the emerging new science of genomics (Figure 1.1). The application of genomics technologies and gene microarrays, in parallel with the availability of the complete sequence of the human genome, will lead to the discovery of thousands of new gene targets, and thousands of new secreted proteins. These discoveries will enable the development of new protein drugs, antisense drugs, and gene therapy. The future will show that large molecule drugs are more likely to be curative medicines, as opposed to the largely palliative effects of small molecule drugs. Thus, the change from chemistry-driven discovery of small molecules to biology-driven large molecule drugs will be paralleled by the development of drugs that actually cure cancer or chronic disease, as opposed to simple amelioration of disease symptoms and marginal prolongation of life.

The small molecule paradigm emanated from the success of penicillin treatment

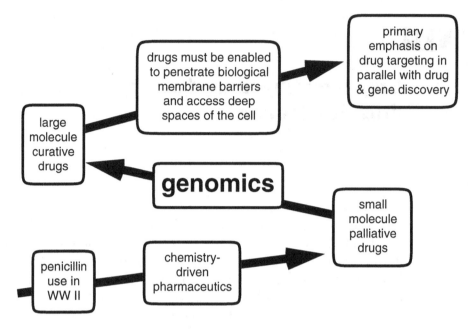

Figure 1.1   The emergence of large molecule therapeutics is driven by the new genomics sciences, and the availability of the human genome sequence. Large molecule drugs offer the opportunity of virtually eliminating the signs and symptoms of disease, but these large molecules must be targeted to the deep spaces (nucleus, cytosol) within the cell. Drug-targeting systems enable the development of large molecule therapeutics. In the new paradigm of drug development, drug targeting is a primary focus of overall drug development.

of severe infections in World War II. Over the next 50 years, numerous small molecule drugs were discovered and proved to be useful, palliative medicines. However, no chronic diseases of the brain, or for that matter any chronic diseases other than infections or vitamin deficiencies, have been cured by small molecule therapy. Some cancers are cured by small molecule chemotherapeutics discovered in the 1960s, but there have been few advances in the last 40 years, and there has been no dramatic decrease in either mortality from cancer or morbidity from chronic disease. The vast majority of people treated with small molecule chemotherapeutics still die from cancer, and there is not a single chronic disease of the brain, or any other organ, that has been cured by small molecule therapeutics. The singular focus on small molecules, and the belief that small molecules can readily traverse biological membranes, is the reason that drug targeting science is so underdeveloped.

The need to develop curative, not palliative, medicines for the brain is derived from the enormity of the impact of brain diseases. Chronic diseases of the brain are the principal cause of morbidity and the number of individuals that suffer from

Table 1.1 Brain disorders in the United States

Disorder	Affected individuals
Migraine headache	25 000 000
Alcohol abuse	25 000 000
Anxiety/phobia	25 000 000
Sleep disorders	20 000 000
Depression/mania	12 000 000
Obsessive-compulsive disorder	10 000 000
Alzheimer's disease	4 000 000
Schizophrenia	3 000 000
Stroke	2 000 000
Epilepsy	2 000 000
HIV infection	1 500 000
Parkinson's disease	500 000

Notes:
HIV, human immunodeficiency virus.
From Pardridge (1991) with permission.

chronic diseases of the brain dwarfs the number of people stricken with cancer and heart disease combined. In the United States alone, over 80 million individuals have some disorder of the brain (Table 1.1). A National Institute of Mental Health (NIMH) epidemiological study showed that one out of three individuals in the United States has a brain disorder in a lifetime (Regier et al., 1988). The economic impact of chronic brain disorders is large. In the case of Alzheimer's disease (AD) alone, the annual cost in the United States is between $70 billion and $90 billion a year for doctors, drugs, and other medical therapy. This situation will only worsen in the twenty-first century when more individuals live to 85 years and beyond, a point where approximately 50% of the population develops AD.

The large number of individuals suffering from chronic brain diseases underlies the enormous potential growth of the neuropharmaceutical market. However, >98% of all potential new brain drugs do not cross the BBB. As discussed in Chapter 3, the BBB is formed by epithelial-like tight junctions, which are expressed by the brain capillary endothelial cell. The formation of tight junctions in the brain capillary endothelium is an example of tissue-specific gene expression, and other examples of tissue-specific gene expression within the brain capillary endothelium are discussed in Chapter 10. The BBB is laid down in the first trimester of human fetal life, and is present in the brains of all vertebrates. The failure of histamine, a small molecule of 111 Da, to cross the BBB in brain or spinal cord is illustrated in Figure 1.2. The absence of brain uptake of histamine (Figure 1.2) is mimicked by

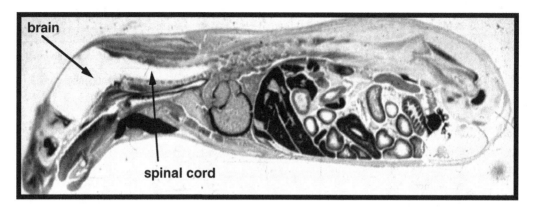

brain

spinal cord

Figure 1.2   Film autoradiogram of a mouse sacrificed 15 min after the intravenous injection of radiolabeled histamine, a small molecule of 111 Da. Histamine does not cross the blood–brain barrier in the brain or spinal cord. Conversely, this molecule readily traverses the capillary bed and enters all other tissues of the body.

hundreds of new CNS drugs discovered every year. These drug programs are terminated because of the BBB problem.

Despite the facts that (a) more than 80 million individuals in the United States alone have some disorder of the brain, and (b) >98 % of all new brain drugs do not cross the BBB, there is not a single pharmaceutical company in the world today that has a BBB drug-targeting program. This is the fundamental paradox in the neuropharmaceutical industry (Figure 1.3). A vice president of a large pharmaceutical firm in the United States once called to ask if the author's laboratory could measure whether a given drug crossed the BBB. The author suggested that the CNS section of this large pharmaceutical firm could perform such a measurement. The vice president of that firm replied that "no, they could not," owing to the lack of sufficient expertise within the company in the BBB field. This company, which is in the top three of US pharmaceutical companies, spends millions of dollars each year in developing new drugs for the brain yet lacks the expertise within the company to measure drug transport across the BBB accurately.

The pharmaceutical industry does not develop BBB drug-targeting programs because it is believed that small molecules freely cross the BBB. However, as discussed in Chapter 3, this is a misconception. Small molecules cross the BBB in pharmacologically significant amounts if the molecule has the dual molecular characteristics of (a) lipid-solubility, and (b) a molecular weight <400–600 Da (Pardridge, 1998a). Virtually all small molecule drugs that emanate from receptor-based high-throughput drug-screening programs will lack these dual molecular characteristics, and will not cross the BBB in the absence of brain drug-targeting

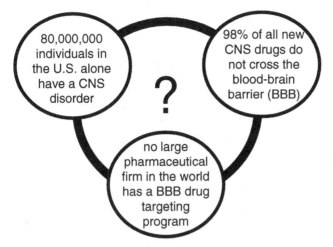

Figure 1.3   The fundamental paradox of the neuropharmaceutical industry is that no large pharmaceutical firm in the world has a blood–brain barrier (BBB) drug-targeting program despite
the fact that >98% of all new drugs for the central nervous system (CNS) do not cross
the BBB.

strategies. In this event, the fate of the CNS drug development program is termination (Figure 1.4).

The large pharmaceutical firms focus on small molecule drugs, and biotechnology companies develop large molecule therapeutics. However, none of the large
molecule pharmaceutical products of biotechnology, i.e., peptide or protein therapeutics, monoclonal antibodies, antisense or gene medicines, cross the BBB (Table
1.2). Peptide and protein therapeutics are presently a >$10 billion annual market
in the pharmaceutical industry and none of these drugs is, or will be, used for the
treatment of brain disorders, because peptides do not cross the BBB. The neurotrophic factors are a case study of the failure of protein-based therapeutics for the
treatment of brain diseases (see below). Monoclonal antibodies are the largest
group of biotechnology drugs either presently in clinical trials or before the Food
and Drug Administration (FDA) and none of these monoclonal antibodies is
used for brain disorders because monoclonal antibodies do not cross the BBB
(Pardridge et al., 1995c). The human genome is now fully sequenced and will give
rise to new antisense or gene medicines that could be applied to the treatment of
brain disorders. However, antisense and gene medicines do not cross the BBB and
these new therapeutics will not be used to treat brain disorders.

The consequences of the lack of even a rudimentary expertise in brain drug targeting in the biotechnology or large pharmaceutical companies are profound, as
illustrated below.

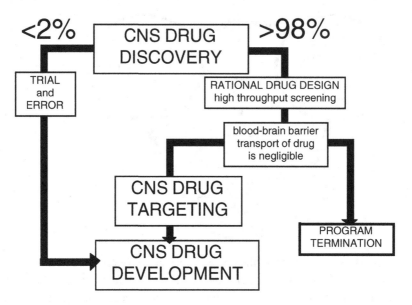

Figure 1.4   Central nervous system (CNS) drug discovery, drug targeting, and drug development. More than 98% of all drugs originating in a CNS drug discovery program do not cross the BBB. Therefore, in the absence of a BBB drug-targeting program, the CNS drug development ends in program termination.

- In the mid-1990s, the neurotrophins were held as promising new treatments of stubborn neurological diseases, such as Lou Gehrig's disease (amyotrophic lateral sclerosis, ALS) or AD, and clinical trials were initiated for the treatment of neuro-degenerative diseases (The BDNF Study Group, 1999). These "large molecule" protein drugs do not cross the BBB, and because the drugs never reached the target neurons, the phase III clinical trials failed. In general, the neurotrophins are no longer developed by the pharmaceutical or biotechnology industry for CNS disorders.
- The three drugs that form the "triple therapy" of acquired immune deficiency syndrome (AIDS) were hailed as a cure for this disease (Hogg et al., 1998). However, the human immunodeficiency virus (HIV) strongly infects the brain early in the course of the infection in virtually all subjects, and none of the three drugs forming the triple therapy of AIDS cross the BBB. Therefore, the virus is harbored within the sanctuary of the brain behind the BBB, and the virus cannot be effectively eradicated from the brain with present-day AIDS triple therapy.
- The gene for Huntington's disease (HD) was identified several years ago and shown to have CAG repeats which cause glutamine repeats in the huntingtin protein (Gutekunst et al., 1995). This classical genetic disease of the brain could be treated with antisense therapy designed selectively to block the huntingtin

Table 1.2 Neuropharmaceuticals and blood–brain barrier (BBB) transport

Drug class	BBB transport
Peptides, proteins	No
Monoclonal antibodies	No
Antisense drugs	No
Gene medicine	No
Small molecules	
Lipid-soluble, MW <600 Da	Yes
Lipid-insoluble, MW >600 Da	No

Note:
MW, molecular weight.

transcript containing the CAG repeats. However, no antisense therapy can be developed for HD because antisense drugs do not cross the BBB.

- Gene therapy for human brain tumors was pronounced as a potential cure for this disease, despite the fact that no system existed for safely targeting the new gene medicines through the BBB (Weyerbrock and Oldfield, 1999). Recently, virtually all efforts by the pharmaceutical industry to treat brain tumors with gene therapy have been terminated.
- There are numerous single-gene defect diseases that have devastating effects on the children of adult carriers, such as Rett's syndrome, fragile X syndrome, Canavan's disease, the mucopolysaccaridoses, Tay–Sachs disease, and many others. All of the diseases have support groups formed by the parents of afflicted children. In all cases, the mutated gene is known and cloned. But, copies of these potentially life-saving genes sit in bottles in research laboratories because there is no means of expressing an exogenous gene throughout the brain.
- Monoclonal antibodies or peptide radiopharmaceuticals offer the promise of diagnosing a wide variety of brain disorders, but no such tests have been developed because the imaging agents do not cross the BBB. The most glaring shortfall in this area is the lack of a diagnostic test for AD. AD is caused by the deposition within the brain of amyloid, which is formed by a 43 amino acid peptide, designated $A\beta^{1-43}$. Amyloid imaging agents, including truncated forms of $A\beta^{1-43}$, exist and could be used for the development of an AD amyloid brain scan, but these agents do not cross the BBB (Wu et al., 1997b).
- The development of new drugs and neuroprotective agents for the treatment of stroke or brain trauma has been slow, because most of the new agents discovered do not cross the BBB, as illustrated by one neurotrophin, brain-derived neurotrophic factor (BDNF) (Wu and Pardridge, 1999b).

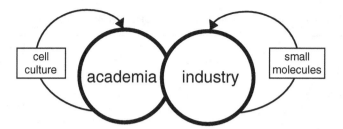

Figure 1.5   The two principal platforms underlying present-day brain drug development are academia
and industry. Owing to a primary emphasis of academic research on tissue culture model
systems, brain drug-targeting strategies are not required. There are few, if any, significant
biological barriers to drug transport in a cell culture system. In industry, the focus is
primarily on the development of small molecules, owing to the belief that small
molecules do not require membrane barrier drug-targeting systems.

• The imaging of gene expression in the brain with antisense radiopharmaceuticals
is not possible, because antisense drugs do not cross the BBB (Pardridge et al.,
1995a). Without the capability of imaging gene expression, genetic counseling
will be based solely on testing for the presence of a gene in an individual, not
whether that particular gene is actually expressed at a given time. The need to
develop technology that enables imaging gene expression in vivo in humans will
become even more acute in the future as the human genome sequence is further
analyzed. Genomics programs will identify thousands of genes that are uniquely
expressed in a given condition, and >99% of these uniquely expressed genes will
be unknown genes. The only way to image gene expression in vivo is with antisense radiopharmaceuticals (Chapter 8).

  The chronic underdevelopment of brain drug-targeting science is rate-limiting
for overall brain drug development (Figure 1.4). It is difficult to pinpoint the origin
of the underdevelopment of brain drug-targeting science, but this certainly parallels the chronic underdevelopment of the molecular and cellular biology of the
BBB within the overall neurosciences. The two sectors that might give rise to the
development of effective brain drug-targeting science are industry and academia
(Figure 1.5). However, brain drug development in industry is focused solely on the
development of small molecule drugs. Given the belief that small molecules freely
cross biological membranes, including the BBB, and do not need targeting mechanisms, industry has not developed brain drug-targeting science. The development
of brain drug-targeting science within academia has been hindered by the oftentimes sole reliance of academic research on cell culture systems. In cell culture there
is no endothelial barrier or BBB, and targeting science is not needed. The chronic

underdevelopment of the molecular and cellular biology of the brain capillary endothelium within the overall neurosciences has led to the present-day situation where there are very few scientists trained worldwide in BBB research on an annual basis. Large pharmaceutical firms lack individuals trained in BBB science, so BBB issues are rarely articulated within the company. Even if a large pharmaceutical firm desired to establish a free-standing BBB drug-targeting program, it would be very difficult to recruit a sufficient number of BBB-trained scientists to that program. All of these factors help promote the perception that the BBB is an insoluble problem, and oftentimes new treatments for brain disorders are discussed within a context that never even mentions the BBB problem.

The suppression of BBB drug-targeting research characterizes present-day brain drug development and is illustrated as a case study with the neurotrophins (Figure 1.6).

- Advances in the molecular neurosciences during the Decade of the Brain of the 1990s led to the cloning, expression and purification of >30 different neurotrophic factors (Hefti, 1997). These natural substances have powerful restorative and neuroprotective effects when injected directly into the brain. The neurotrophic factors are peptide and protein-based therapeutics that do not cross the BBB. Therefore, it is not expected that neurotrophic factors will have beneficial effects on brain disorders following the peripheral (intravenous, subcutaneous) injection of these substances.
- During the 1990s, several pharmaceutical companies spent several hundred million dollars to develop neurotrophic factors for a single neurological disease, ALS. All the protocols administered the neurotrophic factor by peripheral (subcutaneous) administration, even though the preclinical research showed the neurotrophic factors do not cross the BBB. Nevertheless, the clinical trials went forward, and all the phase III ALS trials failed.
- The direct intracerebral injection of genetically engineered cells secreting neurotrophic factors was attempted, but this strategy, in the main, proved unsuccessful, owing to the very small effective treatment volume (<1 mm³) around the cerebral implants (Krewson and Saltzman, 1996) (see Chapter 2).
- The intracerebroventricular (ICV) infusion of neurotrophic factors was attempted, but this approach also failed. The ICV infusion of drugs is comparable to an intravenous injection because drug infused into the ventricular space rapidly distributes into the venous circulation (Aird, 1984). Drug injected directly into the lateral ventricle distributes largely only to the *surface* of the brain and does not penetrate into brain (Figure 1.6). The invasive approaches such as intracerebral implants or ICV infusion cost in excess of $15 000 per patient just for the neurosurgical procedure. This would cost >$7.5 billion just to begin

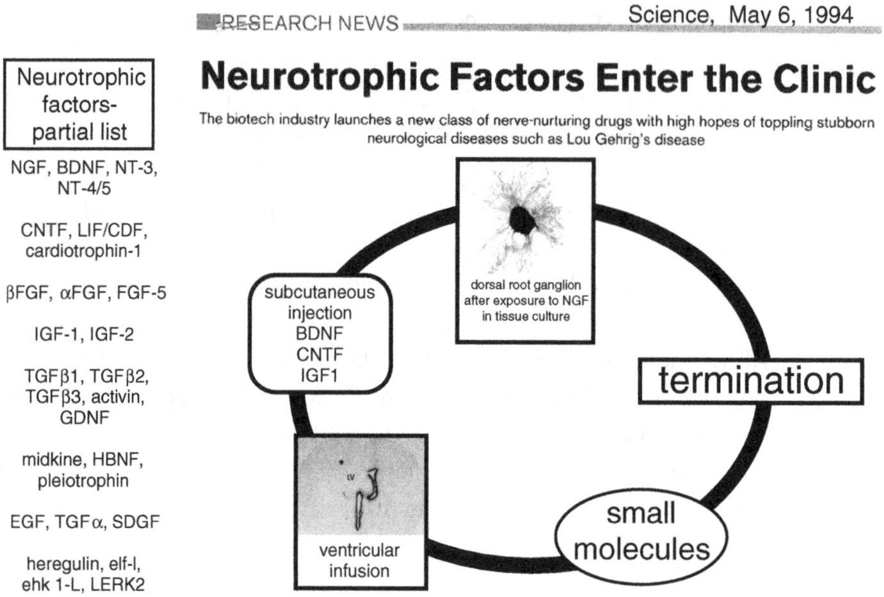
RESEARCH NEWS
Science, May 6, 1994
Neurotrophic Factors Enter the Clinic
The biotech industry launches a new class of nerve-nurturing drugs with high hopes of toppling stubborn neurological diseases such as Lou Gehrig's disease
Neurotrophic factors- partial list
NGF, BDNF, NT-3, NT-4/5
CNTF, LIF/CDF, cardiotrophin-1
βFGF, αFGF, FGF-5
IGF-1, IGF-2
TGFβ1, TGFβ2, TGFβ3, activin, GDNF
midkine, HBNF, pleiotrophin
EGF, TGFα, SDGF
heregulin, elf-l, ehk 1-L, LERK2
dorsal root ganglion after exposure to NGF in tissue culture
subcutaneous injection BDNF CNTF IGF1
termination
ventricular infusion
small molecules

Figure 1.6 There are >30 different neurotrophic factors that have remarkable neuroprotective and restorative effects when injected directly into the brain (Hefti, 1997). However, these molecules do not cross the BBB. Preclinical research and brain drug development of the neurotrophins was largely restricted to cell culture (Hefti, 1997), and the effects of nerve growth factor (NGF) on the dorsal root ganglion in cell culture are shown (Apfel, 1997). Largely on the basis of tissue culture studies, large clinical trials for neurotrophic factors such as brain-derived neurotrophic factor (BDNF), ciliary neurotrophic factor (CNTF), or insulin-like growth factor (IGF)-1, were initiated wherein the neurotrophic factor was administered by subcutaneous injection. None of these neurotrophic factors cross the BBB and the phase III clinical trials failed. Subsequently, pharmaceutical companies attempted to administer neurotrophic factors to the brain by ventricular infusion. However, as shown in the autoradiogram, the distribution of a neurotrophic factor into brain following administration into a lateral ventricle is restricted to the ipsilateral ependymal surface of the brain at 24 h after administration (Yan et al., 1994). The underlying physiologic reasons for the poor penetration of drug into brain parenchyma following intracerebroventricular (ICV) infusion are discussed in Chapter 2. Given the poor penetration into the brain of neurotrophic factors following either peripheral or ICV administration, these drug development programs were halted. It was believed that neurotrophic factor small molecules would be discovered and that these small molecules would cross the BBB. However, as discussed in Chapter 3, peptidomimetic small molecules, should they be discovered, would still need brain drug-targeting systems. Therefore, the fate of the neurotrophic factor drug development program ultimately is termination, because no BBB drug-targeting strategy was available. Abbreviations: NT, neurotrophin; FGF, fibroblastic growth factor; TGF, transforming growth factor; GDNF, glial-derived neurotrophic factor; HBNF, heparin-binding growth factor; EGF, epidermal growth factor; SDGF, Schwannoma-derived growth factor; LIF, leukemia-inhibitory factor; CDF, cholinergic neuron differentiation factor. The partial list of neurotrophic factors is adapted from Hefti (1997).

treatment of the 500 000 people with Parkinson's disease in the US alone. It is doubtful that third parties can pay for this.

At present, virtually all clinical trials of neurotrophic factors for CNS diseases have been abandoned by US pharmaceutical companies. The present focus is on the development of neurotrophic factor peptidomimetic *small molecules*. However, peptidomimetic small molecules tend to be antagonists, not agonists (Hefti, 1997). Moreover, small molecules cross the BBB only when the molecule is both lipid-soluble and has a molecular weight <500 Da threshold. Virtually all peptidomimetic small molecules will lack these molecular criteria and will still not cross the BBB without a drug-targeting strategy (see Chapter 3).

If most small molecule drugs still require a BBB drug-targeting system, then it is important to view brain drug development as comprised of two parts: brain drug discovery and brain drug targeting. This book focuses on the idea that innovation in brain drug-targeting strategies follows naturally from the investigation of the molecular and cellular biology of endogenous transport systems localized within the brain capillary endothelium that forms the BBB in vivo (Pardridge, 1991). Despite the success of L-DOPA treatment for Parkinson's disease, the targeting of endogenous BBB transport systems as a means of solving the BBB drug delivery problem has not been pursued by a critical mass of investigation. Rather, the history of drug (or gene) development for the brain has followed the same pathway (Figure 1.7). The primary emphasis has been historically devoted to the bypass of the BBB via craniotomy-based brain drug delivery, with a parallel effort at the disruption of the BBB (Figure 1.7). These invasive brain drug delivery strategies are reviewed in Chapter 2.

This book advances the theme that drugs must be administered to the brain by routes of administration no more invasive than an intravenous injection. This can be achieved by brain drug-targeting systems that utilize endogenous transporters at the BBB. The endogenous carrier-mediated transport (CMT) systems are discussed in Chapter 3. The receptor-mediated transcytosis (RMT) systems are discussed in Chapter 4. Endogenous peptides or peptidomimetic monoclonal antibodies, that bind specific receptor transport systems within the BBB (Chapter 4), may be used as molecular Trojan horses to deliver drugs across the BBB via endogenous peptide transport systems within the BBB (Chapter 5). The conjugation of the therapeutic to the targeting vector must be performed in such a way that the biological activity of both the drug and the vector are retained, and the linker strategies available for drug/vector conjugation are reviewed in Chapter 6. Peptide and protein therapeutics are potential new agents for both the treatment of neurologic disease, and the diagnosis of brain disorders with receptor-specific peptide radiopharmaceuticals, and these are discussed in Chapter 7. Antisense agents have the potential for arresting cancer and chronic disease by targeting tumor-specific

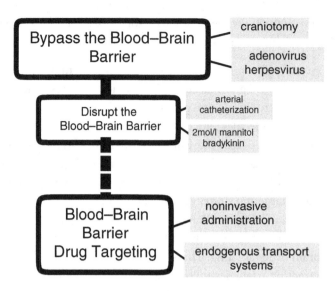

Figure 1.7   Drug or gene development for the brain has historically emphasized neurosurgical-based approaches that are invasive and require either craniotomy or arterial catheterization. In contrast, strategies for the noninvasive drug targeting to the brain emanate from the study of the biology of the endogenous transport systems within the BBB.

or viral-specific transcripts. Strategies for the brain targeting of antisense agents through the BBB in vivo are discussed in Chapter 8. Antisense radiopharmaceuticals also offer the promise of diagnosing brain diseases based on the expression of specific gene products in vivo, and the development of antisense radiopharmaceuticals for imaging gene expression in the brain in vivo is also discussed in Chapter 8. The ability to image gene expression in living subjects can greatly augment genetic counseling and inform individuals when a given pathologic gene is expressed in their lifetime. The promise of gene therapy of the brain will be realized when gene medicines can be targeted through the BBB following methods of administration no more invasive than an intravenous injection. The targeting of gene medicines to the brain is reviewed in Chapter 9. Finally, brain vascular genomics or "BBB genomics" is discussed in Chapter 10. The discovery of BBB-specific genes provides the platform for the discovery of new endogenous transport systems or endogenous receptor systems within the BBB. The discovery of such systems can provide the basis for future innovation in brain drug-targeting science and ultimately lead to the development of brain-specific drug-targeting systems.

2

Invasive brain drug delivery

- Introduction
- Neurosurgical implants
- Blood–brain barrier disruption

Introduction

Invasive brain drug delivery strategies have been the most widely used for circumventing the blood–brain barrier (BBB) drug delivery problem. The invasive strategies require either a craniotomy by a neurosurgeon or access to the carotid artery by an interventional radiologist. The neurosurgery-based strategies include intracerebroventricular (ICV) infusion of drugs, or intracerebral implants of either genetically engineered cells or biodegradable polymers. Thus, the neurosurgical-based strategies fundamentally emanate from the material sciences and employ controlled-release formulations, which is a classical drug delivery strategy (Figure 2.1). In contrast, the theme of this book is that brain drug targeting emanates from transport biology science, and is focused on the endogenous BBB transport systems (Figure 2.1). In the absence of brain drug-targeting strategies that allow drugs to be transported *through* the BBB, then it is necessary to employ invasive strategies. These approaches either deliver drug *behind* the BBB, as with either ICV infusion or intracerebral implants, or physically *disrupt* the BBB following the intracarotid arterial infusion of noxious agents.

Neurosurgical implants

Intracerebroventricular infusion

Cerebrospinal fluid (CSF) physiology

The failure of a blood-borne agent to cross the brain capillary endothelial wall, which forms the BBB in vivo, is illustrated with the light microscopic histochemical study (Brightman, 1977), as shown in Figure 2.2. In this study, horseradish peroxidase (HRP) was injected either intravenously or by ICV injection. Following intravenous injection, the HRP fills the plasma compartment at the capillary level,

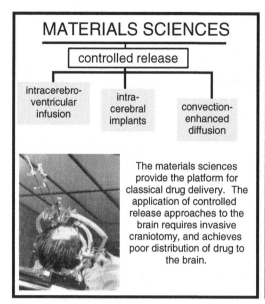

MATERIALS SCIENCES

controlled release

intracerebro-ventricular infusion

intra-cerebral implants

convection-enhanced diffusion

The materials sciences provide the platform for classical drug delivery. The application of controlled release approaches to the brain requires invasive craniotomy, and achieves poor distribution of drug to the brain.

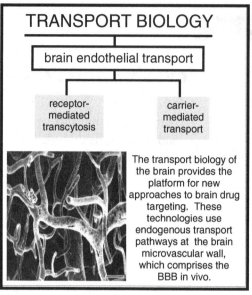

TRANSPORT BIOLOGY

brain endothelial transport

receptor-mediated transcytosis

carrier-mediated transport

The transport biology of the brain provides the platform for new approaches to brain drug targeting. These technologies use endogenous transport pathways at the brain microvascular wall, which comprises the BBB in vivo.

Figure 2.1   Two pathways to solving the brain drug delivery problem. Left: The neurosurgical-based strategies employ controlled-release drug delivery systems that are derived from the materials sciences. Reprinted from *Pharm. Sci. Technol. Today*, **2**, Pardridge, W.M., Non-invasive drug delivery to the human brain using endogenous blood–brain barrier transport systems, 49–59, copyright (1999), with permission from Elsevier Science. Right: Brain targeting utilizes the endogenous transport systems within the brain capillary endothelium, which forms the BBB in vivo. Brain drug-targeting is derived from the transport biology of either receptor-mediated transport or carrier-mediated transport across the brain capillary endothelium. The scanning electron micrograph of a vascular cast of the human cerebellar cortex is from Duvernoy et al. (1983). The magnification bar is 40 μm.

but does not traverse the BBB and does not enter brain parenchyma (Figure 2.2A). The exception to this rule is the median eminence at the base of the third ventricle. The median eminence is one of a half-dozen tiny areas of the brain around the ventricular system that lack a BBB, and these areas are called the circumventricular organs (CVO), as discussed below. When the HRP is injected into the ventricle, the protein distributes freely across the porous ependymal epithelial lining of the ventricle and diffuses into the subependymal space of brain parenchyma (Figure 2.2B).

BBB and blood–CSF barrier

There are two barriers in brain: the BBB and the blood–CSF barrier. The BBB is formed by endothelial tight junctions in capillaries perfusing brain (Brightman et al., 1970). The BBB segregates blood from brain interstitial fluid (ISF). The blood–CSF barrier is at the choroid plexus and other CVOs and is formed by apical

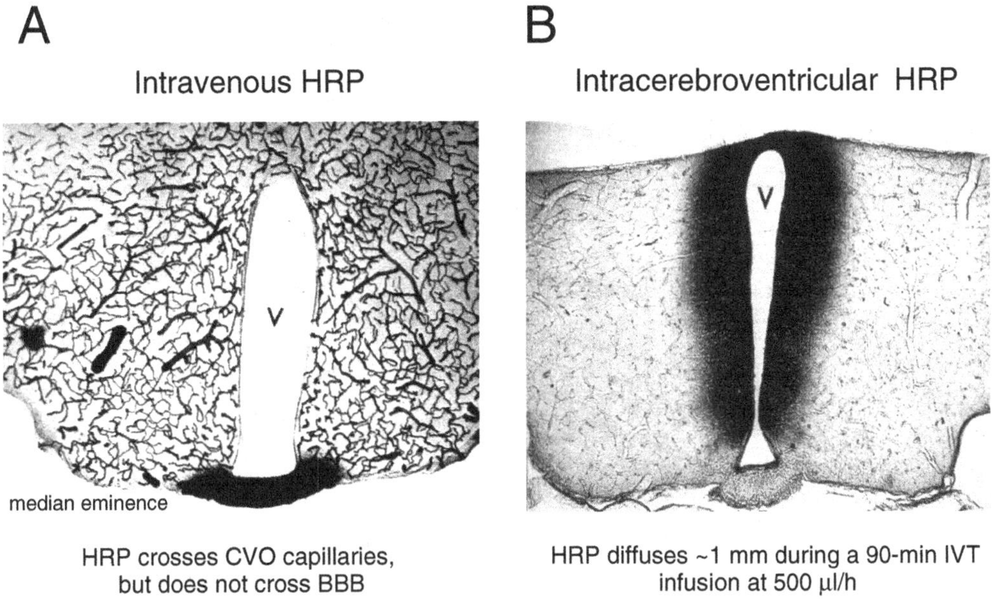

A

Intravenous HRP

median eminence

HRP crosses CVO capillaries,
but does not cross BBB

B

Intracerebroventricular HRP

HRP diffuses ~1 mm during a 90-min IVT
infusion at 500 µl/h

Figure 2.2   Light microscopic histochemistry following the injection of horseradish peroxidase (HRP)
in the mouse by either the intravenous (A) or the intracerebroventricular (B) route.
Following intravenous administration, the HRP is trapped within the capillaries of brain
parenchyma. HRP readily crosses the capillaries perfusing the median eminence at the
base of the third ventricle (V) and this circumventricular organ (CVO) lacks a BBB.
Following the ICV injection of the HRP, the protein diffuses approximately 1 mm during a
90-min period, a distance predicted from the laws of diffusion (see text). Further diffusion
into brain is restricted, because diffusion decreases with the square of the diffusion
distance. From Brightman et al. (1970) with permission. © 1970 The Alfred Benzon
Foundation, DK-2900, Hellerup, Denmark.

tight junctions in the epithelium of the choroid plexus (Brightman et al., 1970).
The blood–CSF barrier segregates blood from CSF. The BBB and blood–CSF
barrier are anatomically and functionally distinct (Figure 2.3). The tissue-specific
gene expression at the choroid plexus epithelium is markedly different from the
tissue-specific gene expression at the brain capillary endothelium. Consequently,
the type of transporters expressed on the plasma membranes at these two barrier
systems is quite different and a given drug may cross the blood–CSF barrier, and
enter CSF readily, but may not cross the BBB or enter brain ISF.

Drug entry and BBB permeability

Drug entry into CSF is not an index of BBB permeability. The entry of drug into
CSF following systemic administration is frequently taken as an index of BBB
permeability (Hengge et al., 1993; Owens et al., 1999). However, drug entry into
CSF is only a measure of blood–CSF barrier permeability, and is not a measure of

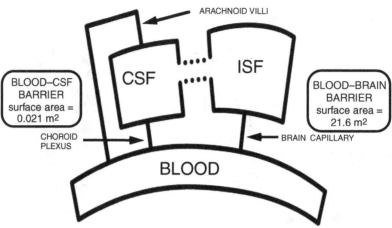

TWO BARRIERS IN BRAIN

Figure 2.3   The two barriers in brain are the blood–cerebrospinal fluid (CSF) barrier at the choroid plexus and the blood–brain barrier at the brain capillary. The blood–CSF barrier separates blood from CSF and has a surface area in the human brain of 0.021 m². The blood–brain barrier separates blood and brain interstitial fluid (ISF) and has a surface area of 21.6 m² in the human brain. Therefore, the surface area of the blood–brain barrier is >1000-fold greater than the surface area of the blood–CSF barrier. There is no anatomic barrier separating CSF and ISF, but there is a functional barrier owing to the continuous absorption of CSF into the general circulation at the arachnoid villi.

BBB permeability. An example of the distinct membrane transport properties at these two membranes is provided in the case of azidothymidine (AZT). As shown in Figure 2.4, systemically administered radiolabeled AZT does not cross the BBB and does not enter brain parenchyma (Terasaki and Pardridge, 1988; Ahmed et al., 1991). However, systemically administered AZT readily crosses the blood–CSF barrier at the choroid plexus and enters human CSF (Figure 2.4) (Yarchoan and Broder, 1987). Foscarnet is another example of a drug that readily distributes into CSF (Hengge et al., 1993), but does not cross the BBB. Therefore, it cannot be inferred that a given drug crosses the BBB just on the basis of its distribution into CSF.

The human immunodeficiency virus (HIV) causes acquired immune deficiency syndrome (AIDS), and the HIV infects the central nervous system (CNS). The dementia of AIDS improves on AZT therapy (Sidtis et al., 1993), but this is secondary to the decrease in viral burden in the blood. AZT therapy does not block viral replication within the brain. This is because AZT does not penetrate the BBB and does not enter brain parenchyma following systemic administration, as shown by the autoradiography studies in Figure 2.4. As discussed in Chapter 3, AZT is a rel-

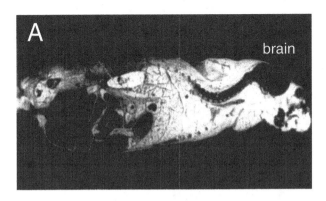

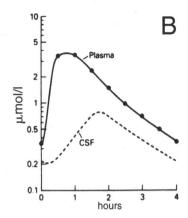

Restricted transport of AZT into brain   Rapid transport of AZT into CSF

Figure 2.4   Azidothymidine (AZT) crosses the blood–cerebrospinal fluid (CSF) barrier and enters CSF
but does not cross the blood–brain barrier and does not enter brain. (A) Film
autoradiogram of a mouse taken 2 min following the intravenous administration of
^{14}C-AZT. This small molecule readily traverses the capillary barrier in all organs except for
the brain or spinal cord. From Ahmed et al. (1991) with permission. (B) The concentration
of AZT in plasma and CSF in humans is shown following oral administration of 200 mg
AZT in adult humans every 4 h. From Yarchoan and Broder (1987) with permission.
Copyright © 1987 Massachusetts Medical Society. All rights reserved.

atively lipophilic molecule that enters CSF by transport across the choroid plexus
barrier via lipid mediation (Thomas and Segal, 1997). A similar transport across
the BBB does not occur because AZT is a substrate for active efflux systems at the
BBB (Galinsky et al., 1990; Dykstra et al., 1993; Takasawa et al., 1997). Any AZT
that passively influxes into brain is rapidly extruded from brain back to blood by
BBB active efflux systems (Chapter 3).

Brain barrier surface area

The two barriers in brain have vastly different surface areas. The surface area of the
BBB is 180 cm^2 per gram brain (Crone, 1963). For a 1200-g human brain, there is
a total BBB surface area of 21.6 m^2 (Figure 2.3). In contrast, the surface area of the
choroid plexus epithelia is 0.021 m^2 in the human brain (Dohrmann, 1970).
Therefore, the surface area of the BBB is >1000-fold greater than the surface area
of the choroid plexus epithelium, which forms the blood–CSF barrier. The large
BBB surface area means the extent to which a given molecule in blood enters brain
parenchyma is determined solely by the permeability characteristics of the BBB.
The distribution of circulating drug into brain via the transport through the
blood–CSF barrier followed by diffusion into brain is minimal, owing to rapid
export of drugs and solutes from CSF to blood.

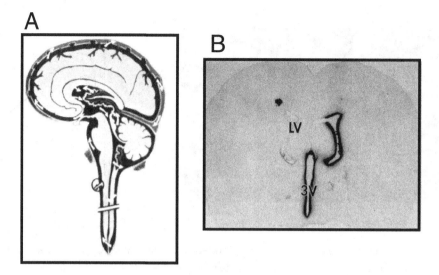

Figure 2.5   (A) Anatomy of CSF flow tracks in human brain. The CSF is produced at the choroid plexus at the two lateral ventricles, the third ventricle, and the fourth ventricle. The CSF then flows over the convexities of the brain and is absorbed into the superior sagittal sinus across the arachnoid villi. From Fishman (1980) with permission. (B) Film autoradiogram of rat brain 20 h after the intracerebroventricular injection of ^{125}I-brain-derived neurotrophic factor (BDNF). BDNF does not diffuse into the brain and is confined to the subependymal area in the ipsilateral lateral ventricle (LV) and the third ventricle (3V). There is minimal movement of the BDNF to the contralateral brain. From Yan et al. (1994) with permission.

Molecules in CSF are rapidly exported

Although circulating molecules only slowly gain access to CSF from the blood compartment, molecules that are injected into the CSF compartment are rapidly exported to blood (Rothman et al., 1961). CSF is produced at the choroid plexus of the two lateral ventricles, the third ventricle, and the fourth ventricle and the CSF is rapidly moved by bulk flow over the cerebral convexities and absorbed into the general circulation at the superior sagittal sinus across the arachnoid villi (Figure 2.5A). There are 100–140 ml of CSF in the adult human brain and approximately 50 ml of CSF in the infant human brain. The rate of CSF production, which is comparable to the rate of CSF absorption into the peripheral blood stream, in the human brain is about 20 ml/h. Therefore, the entire CSF volume in human brain is cleared every 5 h or 4–5 times in a day (Pardridge, 1991). This turnover is even faster in smaller animals and the CSF volume in a mouse brain is turned over every 2 h or approximately 12 times per day. Owing to the rapid exit of drug from the CSF compartment to the blood stream, an ICV injection is like a slow intravenous infusion (Fishman and Christy, 1965). Aird (1984) has shown that the dose of barbiturates that induce anesthesia in the dog is identical whether the drug is given by the intravenous route or by the ICV route. After the drug administration by the ICV route, the drug is rapidly exported from the brain via absorption across the arachnoid villi into the general circulation at the superior sagittal sinus (Pardridge, 1991). The drug then passes through the arterial system to reenter brain via transport across the BBB and the barbiturate then induces anesthesia (Aird, 1984). The rapid export of CSF to the blood is also illustrated in the case of a neuropeptide, cholecystokinin (CCK). Following the ICV injection of 5 μg of CCK into the rat, the peripheral blood level of the neuropeptide rises to a 2 nmol/l concentration within 30 min and this is sufficient to inhibit feeding via action on the peripheral nervous system (Crawley et al., 1991). Therefore, the ICV injection of a drug cannot localize a CNS site of action. In fact, an ICV injection is no different from a slow intravenous infusion (Fishman and Christy, 1965), and peripheral action of a drug can follow shortly after ICV administration.

The dual factors of slow drug diffusion into brain parenchyma from the ependymal surface and rapid drug export from the CSF compartment to blood both limit the efficacy of inducing CNS pharmacologic actions by ICV injection of drug. Certain drugs clearly have CNS pharmacologic effects following ICV administration. However, this is because the site of drug action in the brain is contiguous with the CSF flow tracks. For example, opioid peptides induce CNS-mediated analgesia following ICV administration (Bickel et al., 1994c). However the site of opioid action in brain is at the periaqueductal central gray region which surrounds the cerebral aqueduct in the midbrain (Watkins et al., 1992). Autoradiography studies of ICV-injected radiolabeled morphine show that the pharmacologic action in brain occurs in the ventricular wall (Herz et al., 1970). Thus, the distance morphine or opioid peptides must diffuse to the site of action from the ependymal surface is minimal. If CNS pharmacologic effects of a drug or peptide are observed following ICV administration, this suggests that the site of action of the drug within the brain is subependymal.

Circumventricular organs

The CVOs (Weindl, 1973) include the median eminence and the organum vasculosum of the lamina terminalis (OVLT) at the floor of the third ventricle, the subfornical organ (SFO) at the roof of the third ventricle, the subcommissural organ (SCO) and pineal gland at the back of the third ventricle, and the area postrema near the fourth ventricle. The CVOs are mid sagittal specializations of ependymal tissue that lie outside the BBB and appear to be involved in neuroendocrine regulation (Weindl, 1973). For example, there is a dipsogenic action of angiotensin II following the intracarotid arterial infusion of the peptide. This arises from the rapid distribution of the neuropeptide into the interstitial space of the subfornical organ, owing to the high permeability of the capillaries perfusing this CVO (Mangiapane and Simpson, 1980). The chemical triggering zone (CTZ) is in the brainstem and is sensitive to the blood level variety of pharmaceutical agents because this region is situated within the area postrema, a CVO that lacks a BBB (Borison et al., 1984). The cytokine, interleukin-1, induces fever by activation of arachidonic acid metabolism in the brain following systemic administration (Hashimoto et al., 1991). The cytokine is able to distribute into the brain parenchyma of the OVLT owing to the porous nature of the CVO capillaries perfusing this region. While the CVOs can be viewed as "portals to the brain," the surface area of the CVOs is trivial compared to the surface area of the choroid plexus, and as discussed above, the surface area of the BBB is 1000-fold greater than the surface area of the choroid plexus. Therefore, while the CVOs act in neuroendocrine regulation, they are not effective portals of drug targeting to the brain.

The pial membrane and the Virchow–Robin space

The pial membrane and Virchow–Robin space are illustrated in Figure 2.6 (Zhang et al., 1990). The pial membrane, which is leaky to circulating molecules, is equivalent to the ependymal membrane lining the ventricular compartment. The pial membrane extends to the capillary level in brain, where it is replaced by astrocyte foot processes on the arterial side of the circulation (Zhang et al., 1990). There is minimal pial membrane on the venous side of the cerebral circulation. The leakiness of the pial membrane causes a free communication of molecules in the subarachnoid space and the Virchow–Robin or perivascular space around cerebral arterioles that penetrate from the surface of the brain. Evidence was produced by Cserr (Cserr et al., 1981; Szentistvanyi et al., 1984) that tracers injected directly into the brain could pass from brain ISF through the Virchow–Robin space into the subarachnoid space of the frontal and olfactory lobes. In this way, molecules could move into the submucous spaces of the nose and to the cervical lymphatic circulation following intracerebral injection. Bulk flow through the brain principally occurs in white matter at a rate of 10 μl/min in the cat with minimal bulk flow in gray matter (Rosenberg et al., 1980).

The finding that drugs injected into the brain may move out of brain via the Virchow–Robin space suggests there can be rapid drug distribution to all parts of the brain following drug entry into the brain (Rennels et al., 1985). However, when radiolabeled molecules are injected directly into brain tissue, the molecule is generally not detected in CSF or other parts of brain (Leininger et al., 1991; Kakee et al., 1996). In another study, a dialysis fiber was placed in the cerebral cortex and atenolol was injected into the lateral ventricle of the rat (De Lange et al., 1994). However, no drug was found in the dialysis fiber within the cortex. Therefore, fluid

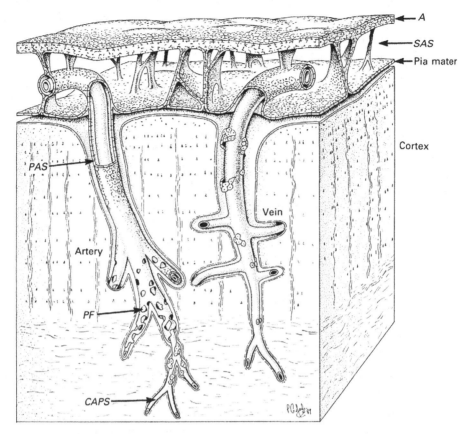

Figure 2.6   The Virchow–Robin space is equivalent to the periarterial spaces (PAS). The subarachnoid space (SAS) is just beneath the arachnoid membrane (A) and is situated between the arachnoid membrane and the pial membrane, also called pia mater, at the surface of the cortex. An artery on the left side is coated by sheath of cells derived from the pia mater and this sheath has been cut away to show the Virchow–Robin space of the intracerebral vessels. The layer of pial cells becomes perforated (PF) and incomplete as smooth muscle cells are lost from smaller branches of the artery. The pial sheath and Virchow–Robin space finally disappear as the perivascular spaces are obliterated around capillaries (CAPS). Reprinted from Zhang et al. (1990) with the permission of Cambridge University Press.

movement may occur along the Virchow–Robin space, but this is not a quantitatively significant pathway for drug or solute equilibration between brain and CSF.

Diffusion within the brain

The effective diffusion distance (x) of a molecule may be calculated from the following equation:

$t = x^2/D$

where t = time for diffusion and D = the diffusion coefficient with units of cm²/s. Diffusion coefficients are inversely related to the molecular weight and size, and the diffusion coefficients for sodium, glucose, myoglobin, and albumin are 20×10^{-6}, 6×10^{-6}, 1.1×10^{-6}, and 0.7×10^{-6} cm²/s, respectively (Pardridge, 1991). The molecular weights of these molecules are 23 Da, 180 Da, 17500 Da and 68 kDa, respectively. With the above equation it can be shown that the time it takes a molecule such as sodium, glucose, myoglobin, or albumin to diffuse 5 mm is 3.5 h, 11.7 h, 2.7 days, and 4.2 days, respectively. These calculations are based on the diffusion coefficients in water or aqueous solution, which are higher than the coefficients of diffusion in brain tissue in vivo (Fenstermacher and Kaye, 1988). A molecule such as HRP, which has a molecular weight of approximately 40 kDa, should diffuse 0.5 mm in 60 min, and this is what is experimentally observed when HRP is injected into the ventricular compartment (Brightman and Reese, 1969; Wagner et al., 1974).

Drug penetration following ICV injection

Drug penetration into brain is minimal following ICV injection. The diffusion equation predicts that the efficacy of molecular diffusion decreases with the square of the distance. This can also be shown when the concentration of drug in brain parenchyma is measured following an ICV injection. This was performed for a series of small molecules by Blasberg et al. (1975) in the rhesus monkey. The concentration of drug in brain parenchyma is only a fraction (<5%) of the drug concentration in the CSF at distances as short as 1–2 mm from the ependymal surface. The poor penetration of drugs into brain parenchyma following ICV injection is also shown in the autoradiography study of brain-derived neurotrophic factor (BDNF) in Figure 2.5B (Yan et al., 1994). In this study, radiolabeled BDNF was injected into one lateral ventricle and the rat was sacrificed 20 h later. This study shows that the BDNF has diffused only into the brain parenchyma immediately beneath the ependymal surface on the ipsilateral side of the brain. The BDNF moves into the third ventricle, then to the fourth ventricle, and then to the systemic circulation at the arachnoid villi with minimal movement into the contralateral brain. Owing to the one-way flow of CSF in the brain (Fishman, 1980), the distribution of drug to both sides of the brain following ICV injection would require the placement of catheters in *both* lateral ventricles. This would yield bilateral drug distribution to the human brain, albeit only to the brain immediately beneath the ependymal surface, as illustrated in Figure 2.5B. A minor amount of drug will be found on the contralateral brain following the injection into the lateral ventricle, but this arises from retrograde transport (Ferguson et al., 1991; Ferguson and Johnson, 1991). The drug that is injected into a lateral ventricle diffuses across the ependymal surface on the ipsilateral side where it is taken up by nerve endings terminating in that region. Following retrograde transport, the drug may be found in the cell bodies on the contralateral brain. However, this is a quantitatively minor pathway of drug delivery within the brain.

Drug delivery to brain after ICV infusion

In an early study, Noble et al. (1967) injected radiolabeled norepinephrine into the lateral ventricle of a rat and within 2 h found the drug in equal concentrations in the ipsilateral and contralateral brain. However, in this study, a volume of 30 μl was injected, which is twice the CSF volume in a lateral ventricle of a rat. Moreover, the ventricles were found to be dilated following this infusion, which was performed at high infusion pressures that distorted the normal physiology of CSF flow in the brain. When drug is infused into the ventricle, the typical finding is minimal penetration into brain on the ipsilateral side, much less the contralateral brain. For example, following the ICV infusion of interferon-α (Greig et al., 1988), the cytokine does not penetrate into brain tissue, owing to rapid export to the blood. Similarly, the ICV injection of a small molecule, 6-mercaptopurine, in the monkey did not result in significant drug entry into brain (Covell et al., 1985). The ICV infusion of insulin in the rat resulted in minimal distribution of the peptide into the brain, and insulin was found only on the ependymal surface (Baskin et al., 1983b). Following the ICV injection of interferon-β in the rhesus monkey, the cytokine was found to distribute rapidly into the blood, but not into the brain tissue (Billiau et al., 1981). The injection of ^{125}I-morphine, a neuroactive small molecule, into the lateral ventricle of humans was followed by brain scanning 60–90 min later (Tafani et al., 1989). These studies showed minimal penetration into the brain and after 90 min, only 5% of the morphine had distributed to the spinal cord and no drug was found lower than the thoracic spinal cord.

Neuropathologic effects of ICV infusion

When basic fibroblast growth factor (bFGF) is given by chronic ICV infusion at a dose of 1 μg/week over a 4-week period, there is astrogliosis in the ipsilateral periventricular area with increased immunoreactivity for glial fibrillary acidic protein (GFAP) (Yamada et al., 1991). The chronic ICV infusion of nerve growth factor (NGF) in the lateral ventricle of a rat for 7 weeks caused Schwann cell hyperplasia in the subpial region immediately contiguous with the site of ICV infusion (Winkler et al., 1997). Intracranial hypertension can be induced following the ICV administration of drugs (Morrow et al., 1990). In humans, the insertion of ICV catheters results in an approximate 6% complication rate that required repeat surgery (Chamberlain et al., 1997). The ICV infusion of human glial-derived neurotrophic factor (GDNF) resulted in a significant neurotoxicity that prompted discontinuation of the infusion in humans (Kordower et al., 1999). The common theme in these studies is that the brain tissue immediately contiguous with the CSF flow tract beneath the ependymal membrane is exposed to extremely high concentrations of drug following ICV infusion. For example, given a gradient of 0.001% at a distance of 2 mm from the ependymal surface, it would be necessary to achieve a ventricular CSF concentration of 500 000 ng/ml to generate a local brain concentration of 5 ng/ml (Pardridge, 1991). Owing to the logarithmic decrease in drug concentration in brain parenchyma with each millimeter removed from the ependymal surface (Blasberg et al., 1975), it is necessary to expose brain tissue around the CSF flow tracts to extremely high drug concentrations. In an animal study, NGF was chronically ICV-infused with a subcutaneously implanted osmotic minipump. The concentration of NGF in brain tissue contiguous with the lateral ventricle was increased fivefold to 5 ng/g, yet the NGF concentration in the reservoir was 200 000 ng/ml (Isaacson et al., 1990). In this study, the drug was infused at a rate of 0.5 μl/h, which is about 3% of the CSF secretion rate in the mouse. Therefore, the CSF concentration of the NGF was approximately 5000 ng/ml of NGF, or 1000-fold higher than the brain concentration of NGF

Intranasal drug administration

Drug delivery directly to the brain following intranasal administration of drugs has been investigated (Cool et al., 1990; Gizurarson et al., 1997). The evaluation of these studies requires a review of the anatomy of solute diffusion from the submucous spaces of the nose to the brain (Kristensson and Olsson, 1971). When dye is injected into CSF, it penetrates the subarachnoid space of the cribriform plate and enters into the submucous spaces of the nose. Moreover, axons originating from the olfactory lobe penetrate the mucosal basement membrane and enter into the submucous spaces of the nose and this may be a conduit for virus infection of the brain from the nasal compartment (Kristensson and Olsson, 1971). However, in order for molecules to enter the olfactory CSF following entry into the submucous spaces of the nose, the molecule must cross the epithelial barrier of the arachnoid membrane, which has tight junctions (Kristensson and Olsson, 1971). Thus, the entry of the molecules from the nose into olfactory lobe CSF is restricted by the same factors that control drug transport across a typical biological epithelial barrier. Drug or solute diffusion across any biological membrane occurs via one of two mechanisms: lipid-mediated transport of small lipid-soluble molecules or receptor-mediated transport. Sakane et al. (1991) have shown that the distribution of drugs into olfactory lobe CSF following intranasal administration is directly proportional to the lipid-solubility of a variety of small molecule drugs. However, in the case of peptides, it would be necessary for the peptide to access a receptor-mediated transcytosis system in order to traverse the arachnoid membrane. For example, when a conjugate of HRP and wheat germ agglutinin (WGA) was administered by intranasal administration, the HRP–WGA conjugate was found in the olfactory bulb (Thorne et al., 1995). Conversely, when HRP alone was administered, there was no HRP detected in the olfactory bulb (Thorne et al., 1995). This is because HRP does not cross biological membranes by active processes. The HRP–WGA conjugate binds to WGA lectin receptors, which triggers an absorptive-mediated transcytosis across either the arachnoid membrane (Thorne et al., 1995) or the BBB (Broadwell et al., 1988). In summary, unless there are specific receptors for the neuropeptide at the arachnoid membrane, it is unlikely that the intranasal administration of peptide-based drugs or other large molecule therapeutics would gain access to olfactory lobe CSF.

Lipid-soluble small molecules that are administered by intranasal administration will distribute to olfactory lobe CSF in proportion to lipid-solubility (Sakane et al., 1991). However, this is actually a mode of delivery to olfactory lobe CSF, and not to brain tissue per se. The olfactory CSF equilibrates with the remainder of CSF before undergoing rapid export from the CSF flow tracts to the systemic circulation via absorption at the arachnoid villi. Therefore, intranasal administration is analogous to an ICV injection, which is similar to a slow intravenous infusion. In either case, there is a nearly complete bypass of brain parenchymal tissue, with the exception of the olfactory lobe surface, following intranasal administration of lipid-soluble small molecules.

Intracerebral implants and convection-enhanced diffusion

Intracerebral implants

Similar to ICV infusion, there is minimal penetration of drug into brain parenchyma following release from an intracerebral implant of either genetically engineered cells or biodegradable polymers. The maximum distance of drug penetration into brain is approximately 1 mm following ICV infusion, microdialysis or intracerebral implantation (Mak et al., 1995). The concentration of a small molecule, 1,3-bis(2-chloroethyl)-1-nitrosourea (BCNU), is decreased by >90% at only 500 μm from the depot site following intracerebral implantation of a biodegradable polymer (Fung et al., 1996). The very circumscribed localization of drug following intracerebral implants is shown in the autoradiographic study for nerve growth factor (NGF), as illustrated in Figure 2.7A. This shows limited diffusion of NGF from the polymer site following intracerebral implantation of a polymer comprised of poly(ethylenecovinyl acetate) (EVAC). The use of intracerebral implants as vehicles for drug delivery to the brain is discussed further in Chapter 9 on the targeting of gene medicines to the brain.

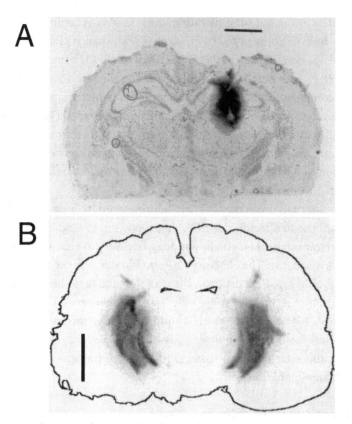

Figure 2.7   (A) Film autoradiogram of rat brain taken after the intracerebral implantation of a
biodegradable polymer comprised of poly(ethylenecovinyl acetate) (EVAC) embedded
with 10 mg of [^{125}I]nerve growth factor (NGF). The EVAC was implanted into the brain as a
disk with a diameter of 2 mm. The bar is a distance of 2.5 mm. Therefore, there has been
minimal diffusion of the NGF from the site of implantation at 48 h after administration.
Reprinted from *Brain Res.*, **680**, Krewson et al., Distribution of nerve growth factor
following direct delivery to brain interstitium, 196–206, copyright (1995), with permission
from Elsevier Science. (B) Film autoradiogram of cat brain following the intracerebral
infusion of [^{111}In]transferrin via convection-enhanced diffusion at a rate of 1.15 μl/min for
a total infusate volume of 75 μl. Bilateral cannulas were positioned stereotactically in the
corona radiata. The magnification bar is 5 mm. From Morrison et al. (1994) with
permission.

Convection-enhanced diffusion

The administration of drug to the brain following either ICV infusion (Figure 2.5B)
or intracerebral implantation (Figure 2.7A) is minimal owing to the poor penetration into tissue of drugs by diffusion. This is predicted by the equation for diffusion
(see above). The efficacy of diffusion decreases with the square of the distance from
the depot site. In contrast to diffusion, bulk flow (convection) is an effective drug
delivery vehicle. Convection-enhanced diffusion of drug delivery in the brain

involves the intracerebral infusion of fluid through the brain tissue at a rate of approximately 1 μl/min in the cat and 10 μl/min in humans (Morrison et al., 1994; Laske et al., 1997). Convection-enhanced diffusion has been used to treat human brain tumors with a 2-week intratumoral infusion of a conjugate of transferrin and a genetically modified diphtheria toxin (Laske et al., 1997). Convection-enhanced diffusion results in significant distribution of drug into brain tissue (Figure 2.7B). For example, in the cat, there is a mean radial spread of 3.2 mm following the infusion of 75 μl of transferrin labeled with ^{111}In at a rate of 1.2 μl/min (Morrison et al., 1994). Thus, convection-enhanced diffusion is the most effective of the neurosurgical-based strategies for delivering drug into brain parenchyma and seems particularly suited for the treatment of human brain tumors. However, even with this device, it would not be possible to deliver drug throughout brain parenchyma. This is also a highly invasive procedure that would require repeated craniotomy for subsequent administration of drug.

Blood–brain barrier disruption

Mechanisms of blood–brain barrier disruption

Brain capillary endothelium ultrastructure

BBB disruption results in generalized changes in brain microvascular permeability to circulating substances. The mechanism of BBB disruption may involve either opening of tight junctions, i.e., the paracellular pathway, or enhancement of endothelial pinocytosis, i.e., the transcellular pathway. The unique anatomic specializations of the vertebrate brain microvasculature are shown in Figure 2.8. These include epithelial tight junctions that are found in the BBB of all vertebrate brains and are laid down in the first trimester of human fetal life (Mollgard and Saunders, 1975). The evolution of the BBB tight junctions parallels the evolution of the myelination of brain, since both myelin and the BBB are found in all vertebrate brains. The presence of these very high-resistance endothelial tight junctions means there is no paracellular pathway for free diffusion of solutes through the BBB from the circulation. The BBB even restricts the transport of urea, which has a molecular weight of only 60 Da. When microperoxidase, a heme peptide of only 1800 Da, is injected intravenously, the molecule cannot enter brain because of the endothelial tight junction (Figure 2.8). The tight junctions also reduce the pinocytosis across the endothelium, i.e., the transcellular pathway (Figure 2.8). Therefore, the only way that circulating molecules can enter brain is to move through the endothelial plasma membranes via lipid mediation or catalyzed transport (carrier or receptor mediation), as reviewed in Chapter 3. Another anatomic specialization of the BBB is the presence of the astrocyte foot process, which envelopes >99% of the brain surface of the capillary endothelium (Figure 2.8), as reviewed in Chapter 3.

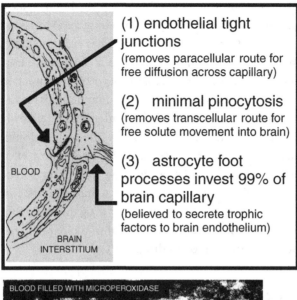

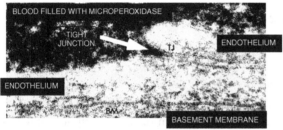

Figure 2.8   Top: The anatomic specializations of the brain capillary endothelium that form the blood–brain barrier (BBB) include endothelial tight junctions, minimal endothelial pinocytosis, and full investment of the abluminal side of the capillary endothelium by astrocyte foot processes. From Pardridge (1998a) with permission. Bottom: Electron microscopic histochemical study shows the anatomical basis of the BBB is the endothelial tight junction. In this experiment, a mouse was injected with microperoxidase intravenously, and the small heme peptide of molecular weight of only 1800 Da was confined to the vascular compartment. The entry of the heme peptide into the brain interstitial fluid was blocked at the endothelial tight junction. From Brightman et al. (1970) with permission.

Differentiation of paracellular and transcellular pathways

The paracellular and the transcellular pathways of BBB disruption can be distinguished ultrastructurally with electron microscopy. Alternatively, the two pathways can be differentiated with the measurement of the transport of solutes of varying molecular weight while the BBB is disrupted. If molecules of high and low molecular weight are transported through the disrupted BBB at equal rates, then the mechanism is molecular weight-independent and this is indicative of bulk flow via pinocytosis. Conversely, if the transport through the disrupted BBB is inversely related to the molecular weight of the drug or solute, then the mechanism is molecular weight-dependent and this is indicative of diffusion through pores of finite size, i.e., opening of tight junctions.

Biochemical mechanisms of blood–brain barrier disruption

The underlying biochemistry of BBB disruption may involve the action of nitric oxide (NO), which appears to play an important role in BBB disruption caused by certain vasoactive molecules such as histamine. L-NMA, an inhibitor of nitrous oxide synthase (NOS), blocks the histamine-mediated BBB disruption (Mayhan, 1996). NO donors block the BBB disruption of hyperosmolarity (Chi et al., 1997). Excitotoxic amino acids, such as glutamate, cause BBB disruption via an NO mechanism (Mayhan and Didion, 1996). Inhibitors of the receptor for *N*-methyl D-aspartic acid (NMDA) block the BBB disruption in cerebral ischemia (Belayev et al., 1995). The administration of intravenous kainic acid causes BBB disruption via an excitotoxic mechanism. In addition to signal transduction pathways, BBB disruption is also mediated by changes in endothelial cytoskeletal proteins. The intracarotid arterial infusion of cytochalasin B, which binds cellular microfilaments, results in BBB disruption by enhancing pinocytosis without changing endothelial tight junctions (Nag, 1995).

Osmotic BBB disruption

The intracarotid arterial infusion of hyperosmolar solutions of membrane-impermeant drugs causes disruption of the BBB, as first noted in the 1940s by Broman (1949). It was subsequently shown that the intracarotid arterial infusion of 1.7 mol/l mannitol causes BBB disruption in rats (Rapoport et al., 1980). The hypertonicity causes an osmotic shift in water flux at the endothelial–plasma interface and this results in shrinkage of endothelial cells and opening of endothelial tight junctions. Hyperosmolar disruption of the BBB has been used to increase the uptake of chemotherapeutic agents for the treatment of brain tumors (Neuwelt et al., 1982). However, the intracarotid infusion of hyperosmolar agents results in a greater disruption of the BBB in the normal brain relative to the brain tumor region (Hiesiger et al., 1986; Shapiro et al., 1988; Zünkeler et al., 1996). Conversely, BBB disruption mediated by a vasoactive molecule such as bradykinin is greater in brain tumors, relative to normal brain, in both experimental (Inamura and Black, 1994) and human brain tumors (Black et al., 1997).

Vasoactive blood–brain barrier disruption

Bradykinin

Vasoactive molecules such as bradykinin, histamine, serotonin, or vascular endo-thelial growth factor (VEGF) all cause BBB disruption (Gross et al., 1981; Unterberg et al., 1984; Winkler et al., 1995; Dobrogowska et al., 1998). After the initial observations that the application of bradykinin to pial vessels causes BBB disruption (Unterberg et al., 1984), it was subsequently shown that bradykinin analogs cause BBB disruption in brain tumors when infused directly into the carotid artery (Inamura and Black, 1994). Moreover, the intracarotid arterial infu-sion of bradykinin analogs resulted in the selective disruption of the BBB in experi-mental brain tumors and in human brain tumors relative to normal brain (Inamura and Black, 1994; Black et al., 1997). This presumably occurs because bra-dykinin does not normally cross the BBB in normal brain, but does cross the BBB of brain tumors, which is partially permeable compared to the BBB in normal brain. The bradykinin receptor mediating the BBB disruption is presumably on the abluminal side of the BBB and is exposed to circulating bradykinin analogs in a par-tially disrupted BBB within the brain tumor.

Histamine and serotonin

The intracarotid arterial infusion of histamine results in an increase in BBB perme-ability, and this increase is inhibited by H_2 antagonists, but not by H_1 antagonists (Gross et al., 1981). The intravenous infusion of serotonin causes BBB disruption, and this is neutralized by cyproheptadine, a $5HT_2$ blocker (Winkler et al., 1995). Since blood-borne vasoactive agents such as histamine or serotonin cause BBB dis-ruption, but do not cross the normal BBB (Oldendorf, 1971), the brain capillary endothelium must have receptors for these monoamines on the luminal membrane.

BBB disruption and artifacts in data interpretation

The intravenous coadministration of a vasoactive modulator of BBB permeability, e.g., bradykinin, and a radiolabeled marker of BBB permeability, e.g., sucrose or inulin, may result in an increase in brain radioactivity, measured as a percentage of injected dose per gram brain (%ID/g). The increase in %ID/g could be interpreted as being representative of biochemical BBB disruption caused by the vasoactive substance. In this case, the use of the %ID/g parameter as an index of BBB perme-ability assumes the %ID/g is proportional to the BBB permeability–surface area (PS) product, which is a quantitative measure of BBB disruption. As reviewed in Chapter 3, the relationship between PS and %ID/g is found in the "pharmaco-kinetic rule", i.e.:

$$\%ID/g = (PS) \times AUC$$

where AUC = plasma area under the concentration curve for the sucrose or inulin. If a vasoactive substance has an effect on peripheral distribution of the labeled compound, e.g., inhibition of glomerular filtration, then the plasma AUC of the labeled sucrose or inulin will increase, and this will yield a proportional increase in the %ID/g, with no change in the BBB PS product. Artifacts in interpretation of brain uptake data can be eliminated by quantitative methods that measure BBB permeability by converting the measurement of %ID/g into the PS product. Such quantitative methods necessarily involve measurement of the plasma AUC, and this can either be done graphically from serial samples of plasma radioactivity, or can be done with the external organ technique. In the latter method, a catheter is placed in the femoral artery, and blood is withdrawn at a constant rate during the experimental time period. Measurement of solute radioactivity in the arterial plasma blood sample provides instant integration of the plasma AUC for the experimental time period.

Cytokine-mediated blood–brain barrier disruption

The intracerebral injection of CXC chemokines results in BBB disruption and this is greater in suckling rats as compared to adult rats (Anthony et al., 1998a). The intracerebral injection of the cytokine, interleukin-1β, causes a loss in immunoreactive zonula occludin (ZO)-1 and occludin at BBB tight junctions. The interleukin-1β also causes an increase in brain capillary endothelial immunoreactive phosphotyrosine, and this is associated with an increase in adhesion to the brain endothelial cell of circulating polymorphonuclear leukocytes (Bolton et al., 1998). The activation of BBB protein phosphorylation with BBB disruption is of interest, because the activity of protein phosporylation at the BBB is as high as that at brain synaptosomes (Pardridge et al., 1985b), as reviewed in Chapter 4. Activated lymphocytes, even those lymphocytes activated against nonneural antigens, can cause BBB disruption (Westland et al., 1999). The administration of immune adjuvants, such as complete Freund's adjuvant or incomplete Freund's adjuvant, can cause disruption of the BBB in mice with increased brain uptake of immunoglobulin G peaking 2–3 weeks after administration of the adjuvants (Rabchevsky et al., 1999). The disruption of the BBB following the administration of the immune adjuvants may play a role in the beneficial effects caused by immunization of mice to Aβ synthetic peptides (Schenk et al., 1999). In this study, transgenic mice overproducing human Aβ amyloidotic peptide were immunized with Aβ Freund's adjuvants to generate a blood titer of anti-Aβ antibodies. The intent was to deliver these antibodies to the brain to inhibit or reverse the deposition of Aβ amyloid deposits. Since antibody molecules do not cross the BBB, it is not clear how the anti-Aβ antibodies in the blood can gain access to the brain to neutralize Aβ peptide deposited in the brain. However, the administration of Freund's adjuvants to mice results in prolonged disruption of the BBB (Rabchevsky et al., 1999), which would allow circulating antibody to enter the brain.

Miscellaneous forms of blood–brain barrier disruption

Matrix metalloproteinases (MMPs)

The intracerebral injection of MMPs, which are collagenase-like enzymes, results in BBB disruption (Anthony et al., 1998b; Mun-Bryce and Rosenberg, 1998). This effect is blocked by MMP inhibitors. The brain production of MMPs increases in stroke and the administration of anti-MMP monoclonal antibodies reduces the stroke volume in permanent middle cerebral artery occlusion in the rat (Romanic et al., 1998).

Cold or acidic solutions

The intracarotid arterial infusion of a variety of different agents can result in disruption of the BBB. These treatments are generally harsh biochemical applications, and include the intracarotid arterial infusion cold saline, detergents such as sodium dodecylsulfate (SDS), free fatty acids such as oleic acid perfused without albumin, or low-pH solutions (Sztriha and Betz, 1991; Oldendorf et al., 1994; Oztas and Kucuk, 1995; Saija et al., 1997).

Excitotoxic agents

Like kainic acid (Saija et al., 1992), systemic administration of the sugar cane toxin, 3-nitropropionic acid (3-NPA), which is an inhibitor of succinic dehydrogenase, causes encephalopathy and a lesion of the caudate putamen nucleus (Nishino et al., 1997). It also causes BBB disruption and infiltration of the brain by circulating polymorphonuclear leukocytes and a loss of local immunoreactive GFAP. The toxic effects are decreased by D_2 dopamine agonists and are enhanced by D_2 dopamine antagonists (Nishino et al., 1997).

Solvents

High systemic doses (1 g/kg) of ethanol or dimethylsulfoxide (DMSO) can cause BBB disruption, presumably by solubilizing the endothelial membrane (Brink and Stein, 1967; Hanig et al., 1972). These solvents are frequently used to solubilize drugs that are then given systemically. When administered to small animals, such as mice or rats, the dose of the ethanol or DMSO can equal or exceed 1 g/kg, which can cause BBB disruption. A given drug, that normally does not cross the BBB, may then enter brain via the disrupted BBB, and exert pharmacologic actions in the brain following systemic administration of the drug/solvent mixture. The solvent-mediated disruption of the BBB is discussed further in Chapter 3.

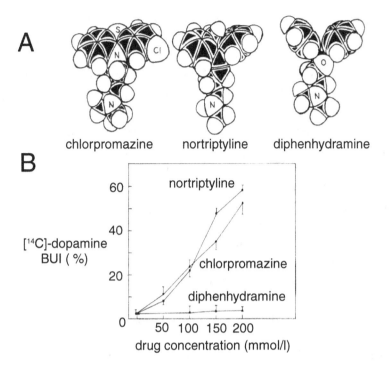

Figure 2.9   (A) Three-dimensional structure for chlorpromazine, nortriptyline, and diphenhydramine is shown. (B) The brain uptake index (BUI) for [^{14}C]dopamine for whole rat brain hemisphere is plotted versus the arterial concentration of nortriptyline, chlorpromazine, or diphenhydramine. Data are mean ± SE ($n = 3$–5 rats per point). The internal reference used in these studies was [^{3}H]water. From Pardridge et al. (1973) with permission.

Micelle-forming molecules

Tricyclic drugs, such as chlorpromazine or the tricyclic antidepressants, cause BBB disruption when infused into the carotid artery at concentrations that exceed a critical threshold, or critical micellar concentration (Pardridge et al., 1973). The formation of micelles by the drug is suggested by the observation that the experimentally observed osmolarity of the solution is much less than that predicted on the basis of the drug concentration. In the presence of these drug micelles, small molecules such as dopamine or mannitol, and to a lesser extent, inulin, cross the BBB via a molecular weight-dependent mechanism (Pardridge et al., 1973). The three-dimensional structures of these neuroactive drugs, chlorpromazine, nortriptyline, and diphenhydramine, are shown in Figure 2.9A. The two phenyl rings of both chlorpromazine and nortriptyline form a tricyclic molecule. Conversely, the two phenyl rings of diphenhydramine are not bridged and do not form a tricyclic structure. Otherwise the structures of these three molecules are similar, with two phenyl rings and an aliphatic amine tail. The three drugs were injected into the common carotid artery with [^{14}C]-dopamine, and the brain uptake index (BUI) for dopamine was measured (Figure 2.9B). There is marked difference in the transport behavior in the presence of either chlorpromazine or nortriptyline versus diphen-hydramine, as shown in Figure 2.9B. The BUI for [^{14}C]-dopamine is at the background level in the presence of all concentrations of diphenhydramine. However, the BUI for dopamine increases progressively with increasing concentrations of either nortriptyline or chlorpromazine. At the highest drug concentrations, the first-pass extraction of dopamine by the brain is 50%. These concentrations of nor-triptyline or chlorpromazine have a generalized effect on BBB permeability, and cause increased BBB permeability of other compounds such as mannitol or inulin, although the effect on inulin is decreased more than 50% relative to mannitol (Pardridge et al., 1973). The tricyclic BBB disruption is molecular weight-dependent, indicating the tricyclic structures cause holes or pores in the plasma membrane of the brain capillary endothelium. The formation of micelles in the nortriptyline or chlorpromazine solutions, but not the diphenhydramine solu-tions, was inferred on the basis of osmolarity measurements of these concentra-tions (Pardridge et al., 1973). The experimentally observed osmolarity of the nortriptyline or chlorpromazine solution was 100 mosmol less than the predicted osmolarity, which is indicative of the formation of micellar structures, which effectively reduces the osmolarity of the solution. These observations are in accord with those of Remen et al. (1969), who showed that the extent to which membrane lytic agents form micellar aggregates in solution is the critical factor in determin-ing membrane destabilization by drugs present in millimolar concentrations.

Alkylating agents

Many chemotherapeutic agents work by alkylating nuclear DNA, and these drugs can at higher concentrations also alkylate proteins, including BBB surface proteins following intracarotid arterial infusion. BBB disruption has been caused by the infusion of etoposide, 5-fluorouracil, and cisplatin (Spigelman et al., 1984). Melphalan is phenylalanine mustard and is a neutral amino acid. Low concentra-tions of melphalan inhibit BBB neutral amino acid transport (see Chapter 3), and higher concentrations of melphalan cause BBB disruption (Cornford et al., 1992).

Blood–brain barrier disruption has chronic neuropathologic effects

The disruption of the BBB is associated with chronic neuropathologic changes (Salahuddin et al., 1988), which is probably expected since circulating albumin is toxic to astrocytes (Nadal et al., 1995). The enhancement of brain uptake of drug by BBB disruption is not an optimal form of drug targeting to the brain since BBB disruption also results in the brain uptake of a variety of circulating molecules and plasma proteins. BBB disruption is also associated with a severe brain vasculopathy (Lossinsky et al., 1995). The intracarotid arterial infusion of 1.6 mol/l mannitol is associated with a 25–60% mortality in the rat (Blasburg and Groothuis, 1991), and with seizures in the dog (Neuwelt and Rapoport, 1984). Osmotic disruption of the BBB, in conjunction with either intravenous or intracarotid methotrexate, worsened survival of rats with experimental brain tumors, as compared to methotrexate alone (Cosolo and Christophidis, 1987).

3

Lipid-mediated transport and carrier-mediated transport of small molecules

- Introduction
- Lipid-mediated transport
- Carrier-mediated influx
- Carrier-mediated efflux
- Plasma protein-mediated transport

Introduction

Central nervous system (CNS) drug development is derived from CNS drug discovery (Chapter 1), and CNS drug discovery is based on structure–activity relationships (SAR), which determine the affinity of the drug for its cognate receptor. However, the typical CNS drug discovery program leads to a drug candidate that is highly active in vitro with very favorable SAR, but has little biologic activity in the brain in vivo, because of poor transport through the blood–brain barrier (BBB). The drug discovery program is then terminated. Since >98% of all drug candidates that emanate from a high-throughput screening drug discovery program do not cross the BBB (Pardridge, 1998a), the inherent efficiency of the CNS drug development program is low. This efficiency could be increased by incorporating structure–transport relationships (STR) early in the drug discovery phase in parallel with SAR (Figure 3.1). The STR are derived from CNS drug-targeting principles.

The STR factors controlling small molecule transport through the BBB are shown in Figure 3.2. The STR of a given drug will allow for prediction of the BBB permeability–surface area (PS) product. The in vivo CNS pharmacologic effect of a drug is proportional to the brain uptake of the drug, expressed as a percentage of injected dose per gram brain (%ID/g). The %ID/g is an equal function of both the BBB PS product and the plasma area under the drug concentration curve (AUC), as shown in Figure 3.2. While the BBB PS product is *directly* proportional to the membrane permeation of the drug, the plasma AUC is *inversely* related to the membrane permeation of the drug. Since membrane permeation is predicted from the STR, the consideration of STR early in the drug discovery process will enable

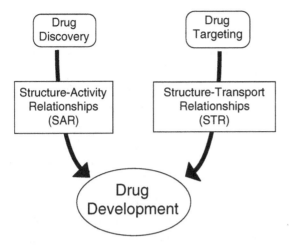

Figure 3.1   Brain drug discovery, drug targeting, and drug development.

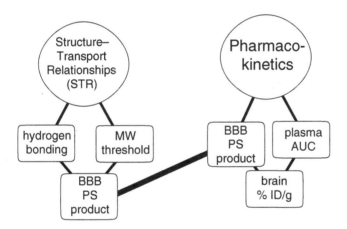

Figure 3.2   The factors controlling small molecule transport through the blood–brain barrier (BBB) are the permeability–surface area (PS) product and the plasma area under the concentration curve (AUC). These factors control the brain uptake or percentage of injected dose per gram brain (%ID/g). The BBB PS product is determined by the hydrogen bonding of the drug and the molecular weight (MW) of the drug which are the two principal determinants of the structure–transport relationships (STR).

predictions of both the PS product and the plasma AUC. Predictions of the BBB PS product are made by measurement of the 1-octanol/saline lipid partition coefficient (P) of the drug (Hansch and Steward, 1964). However, the STR of a drug can also be predicted by visual inspection of the structure of the drug, which leads to calculation of (a) the hydrogen bonding of the drug and (b) the molecular weight

(MW) of the drug (Figure 3.2). These factors are discussed below in the analysis of lipid mediation of drug transport through the BBB.

CNS drug discovery was performed in the past by the "trial and error" approach, wherein thousands of molecules were tested in bioassays and, in so doing, the SAR and STR were empirically assessed in parallel. However, modern methods of CNS drug discovery employ receptor-based high-throughput screening (HTS) programs that focus strictly on the SAR of the drug with little attention paid to the STR (Kuntz, 1992). Since >98% of all drugs that emanate from the CNS drug discovery program, including small molecules, do not cross the BBB, even small molecule drug candidates require a BBB drug-targeting system, if program termination is to be avoided. This chapter outlines approaches for BBB drug targeting of small molecules using either strategies designed to increase the lipid solubility of the drug (lipid-mediated transport), or strategies designed to employ endogenous BBB transport systems (carrier-mediated transport; CMT). Finally, this chapter discusses plasma protein-mediated drug transport at the BBB. Many drugs are avidly bound by plasma proteins, such as albumin or α_1-acid glycoprotein (AAG), and AAG binds many lipophilic amine drugs. While it is traditionally taught that only the free drug is available for transport through the BBB, other studies show that plasma protein-bound drug is available for transport through the BBB (Pardridge and Landaw, 1985). Plasma protein-mediated drug transport involves enhanced dissociation of drug from the plasma protein binding site with no exodus of the plasma protein per se from the brain capillary compartment. Since many small molecule drug candidates are strongly plasma protein-bound, a consideration of plasma protein-mediated drug transport will aid in the selection of drugs that are pharmacologically active in the brain in vivo.

Lipid-mediated transport

Blood–brain barrier membrane transport biology

Lipid-solubility

The goal of BBB drug targeting is to maximize the brain uptake of a drug, i.e., the %ID/g (Figure 3.2). Brain drug uptake is maximized in two ways. First, the plasma pharmacokinetics are optimized, which increases the plasma AUC (see below). Second, the BBB PS product is increased to the level which enables pharmacologic effects to take place in the brain. In an attempt to predict the BBB PS product of a given drug, the log P is determined. The log PS product for drug transport at the BBB is plotted versus the log P of the drug and this gives a linear relationship for 14 different drugs, as shown in Figure 3.3 (Pardridge, 1998a). In the absence of CMT processes, there is a linear relationship between the log PS and the log P, pro-

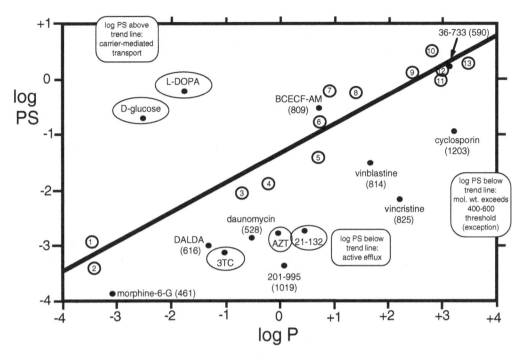

Figure 3.3   The log of the BBB permeability–surface area (PS) product is plotted versus the log of the 1-octanol/saline partition coefficient (P) for over 20 different drugs of varying molecular weight. See text for details. From Pardridge (1998a) with permission.

viding the molecular mass of the molecule is under a threshold of 400–600 Da (Figure 3.3). There are some exceptions to the molecular weight threshold rule, as illustrated by molecule 36–733, which has a molecular mass of 590 Da (Pardridge et al., 1990c), and BCECF-AM, which has a molecular mass of 809 Da, where BCECF-AM is 2′,7′-bis(2-carboxyethyl)-5(6)-carboxyfluorescein acetoxymethyl ester (Hirohashi et al., 1997). Molecules such as 36–733 and BCECF-AM likely assume a compact molecular conformation that enables drug movement through the lipid bilayer. The actual determinant of the BBB PS product of the drug is the molecular volume of the drug and molecular weight is only one determinant of this volume.

Drugs that cross the BBB by CMT, such as D-glucose or L-DOPA, have log PS products that are 4–5 log orders of magnitude *above* the lipid-solubility trendline (Figure 3.3). D-Glucose is transported by the *Glut1* glucose transporter, and L-DOPA is transported by the LAT1 large neutral amino acid transporter, as discussed below. Conversely, several drugs have PS products that are several log orders of magnitude *below* the lipid-solubility trendline and there are two classes of such drugs. The first class is represented by drugs such as azidothymidine (AZT) or 3TC

(Figure 3.3), and these drugs are substrates for carrier-mediated efflux at the BBB (see below). The other drugs with BBB PS products that fall log orders below the lipid-solubility trendline are those drugs with a molecular weight above the 400–600 Da threshold (Pardridge, 1998a). These include cyclosporin (1203 Da), vinblastine (814 Da), vincristine (825 Da), daunomycin (528 Da), DALDA (616 Da), 201–995 (1019 Da), and morphine-6-glucuronide (461 Da), as shown in Figure 3.3. The log PS products for these drugs is below the lipid-solubility trendline because the size of these drugs exceeds the 400–600 molecular weight threshold for drug transport through the BBB (Pardridge, 1998a).

Molecular weight threshold

The concept of a molecular weight threshold for drug transport at the BBB was advanced by Levin (1980) and subsequently confirmed by a number of laboratories (Eibl, 1984; Greig et al., 1990b; Xiang and Anderson, 1994). The biophysical basis of a molecular weight threshold for drug or solute transport across the BBB has not been adequately analyzed to date, although recent studies are attempting to build models of the "nanophysics" of solute permeation through biological membranes (Mouritsen and Jorgensen, 1997). The most plausible model describing the biophysical basis of the molecular weight threshold is that of Träuble (1971), who advanced a molecular theory for solute movement across lipid membranes. Träuble (1971) proposed a "molecular hitchhiking" or kink mediation transport model, whereby drug and solute transport through the lipid bilayer arises from constant conformational changes in the fatty acid hydrocarbon chain of the membrane phospholipids (Figure 3.4). These "holes" in the membrane are formed by kinks that extend only a few chain segments of the fatty acyl side chain. Therefore, there are no actual holes that traverse the entire depth of the lipid bilayer, but merely potential volumes that a molecule may access to penetrate the membrane. Träuble estimates the concentration of the kinks within a lipid bilayer is approximately 10 mmol/l and this concentration may vary depending on the molecular conformation of the membrane phospholipids. The concentration of the kinks increases with the increased abundance of unsaturated free fatty acids in the membrane and decreases with increasing cholesterol content in the lipid bilayer. Thus, lipid-mediated drug transport is a direct function of membrane fluidity. The kink model of lipid-mediated transport cannot be applied to large molecules that have a molecular weight in excess of 600 Da because these molecules have a molecular volume that is too large to occupy the volume created by the kink in the fatty acyl side chains (Figure 3.4).

The Träuble model is of interest not only because it predicts a molecular weight threshold for BBB lipid-mediated transport, but it also predicts a saturability of BBB lipid-mediated transport. The free diffusion of drug or solute through biological

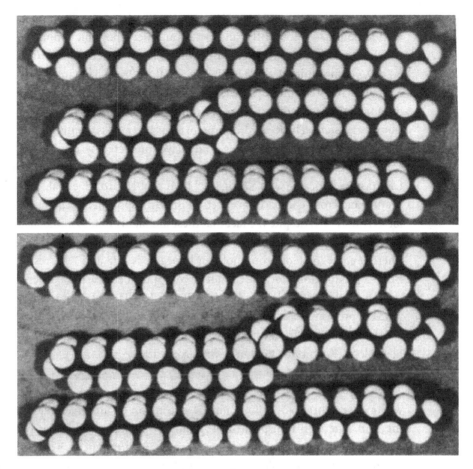

Figure 3.4   Kinks in the membrane phospholipid are formed by rotations about the carbon–carbon bonds which are separated by one carbon unit. These kinks form transient potential spaces in the membrane and this underlies the physical basis of lipid-mediated movement of solutes and drugs through biological membranes. From Träuble (1971) with permission.

membranes via lipid mediation is generally regarded as being a nonsaturable process. However, an anomalous finding is that the BBB transport of certain lipid-soluble molecules is saturable in the 5–50 mmol/l concentration range. This was first noted for lipid-soluble drugs such as amphetamine or methylphenidate (Pardridge and Connor, 1973), which have high lipid-solubility partition coefficients and are believed to undergo lipid-mediated transport through the BBB. However, in both cases, BBB transport was saturable. The K_m of D-amphetamine transport across the BBB was 17 mmol/l. The saturable transport of D-amphetamine was also cross-competed with other lipophilic amines such as β-phenethylamine or methylphenidate (Pardridge and Connor, 1973). A similar saturation phenomenon was demonstrated for BBB transport of another lipophilic amine, propranolol, which is transported through the BBB with a K_m of 9.8 ± 1.2 mmol/l and a V_{max} of 5.7 ± 0.7 μmol/min per g (Pardridge et al., 1984). The magnitude of these Michaelis–Menten kinetic parameters of BBB transport for propranolol indicate the drug transport is mediated by a low-affinity (high K_m), high-capacity (high V_{max}) transport system. The K_m of propranolol transport across the BBB is precisely equal to the concentration of kinks in a lipid bilayer predicted by Träuble (1971). Cross-competition was observed as high concentrations of propranolol inhibited BBB transport of lidocaine with a K_i of 8.1 ± 1.9 mmol/l (Pardridge et al., 1984). The saturation and cross-competition effects of BBB transport of lidocaine and propranolol were observed despite the fact that these are highly lipid-soluble molecules. The 1-octanol/Ringers P of propranolol or lidocaine is 19 ± 1 and 54 ± 2, respectively. Therefore, the log P of propranolol or lidocaine is 1.28 and 1.73, respectively. The BBB PS product for lidocaine cannot be computed because the extraction of unidirectional influx of this drug across the BBB is 100%. The extraction of unidirectional influx of propranolol at the BBB is 0.68 (Pardridge et al., 1984). The BBB PS product can be calculated from the Kety–Renkin–Crone (KRC) equation of capillary physiology (Kety, 1951; Renkin, 1959; Crone, 1963):

$$PS = -F(\ln 1 - E)$$

where F = cerebral blood flow, and E = extraction of unidirectional influx across the BBB. The BBB transport of propranolol was measured under pentobarbital anesthesia with a cerebral blood flow rate of 0.59 ml/min per g. Therefore, the BBB PS product for propranolol is 0.67 and the log PS is -0.17. These observations indicate that the log PS and log P relationship for propranolol fall exactly on the lipid-solubility trendline shown in Figure 3.3. If propranolol was, in fact, transported across the BBB by CMT mechanisms, similar to L-DOPA or D-glucose, then the log PS for propranolol should fall several log orders *above* the lipid-solubility trendline shown in Figure 3.3, but this is not observed. These considerations indicate that propranolol undergoes lipid-mediated transport across the BBB in proportion to its lipid-solubility without the intervention of a specialized CMT system. Therefore, the saturation and cross-competition phenomena observed for BBB transport of lipophilic amines is consistent with the kink model of Träuble (Figure 3.4). That is, there is a finite concentration of kinks or potential spaces within the lipid bilayer, and if these spaces are filled by 5–50 mmol/l concentrations of drug, then lipid-mediated drug transport will become saturated. The saturability and cross-competition of lipid-mediated transport at the BBB is direct support for the model of Träuble (1971), which underlies the molecular weight threshold of BBB transport of lipid-soluble small molecules.

Hydrogen bonding

Providing the molecular weight of the drug is under the 400–600 Da threshold, a linear relationship between the log PS and the log P of the drug can be demonstrated (Figure 3.4). Similar predictions about BBB transport can be made from examination of the structure of the drug, and by computation of the number of hydrogen bonds the drug forms with 55 mol/l solvent water. The hydrogen-bonding rules are reviewed by Stein (1967) and by Diamond and Wright (1969). There are two hydrogen bonds formed with each hydroxyl group, one hydrogen bond formed with each ether group, one hydrogen bond formed with each aldehyde group, one-half hydrogen bond formed with each ester group, three hydrogen bonds formed with each primary amine, and four hydrogen bonds formed with each amide group. The high hydrogen bonding of the amide group is the reason peptides, even short di- or tri-peptides, have such restricted transport at the BBB (see Chapter 4). The BBB permeability decreases by one log order of magnitude for each pair of hydrogen bonds added to the drug structure. This relationship between BBB permeability and hydrogen bonding is illustrated in the case of steroid hormones, as shown in Figure 3.5 (Pardridge and Mietus, 1979). Once the total number of hydrogen bonds is >10, then the BBB transport of the drug in pharmacologically significant amounts is minimal.

The masking of polar functional groups on the drug structure increases the lipid-solubility of the drug. If polar groups such as hydroxyl moieties are converted into nonhydrogen-bonding groups, then the BBB transport of the drug will be markedly increased. This is illustrated in the case of morphine, codeine, and heroin, as shown by Oldendorf et al. (1972). The BBB transport of codeine is increased a log order in magnitude, relative to morphine, because one of the two hydroxyl groups on the morphine structure is methylated to form codeine. When the two hydroxyl moieties of the morphine structure are both acetylated to form diacetyl morphine, which is heroin, the BBB transport of the drug is increased 2 log orders of magnitude. The BBB transport of heroin is characterized by a first-pass brain extraction in excess of 50% (Oldendorf et al., 1972), and this is derived from the loss of four hydrogen bonds created by the acetylation of the two hydroxyl groups on the parent morphine molecule. The conversion of two hydroxyl groups, which form four hydrogen bonds, to two ester groups, which form one-half hydrogen bond each, would be expected to increase BBB transport by 1–2 log orders in magnitude.

There is a considerable amount of effort devoted in present-day CNS drug discovery to quantitative SAR (QSAR). A similar program can be implemented for quantitative STR (QSTR) based on the two structural determinants of molecular weight and hydrogen bonding (Figures 3.1 and 3.2). A program that merges QSAR and QSTR could be a predictor of drugs that have CNS pharmacologic effects in vivo following peripheral (oral, systemic) administration. The QSAR predicts drug

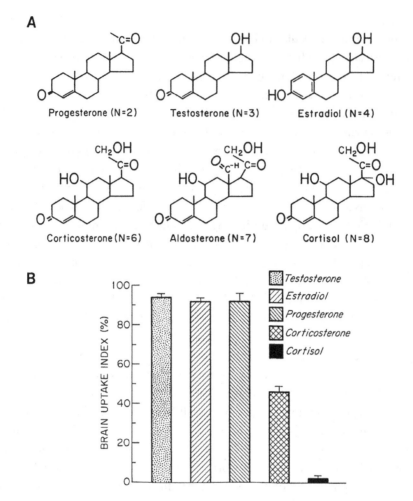

Figure 3.5   (A) Structure of steroid hormones with emphasis on the polar functional groups that form hydrogen bonds with solvent water. The hydrogen bond number (N) is given in parentheses for each steroid hormone and is equal to the total number of hydrogen bonds formed between solvent water and the steroid hormone. (B) The brain uptake index of the [³H]-labeled steroid hormones is shown as mean ± SE (n = 3–5 rats per point). From Pardridge (1998b) with permission.

affinity for the target receptor, and the QSTR predicts the extent to which the drug crosses the BBB in vivo. QSTR can also predict the plasma pharmacokinetics of the drug.

Pharmacokinetic rule

The molecular weight and hydrogen bonding of a drug determine the BBB PS product. However, the brain uptake of a drug (%ID/g) is a dual function of both

The Pharmacokinetic Rule

$$\boxed{\%ID/g} \quad = \quad \boxed{PS} \quad X \quad \boxed{AUC}$$

%ID/g = percentage injected dose delivered per gram brain

PS = blood–brain barrier permeability–surface area product (μl/min per g)

AUC = area under the plasma concentration curve (%ID•min/μl)

Figure 3.6 The pharmacokinetic rule states that the percentage of injected dose per gram brain (%ID/g) is directly proportional to the blood–brain barrier permeability–surface area (PS) product and the plasma area under the concentration curve (AUC). From Pardridge (1997) with permission.

the BBB PS product and the plasma AUC. This is illustrated in the pharmacokinetic rule (Figure 3.6). %ID/g is equally determined by the BBB PS product, which has units of μl/min per g, and the plasma AUC, which has units of %ID·min/μl (Pardridge, 1997). The BBB PS product is a function of the BBB transport properties of the drug and the plasma AUC is a function of the systemic pharmacokinetics, i.e., the degree to which the drug is cleared from the blood stream by organs other than the brain. The pharmacokinetic rule shows that if the BBB PS product and the plasma AUC change in opposite directions, then this can have nullifying effects with minimal change in the %ID/g in brain. This is what happens when BBB transport of a drug is increased by "lipidization." The latter aims to increase the lipid-solubility of the drug by either masking polar functional groups or by attachment of the drug to lipid carriers (see below). While such lipidization efforts may result in substantial increases in the BBB PS product, there is a similar increase in membrane permeation in all peripheral tissues, and this results in increased plasma clearance of the drug and a proportional decrease in the plasma AUC. If the PS product increases and the plasma AUC decreases, then there is minimal change in the %ID/g brain of the drug, as predicted by the pharmacokinetic rule (Figure 3.6). This is illustrated in the case of lipidization of chlorambucil, a chemotherapeutic alkylating agent (Figure 3.7). Esterification of the carboxyl moiety would be predicted to have a marked increase in BBB transport of chlorambucil since this would replace a carboxyl group, which forms three hydrogen bonds with solvent water, with an ester group which forms only one-half hydrogen bond with solvent water. The decrease in two and a half hydrogen bonds would result in an increase

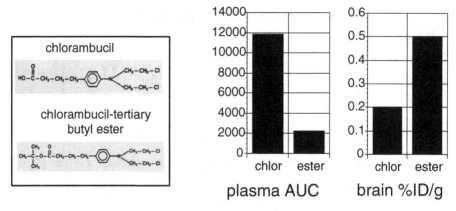

Figure 3.7   Lipidization of chlorambucil: demonstration of the pharmacokinetic rule. Left: Structure of chlorambucil and a tertiary butyl ester of chlorambucil. Right: The plasma area under the concentration curve (AUC) and the brain percentage of injected dose per gram brain %ID/g of chlorambucil (chlor) and the chlorambucil-tertiary butyl ester (ester) are shown. Data are from Greig et al. (1990a).

in BBB permeability in excess of 10-fold (Figure 3.5). The BBB PS product is increased approximately 14-fold when chlorambucil is converted to chlorambucil-tertiary butyl ester (Greig et al., 1990a). However, the brain delivery of the drug is only increased twofold (Figure 3.7), because the plasma AUC of the chlorambucil ester is decreased nearly sixfold compared to the plasma AUC of chlorambucil (Figure 3.7). Maximal BBB penetration for a given drug will be achieved with a targeting strategy that results in parallel increases in *both* the BBB PS product and the plasma AUC. As discussed below, none of the existing lipidization strategies accomplish this, because drug lipidization causes an increase in the BBB PS product and a parallel *decrease* in the plasma AUC.

Lipid carriers

Dihydropyridine

Drugs with limited BBB transport properties have been conjugated to a lipid carrier comprised of dihydropyridine (DHP) (Bodor and Simpkins, 1983). The DHP nucleus is oxidized in tissues to form a quaternary ammonium salt, which results in sequestration of the complex in the tissue followed by the hydrolysis of the drug from the quaternary ammonium DHP carrier. The use of the DHP lipid carrier illustrates the challenges that are presented by attachment of hydrophilic drugs to lipid-soluble carriers. First, lipidization of a drug by conjugation to DHP will increase the lipid-solubility of the molecule and this will result in a proportional *decrease* in the plasma AUC, as predicted by the pharmacokinetic rule (Figure 3.6). A decrease in the plasma AUC will nullify any increases in the BBB PS product, leading to only small increases in the brain %ID/g. This is illustrated in the case of a conjugate of DHP and dideoxycytidine (DDC). There was no change in the brain drug concentration of DDC following administration of the DHP–DDC conjugate, compared to the administration of DDC alone, because of the reduced plasma AUC caused by conjugation of the polar DDC to the lipid DHP carrier (Torrence et al., 1993).

A second limitation to the DHP strategy is that it is necessary not only to conjugate a drug to the DHP carrier, but also to lipidize the drug by blocking polar functional groups. Otherwise, the conjugate is still comprised of a polar drug moiety that will restrict membrane permeation. This is illustrated in the case of an enkephalin pentapeptide, which was attached to the DHP linker at the amino terminus of the peptide; the peptide was further lipidized by conjugation of a cholesterol ester at the carboxyl terminus of the peptide (Bodor et al., 1992). The DHP/enkephalin/cholesterol dual conjugate results in a marked increase in the lipid-solubility of the drug, but this has three effects that impair BBB transport. First, the molecular weight of the drug is now more than doubled to 1128 Da, which exceeds the 400–600 molecular weight threshold of BBB transport. Second, the lipid-solubility of the drug is increased to such an extent that the plasma AUC is decreased such that the plasma residence time of the conjugate following intravenous administration is <5 min (Bodor et al., 1992). Third, the extremely lipidized peptide requires an injection vehicle comprised of 25% dimethylsulfoxide (DMSO) and 50% ethanol (Bodor et al., 1992). The doses of these solvents that are coadministered with the conjugate can approximate 1 g/kg, which results in nonspecific BBB disruption, as reviewed in Chapter 2.

The advantage of the DHP system, relative to other lipid carriers discussed below, is that the DHP moiety is oxidized to the quaternary ammonium salt which results in trapping the conjugate in the tissue. This is analogous to the situation with morphine and heroin (Oldendorf et al., 1972). The diacetylation of the two hydroxyl groups of morphine results in the formation of heroin and this modification causes a nearly 100-fold increase in BBB permeability. Following BBB transport, the heroin is rapidly deacetylated back to morphine owing to the enzymatic action of pseudocholinesterase, which is abundant around the brain microvasculature (Gerhart and Drewes, 1987). The rapid conversion of heroin back to morphine in brain results in the conversion of a drug of high BBB permeability (heroin) to a drug of low BBB permeability (morphine), and this effectively results in an increased brain residence time of morphine relative to the prodrug, heroin.

Free fatty acyl lipid carriers

Dopamine, which has poor BBB membrane permeation, was conjugated to a C_{22} free fatty acid, docosahexanenoic acid (DHA). The highly lipid-soluble conjugate was formulated in 25% propylene glycol and administered to mice at doses of 2–25 mg/kg (Shashoua and Hesse, 1996). The dose of the solvent, propylene glycol, administered in these studies is not known, but may be sufficient to cause solvent-induced BBB disruption (Chapter 2). The maximum brain uptake of the drug by the mouse brain was approximately 1% of injected dose per gram, which is low for the mouse, which has a body weight of only 30 g. (See Chapter 5 for discussion of the inverse relationship between body weight and the brain %ID/g.) The unexpected low BBB permeability of the dopamine–DHA conjugate may result from a variety of factors, including the high molecular weight of the conjugate (608 Da) and the fact that the conjugate will bind to circulating albumin. Although there is some plasma protein-mediated transport of albumin-bound free fatty acids, in general, free fatty acid binding to albumin has a markedly restrictive effect on BBB drug transport (Pardridge and Mietus, 1980). The plasma AUC of this highly lipidized form of dopamine would also be expected to be very low and have offsetting effects on any increase in BBB permeability generated by conjugation of dopamine to the lipid carrier.

Adamantane

Adamantane is the parent nucleus of the antiviral compounds, rimantadine and amantadine (Spector, 1988), and has been used as a lipid carrier for BBB drug transport. A conjugate of adamantane and AZT was constructed. However, the brain level of the AZT following administration of the AZT–adamantane conjugate was no greater than the brain uptake following the administration of the free AZT (Tsuzuki et al., 1994). There was an initial increase in the brain concentration of the AZT–adamantane conjugate, but the conjugate rapidly effluxed from brain back to blood before the ester bond could be hydrolyzed in brain. Therefore, there was no effective sequestration of the AZT–adamantane conjugate in brain. In this regard, the rapid oxidation of the pyridine nucleus of the DHP lipid carrier is an advantage because it results in sequestration in brain that minimizes the rapid efflux of the drug, providing the oxidation of the DHP carrier is, indeed, rapid relative to drug efflux. These considerations illustrate the need to use a lipid carrier prodrug that is rapidly enzymatically modified in brain to promote sequestration within the brain. This sequestration will minimize rapid efflux of the lipid carrier/drug conjugate back to blood.

Blockade of BBB transport of lipid-soluble molecules

A given drug may react with receptors present in both the peripheral nervous system and the CNS and, if the drug is lipid-soluble, the drug will readily cross the

BBB. In some cases, it is desired to have a selective effect in the peripheral nervous system and the aim is to minimize BBB transport of the drug. Strategies aimed at blockade of BBB transport emanate from considerations of hydrogen-bonding rules (Figure 3.5). These involve the addition of polar functional groups to the parent drug in such a way that the affinity of the drug for its cognate receptor is maintained. One strategy is the formation of quaternary ammonium groups on drugs that contain an amine group. This is illustrated in the case of the conversion of zataseron to its corresponding quaternary ammonium salt (Gidda et al., 1995). This results in a drug that is still active in vitro, but is not active in vivo in brain owing to absent transport across the BBB of the drug in the form of the quaternary ammonium salt. The presence of a quaternary ammonium group on a drug will essentially eliminate any BBB transport. The utility of converting tertiary amines to quaternary ammonium amines with respect to inhibition of BBB transport was demonstrated by Oldendorf et al. (1993). It was shown that the conversion of nicotine, which is freely transported across the BBB, to N-methyl nicotine results in the formation of a drug that has minimal BBB transport. Another approach to blocking BBB transport is to add a hydroxyl group to the parent drug, which would be predicted to result in a log order decrease in BBB permeability. This was illustrated in the case of L-663,581 which has a brain uptake index (BUI) of $68 \pm 10\%$ (Lin et al., 1994). However, the monohydroxylated form of 663,581 has a BUI of only $2.5 \pm 0.4\%$. The monohydroxylated form of the drug is active in vitro, but is not active in vivo owing to poor BBB transport. The addition of a single hydroxyl group to the parent drug will cause a log order decrease in BBB permeability and this explains the loss of in vivo CNS action of the drug following hydroxylation.

Liposomes and nanoparticles

Liposomes

Drugs may be incorporated in either small unilamellar vesicles (SUV), which have a diameter of 40–80 nm, or multivesicular liposomes (MVL), which have a diameter of 0.3–2 μm. Liposomes are highly lipid-soluble "sacks" for delivery of drug through the BBB following the initial encapsulation of drug within the liposome. However, if drugs that have a molecular weight in excess of 400–600 Da threshold have restricted BBB transport (Figure 3.3), then it would be predicted that liposomes, even SUVs of 40–80 nm, would not cross the BBB. Although some studies report that liposomes cross the BBB (Chen et al., 1993), these have not been confirmed. For example, sulfatide liposomes were reported to cross the BBB, but this was not confirmed when it was shown that the brain uptake of 50–100 nm sulfatide liposomes required hyperosmolar BBB disruption in order to traverse the BBB (Sakamoto and Ido, 1993). The peripheral administration of MVLs was found to accumulate in brain, but this was due to embolism within the brain microvasculature of these structures, which have a diameter of 0.3–2 µm (Schackert et al., 1989). In the same study, the 40–80 nm SUVs did not cross the BBB. In another study, it was necessary to induce pharmacologic BBB disruption with etoposide (Chapter 2) in order to cause BBB transport of 60 nm liposomes (Gennuso et al., 1993). The encapsulation of superoxide dismutase (SOD) in liposomes was found to promote increased CNS pharmacologic activity of the enzyme in vivo (Chan et al., 1987), but this was in a traumatic brain-injury model, where the BBB is disrupted. In summary, the various studies show that liposomes do not cross the BBB unless the membrane is disrupted using BBB disruption strategies outlined in Chapter 2.

Nanoparticles

Nanoparticles generally have diameters in the 100–400 nm range and are comprised of biodegradable polymers. Like liposomes, nanoparticles are rapidly cleared from the blood following intravenous administration and >90% of the nanoparticle is removed from the blood stream within 5 min in mice. Similar to liposomes, the conjugation of polyethylene glycol (PEG), a process termed pegylation (Chapter 6), can be used to prolong the circulation time in blood (Gref et al., 1994). With this process, the PEG polymers ranging from 5 to 20 kDa in molecular weight are covalently conjugated to the surface of the nanoparticle. This results in a decreased plasma clearance of liposomes or nanoparticles, which increases the plasma AUC of the particles, owing to decreased uptake by the liver, spleen, and other components of the reticuloendothelial system (RES).

Drug encapsulated within nanoparticles has been reported to undergo transport through the BBB (Kreuter et al., 1995; Begley, 1996; Schröder and Sabel, 1996; Alyautdin et al., 1997). These conclusions are based on pharmacologic responses in the brain following peripheral administration of the drug–nanoparticle complex. For example, analgesia was induced in mice following the intravenous administration of the opioid peptide, dalargin, at a dose of 7.5 mg/kg using 230 nm nanoparticles (Kreuter et al., 1995). The BBB transport of the drug embedded in the nanoparticle is somewhat unexpected since the very large size, 230 nm, of the nanoparticle would, by itself, restrict BBB transport. Since 40–80 nm liposomes do not cross the BBB (Schackert et al., 1989; Huwyler et al., 1996), owing to the large size of the structure, it would be expected that 230 nm nanoparticles similarly would not undergo BBB transport. The pharmacologic activity of the nanoparticles may be related to the formulation of these structures, and the need to include stabilizing agents, such as polysorbate 80. Polysorbate 80 is also known as Tween 80 and is a detergent. Detergents can cause solvent-mediated BBB disruption (Chapter 2). Early studies showed that doses of Tween 80 (polysorbate 80) of 3–30 mg/kg intravenous result in BBB disruption owing to solvent destabilization of the BBB (Azmin et al., 1985). In the nanoparticle study, it is necessary to administer relatively large doses of polysorbate 80, up to 200 mg/kg, intravenously to stabilize the nanoparticle (Kreuter et al., 1995; Schröder and Sabel, 1996; Alyautdin et al., 1997). Recent studies show that this detergent present in the formulation is responsible for enhanced BBB transport of the drug/nanoparticle/Tween 80 complex (Olivier et al., 1999). These studies suggest that nanoparticles, like liposomes, do not cross the BBB in the absence of a parallel use of a BBB disruption strategy, as outlined in Chapter 2.

Receptor-mediated targeting of liposomes

Although liposomes, per se, do not cross the BBB, it is possible that immunoliposomes could cross the BBB via receptor-mediated transcytosis (RMT), as discussed in Chapter 4. The construction of immunoliposomes involves the covalent conjugation of specific monoclonal antibodies (MAbs) to the surface of the liposome. However, immunoliposomes, similar to conventional liposomes, are removed rapidly from the blood by the RES. The rapid plasma clearance of liposomes or immunoliposomes can be prevented by the conjugation of PEG polymers to the surface of the liposome (Papahadjopoulos et al., 1991). This results in the formation of "hairy" liposomes and the extended PEG polymers minimize the absorption of plasma proteins to the liposome surface, which triggers rapid uptake by the RES. When MAbs are conjugated to the surface of pegylated liposomes, there is no selective tumor targeting of the structure because the PEG polymers cause steric interference between the MAb and targeted receptor in the tissue (Klibanov et al., 1991; Emmanuel et al., 1996). This problem was solved by conjugation of the MAb to the tip of the PEG tail, which released any steric hindrance caused by the PEG polymers between the MAb and its receptor.

Brain targeting of pegylated immunoliposomes was achieved with the use of peptidomimetic MAbs that target endogenous receptors on the BBB, as discussed in Chapter 5. The structure of the pegylated immunoliposome is outlined in Figure 3.8A and shows the liposome conjugated with PEG of 2000 Da molecular weight, designated PEG^{2000}. A small fraction of the PEG^{2000} polymer attached to the surface of the liposomes contains a maleimide moiety at the tip of the PEG tail (Huwyler et al., 1996). This is made possible with the use of a bifunctional PEG derivative that contains a distearoylphosphatidyl ethanolamine (DSPE) moiety at one end, for insertion into the liposome surface, and the maleimide moiety at the other end, for conjugation to a thiolated MAb, as outlined in Figure 3.8B. The maleimide moiety is conjugated to the thiolated OX26 MAb and this results in the formation of the pegylated OX26 immunoliposome outlined in Figure 3.8A. The liposomes were conjugated to the murine OX26 MAb, which binds the transferrin receptor on the

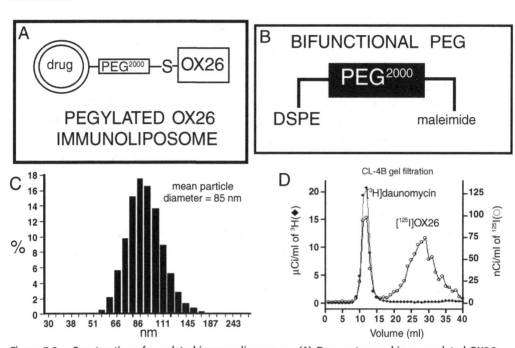

Figure 3.8   Construction of pegylated immunoliposomes. (A) Drug entrapped in a pegylated OX26 immunoliposome. The OX26 monoclonal antibody is conjugated via a thiol–ether bridge to the polyethylene glycol (PEG) strand of 2000 Da molecular weight, which is in turn attached to the surface of the liposome. (B) Synthesis of the pegylated immunoliposomes is made possible with the availability of a bifunctional PEG derivative wherein the PEG^{2000} has a maleimide moiety at one end and a distearoylphosphatidyl ethanolamine (DSPE) moiety at the other end. (C) Size distribution of sterically stabilized liposomes prepared by rapid extrusion shows the mean diameter is 85 nm. (D) Elution profile of the separation of the [^{3}H]daunomycin-loaded immunoliposomes from unencapsulated [^{3}H]daunomycin and unconjugated [^{125}I]-labeled OX26 monoclonal antibody on a gel filtration chromatography. From Huwyler et al. (1996) with permission. Copyright (1996) National Academy of Sciences, USA.

BBB (Chapter 4). The diameter of the pegylated immunoliposome was 85 nm (Figure 3.8C). The OX26 pegylated immunoliposome was separated from unconjugated OX26 with Sepharose CL4B gel filtration chromatography, as shown in Figure 3.8D. These gel filtration studies show comigration of the OX26, which is radiolabeled with [^{125}I], and the [^{3}H]daunomycin, which is incorporated within the interior of the liposome (Figure 3.8D).

A pharmacokinetic analysis was performed following an intravenous injection of [^{3}H]daunomycin administered in one of four formulations (Figure 3.9A). These formulations were: (a) unencapsulated drug (free drug), (b) [^{3}H]daunomycin encapsulated in conventional, nonpegylated liposomes (liposome), (c) [^{3}H]daunomycin encapsulated within pegylated liposomes (PEG-liposome), and (d)

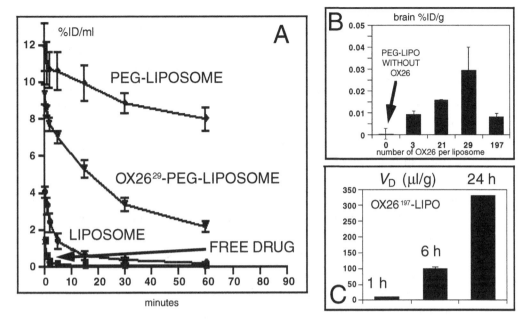

Figure 3.9   (A) The percentage of injected dose per milliliter of plasma of daunomycin is plotted versus the time after intravenous injection of the [³H]daunomycin injected as one of four different formulations: (a) free drug, (b) drug encapsulated in conventional liposomes (LIPOSOME), (c) drug encapsulated within pegylated liposomes carrying no monoclonal antibody (PEG-LIPOSOME), and (d) drug encapsulated within OX26 pegylated in the liposomes, wherein the liposome has 29 OX26 antibody molecules attached at the surface (OX26²⁹-PEG-LIPOSOME). Data are mean ± SE ($n = 3$ rats per point). (B) The brain uptake of the [³H]daunomycin encapsulated within OX26 pegylated immunoliposomes increases with the number of OX26 antibodies attached per liposome in the range of 0–29, but decreases when 197 antibody molecules are attached to the surface. The optimal number of OX26 molecules attached per liposome is 30. (C) The brain volume distribution (V_D) of the daunomycin encapsulated within OX26 pegylated immunoliposomes increases with time after intravenous injection, indicating the pegylated OX26 immunoliposomes are sequestered in brain. From Huwyler et al. (1996) with permission. Copyright (1996) National Academy of Sciences, USA.

[³H]daunomycin encapsulated within OX26 pegylated liposomes that contain 29 OX26 MAb molecules per individual liposome (OX26²⁹-PEG-liposome). The daunomycin is rapidly removed from the blood stream following administration of drug in its free form. Similarly, the daunomycin encapsulated within the conventional liposome is also rapidly removed from blood, owing to uptake of the liposome by the RES. Conversely, the uptake of the daunomycin encapsulated within PEG-liposomes is markedly delayed (Figure 3.9A). The plasma clearance of the free daunomycin is 45 ± 7 ml/min per kg and this is reduced 235-fold following encapsulation of the daunomycin in the PEG-liposome, which has a plasma clearance of 0.19 ± 0.01 ml/min per kg. The attachment of 29 OX26 MAb molecules to the surface of the pegylated immunoliposome results in an increase in plasma clearance from 0.19 ± 0.01 to 0.91 ± 0.11 ml/min per kg and this change in clearance is shown in the comparison of the plasma decay curves (Figure 3.9A). The increased plasma clearance of the OX26 pegylated immunoliposome is caused by the targeting of the liposome to tissues such as liver and brain that express high levels of transferrin receptor (TfR) at the microcirculation (Huwyler et al., 1997). The BBB TfR is freely exposed to circulating plasma because the receptor is on the brain capillary endothelial plasma membrane (Chapter 4). The hepatocyte TfR is freely exposed to the circulating liposome because of the absence of a capillary barrier to liposomes in liver. The TfR on cells in other tissues is not readily available to the circulating OX26 pegylated immunoliposomes because of the capillary barrier to 80 nm structures in tissues other than liver or the BBB.

There is an optimal number of MAb molecules that should be attached to the liposome and this is approximately 30 (Huwyler et al., 1996). As shown in Figure 3.9B, the brain %ID/g increases linearly with the number of OX26 MAb molecules attached in the range of 3–29. However, a log order increase in the number of attached MAb molecules actually results in decreased brain clearance (Figure 3.9B). The brain uptake of the pegylated liposome without OX26 attached (designated as "0" in Figure 3.9B) is zero, and this is indicative of a lack of transport of pegylated liposomes through the BBB in vivo. The brain uptake (%ID/g) of the OX26 pegylated immunoliposome is approximately 10% of the brain uptake of unconjugated OX26 (Chapter 5). These data indicate that the BBB PS product of the OX26 MAb is reduced approximately 10-fold, when the 85 nm pegylated immunoliposome is attached to the MAb. However, only two to four small molecules can be attached to a given OX26 MAb. In contrast >10000 small molecules may be entrapped in a single 100 nm liposome. Lipid/drug ratios of approximately 3 are achieved with 100 nm liposomes (Mayer et al., 1989). Since approximately 100000 lipid molecules occupy the surface of a 100 nm liposome (Huwyler et al., 1997), up to 28000 daunomycin molecules are packaged within a single 100 nm liposome. Therefore, the conjugation of the PEG liposome greatly increases the carrying capacity of OX26 by up to 4 log orders in magnitude and this offsets the decrease in BBB PS product caused by attachment of an 85 nm pegylated liposome to the OX26 MAb. The brain volume distribution (V_D) of the OX26 pegylated immunoliposome increases with time after injection (Figure 3.9C), indicating that the liposomes are sequestered in brain, and not merely absorbed to the luminal membrane of the BBB.

Further evidence that the OX26 pegylated immunoliposome was transported through the brain endothelium was obtained with confocal microscopy (Figure

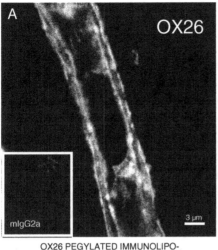

OX26

mIgG2a

3 µm

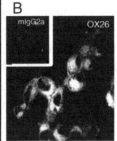

mIgG2a   OX26

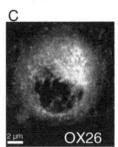

OX26

2 µm   OX26

CONFOCAL MICROSCOPY:
RHODAMINE-LABELED
PEGYLATED
IMMUNO-LIPOSOMES

B   C

OX26 PEGYLATED IMMUNOLIPO-
SOMES ARE BOUND BY BOTH LUMINAL
AND ABLUMINAL MEMBRANES OF
ISOLATED RAT BRAIN CAPILLARIES

OX26 PEGYLATED IMMUNOLIPO-
SOMES ARE ENDOCYTOSED BY RAT
GLIOMA (RG)-2 CELLS

Figure 3.10   Confocal fluorescent microscopy of OX26 pegylated immunoliposomes incubated with either isolated rat brain capillaries (A) or RG2 rat glioma cells (B, C). These liposomes contain rhodamine conjugated at the surface of the phospholipid to allow for visualization by fluorescent microscopy. When the OX26 monoclonal antibody was replaced with the mouse IgG$_{2a}$ isotype control, there was no binding to either the isolated rat brain capillaries (A, inset), or to the RG2 glioma cells (B, inset). The OX26 pegylated immunoliposomes bind to both the luminal and abluminal surface of the isolated rat brain capillary, as shown in (A). The OX26 pegylated immunoliposomes are endocytosed into RG2 glioma cells, as shown at low magnification in (B). The high-magnification view of the RG2 cells shown in (C) reveals liposomes entrapped with intracellular endosomes. There is also diffuse cytoplasmic staining, which indicates that the liposomes fuse with the endosomal membrane and release the contents to the cytoplasm. Figure 3.10A from Huwyler et al. (1997) with permission and Figure 3.10B and C from Huwyler and Pardridge (1998) with permission.

3.10). For the synthesis of fluorescent immunoliposomes, rhodamine-conjugated phosphatidyl ethanolamine (PE) was incorporated in the liposome surface (Huwyler et al., 1997). RG2 rat glioma cells, which express the rat TfR, were exposed to fluorescent OX26 pegylated immunoliposomes for 2 h at 37 °C and the cells were then fixed in paraformaldehyde and viewed with confocal microscopy, as shown in Figure 3.10B and 3.10C. The fluorescent OX26 pegylated immunoliposomes endocytoses into the RG2 cells and then distributes into the cytoplasm (Figure 3.10B). At higher magnification, there is a punctate staining pattern indicative of entrapment of the pegylated immunoliposomes within the intracellular endosomal system (Figure 3.10C). However, there is also diffuse cytoplasmic staining, indicating the liposome fuses with the endosomal plasma membrane and releases the contents to the cytoplasm. Similar confocal microscopy studies were performed with isolated rat brain capillaries, as shown in Figure 3.10A. In these studies, freshly isolated rat brain capillaries were incubated with rhodamine-labeled pegylated immunoliposomes before confocal analysis of the unfixed specimen (Huwyler and Pardridge, 1998). Immunoliposome molecules contained approximately 24 molecules of OX26 MAb conjugated to the tip of the PEG strand. The OX26 immunoliposome is bound to both luminal and abluminal membranes, which could be resolved by confocal microscopy (Figure 3.10A). In both confocal studies with either the RG2 glioma cells or the isolated rat brain capillaries, control studies were performed. In these control experiments, the mouse IgG_{2a} isotype control for the OX26 MAb was conjugated to the tip of the PEG strand, in lieu of the OX26 MAb. Confocal microscopy studies were then performed similar to that done with the OX26 pegylated immunoliposomes. However, there is no confocal fluorescent signal observed with the mouse IgG_{2a} pegylated immunoliposomes in either the RG2 glioma cells (Figure 3.10B, inset) or the isolated rat brain capillaries (Figure 3.10A, inset).

These studies, described in Figures 3.8–3.10, indicate that pegylated immunoliposomes can be targeted to the brain via endogenous BBB receptors (Chapter 4) using specific MAbs that bind to endogenous BBB receptors. One of the more important applications of the pegylated immunoliposomes for brain drug targeting is brain gene therapy and this is discussed in Chapter 9.

Carrier-mediated influx

Glut1 glucose transporter

The first demonstration of saturable CMT of a nutrient across the BBB was reported by Crone (1965) and subsequently confirmed and extended by Oldendorf (1971). These workers employed the arterial single injection technique and Crone used a venous sampling/single arterial injection method called the indicator dilution technique, and Oldendorf invented the tissue sampling/single arterial injection method called the BUI method (Oldendorf, 1970). The BUI technique was a significant advance in BBB methodology since it allowed the rapid acquisition of BBB saturation data for a wide variety of substrates and drugs. The Michaelis–Menten kinetic parameters (K_m, V_{max}) of BBB transport of glucose, or many other substances, were computed from BUI data by merging the principles of capillary physiology and classical enzymology kinetics. This was accomplished by recognizing that the BBB PS product of CMT is equal to the V_{max}/K_m ratio, when the radiolabeled nutrient is injected in tracer concentrations (Pardridge and

Table 3.1 Blood–brain barrier nutrient and thyroid hormone carriers

Carrier	Representative substrate	K_m (μmol/l)	V_{max} (nmol/min per g)
Hexose	Glucose	$11\,000 \pm 1400$	1420 ± 140
Monocarboxylic acid	Lactic acid	1800 ± 600	91 ± 35
Neutral amino acid	Phenylalanine	26 ± 6	22 ± 4
Amine	Choline	340 ± 70	11 ± 1
Basic amino acid	Arginine	40 ± 24	5 ± 3
Nucleoside	Adenosine	25 ± 3	0.75 ± 0.08
Purine base	Adenine	11 ± 3	0.50 ± 0.09
Thyroid hormone	T_3	1.7 ± 0.7	0.19 ± 0.08

Notes:

T_3, triidothyronine.

From Pardridge (1991) with permission.

Oldendorf, 1975b). This allowed for the computation of the Michaelis–Menten parameters of BBB transport of metabolic substrates, and the K_m and V_{max} values for BBB nutrient carriers are listed in Table 3.1 (Pardridge, 1983a). The formal merger of the KRC and Michaelis–Menten equations is as follows:

$$E = 1 - e^{-PS/F}$$

$$PS = \frac{V_{max}}{(K_m + Ca)} + K_d$$

where E is the extraction of unidirectional influx, PS is permeability–surface area, F is cerebral blood flow, V_{max} is the maximal transport rate, K_m is the half-saturation constant, Ca is the arterial substrate concentration, and K_d is the constant of non-saturable transport (Pardridge, 1983a).

The characterization of BBB CMT changed from an analysis of the Michaelis–Menten parameters to a molecular biological analysis when a series of cDNAs for sodium-independent glucose transporters (*Glut*) were isolated and sequenced in the late 1980s. These transporters are designated *Glut1–Glut5*. *Glut1* was originally isolated from a human hepatoma cultured cell cDNA library using an antiserum to the purified *Glut1* glucose transporter obtained from human erythrocyte plasma membranes (Mueckler et al., 1985). Subsequently, *Glut1* was identified in rat brain and was originally known as the brain glucose transporter (Birnbaum et al., 1986). The *Glut1* isoform was shown by Flier et al. (1987) to be enriched at the BBB, but subsequent quantitative studies showed that essentially all of the *Glut1* transcript in brain was derived from the brain microvascular endothelium forming the BBB in vivo (Boado and Pardridge, 1990b; Pardridge et al., 1990a; Farrell and Pardridge, 1991a). The neuronal glucose transporter was identified as the *Glut3* isoform (Nagamatsu et al., 1992). The *Glut1* isoform has also been proposed as the principal glucose transporter in astrocytes in brain in vivo (Maher et al., 1994). However, the widespread expression of immunoreactive *Glut1* in brain astrocytes in vivo under normal conditions has not been observed (Pardridge et al., 1990a; Dermietzel et al., 1992; Farrell et al., 1992; Cornford et al., 1993; Urabe et al., 1996). The *Glut1* gene is expressed in brain cells in cerebral ischemia (Lee and Bondy, 1993). However, in normal conditions, antibodies to the *Glut1* glucose transporter only illuminate the microvascular endothelium in brain, as shown in Figure 3.11B. When in situ hybridization experiments in brain are performed with RNA probes antisense to the *Glut1* transcript, the in situ hybridization signal is found only over the brain microvascular endothelium (Figure 3.11C). When control experiments are performed, the hybridization signal over brain parenchyma with either the antisense or sense probe is identical, indicating the absence of experimentally detectable *Glut1* transcript in brain parenchyma in vivo under normal conditions. The immunoreactive *Glut1* glucose transporter protein may also be detected in brain using the electron microscopic immunogold technique, as shown in Figure 3.11D, which is a study of rat brain (Farrell and Pardridge, 1991a). Unlike human erythrocytes, which contain abundant immunoreactive *Glut1*, rat erythrocytes express minimal immunoreactive *Glut1* (Andersson and Lundahl, 1988), and this accounts for the lack of staining of the erythrocyte plasma membrane in Figure 3.11D. However, the important finding of the immunogold electron microscopic analysis of BBB *Glut1* is the selective distribution of the transporter to the abluminal membrane (Farrell and Pardridge, 1991a). There is threefold more immunoreactive *Glut1* molecules on the abluminal endothelial membrane, as compared to the luminal membrane (Figure 3.11D). When quantitative counting of gold particles over brain parenchyma is performed with electron microscopic immunogold analysis, there is no significant immunoreactive *Glut1* measurable over brain parenchyma (Farrell and Pardridge, 1991a), which is indicative of minimal immunoreactive *Glut1* in astrocytes in vivo.

BBB transport of glucose/drug conjugates is restricted

The high expression of the *Glut1* glucose transporter at the BBB raises the question as to whether the glucose molecule, per se, could be conjugated to drugs, and initiate BBB transport of the drug/glucose conjugate via the BBB *Glut1* glucose transporter. Support for this idea was found in the observation that morphine and morphine-6-glucuronide (M6G) are transported across the BBB at identical rates based on dialysis fiber measurements (Aasmundstad et al., 1995). On the basis of

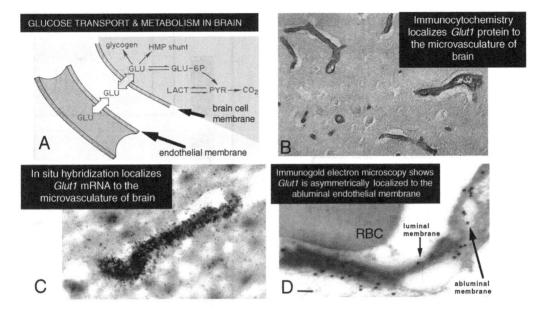

Figure 3.11   Blood–brain barrier (BBB) glucose transport is mediated by the *Glut1* glucose transporter. (A) Glucose transport from blood to brain involves movement through two membranes in series, the endothelial plasma membranes, and the brain cell (neuronal, glial) plasma membrane. Since the surface area of the brain cell membrane is log orders greater than the surface area of the endothelial membrane, the rate-limiting step in glucose movement from blood to brain intracellular spaces is at the endothelial membrane forming the BBB. HMP, hexose monophosphate; GLU, glucose; LACT, lactic acid; PYR, pyruvic acid. (B) Immunocytochemistry of bovine brain with an antiserum directed against the carboxyl terminus of the *Glut1* glucose transporter isoform. The study shows continuous immunostaining of brain microvessels with no measurable immunostaining of brain parenchyma. (C) In situ hybridization of bovine brain with a [^{35}S]antisense riboprobe to the *Glut1* mRNA shows hybridization over brain microvessels with no specific hybridization over brain parenchyma. (D) Electron microscopic immunogold analysis of rat brain with an anti-*Glut1* glucose transporter antibody shows localization of the transporter to the luminal and abluminal membranes of the capillary endothelium with a preferential expression on the abluminal membrane. RBC, red blood cell. From Pardridge et al. (1990a) and Farrell and Pardridge (1991a) with permission.

these studies, "glycopeptides" have been synthesized, wherein peptides are conjugated to glucose in order to facilitate neuropeptide transport through the BBB via the *Glut1* CMT system (Polt et al., 1994; Tomatis et al., 1997; Negri et al., 1998). However, the transport of the "glycopeptide" via the BBB *Glut1* glucose transporter has not been documented. Moreover, subsequent studies demonstrated the apparent high permeability of the BBB to M6G was an artifact, and that the transport of

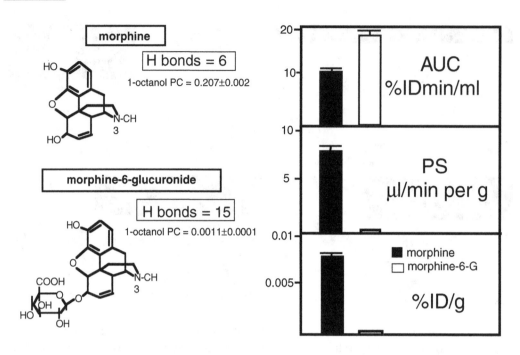

Figure 3.12 Differential blood–brain barrier (BBB) permeability of morphine and morphine-6-glucuronide. Left: Structure of morphine and morphine-6-glucuronide. Right: Plasma area under the concentration curve (AUC), blood–brain barrier permeability–surface area (PS) product, and brain uptake of morphine and morphine-6-glucuronide (morphine-6-G). From Wu et al. (1997a) with permission.

M6G through the BBB is low and in proportion to lipid-solubility (Figure 3.12). The morphine molecule has six hydrogen bonds and has a 1-octanol partition coefficient of 0.207 ± 0.02, and a log $P = -0.68$. In contrast, the M6G molecule forms 15 hydrogen bonds and has a 1-octanol partition coefficient of 0.0011 ± 0.0001 and a log $P = -2.96$ (Figure 3.12). The BBB PS product of M6G is 57-fold lower than that of morphine, 0.14 ± 0.03 versus 8.0 ± 0.3 μl/min per g, respectively (Figure 3.12), which is expected based on the much higher hydrogen bonding with M6G compared to morphine (Figure 3.12). Similar results on BBB transport of morphine or M6G were obtained with either an intravenous injection technique or an internal carotid artery perfusion method (Bickel et al., 1996; Wu et al., 1997a).

The very low BBB permeability of M6G, relative to morphine, is not consistent with the observation that these two molecules enter brain from blood at comparable rates based on measurements with the dialysis fiber method. Subsequent studies by Morgan et al. (1996) with intracerebral dialysis fibers demonstrated why the BBB permeability for morphine and M6G is comparable using the dialysis fiber technique. In agreement with the studies of Westergren et al. (1995), the placement of an intracerebral dialysis fiber within the brain results in traumatic brain injury leading to BBB disruption (Morgan et al., 1996). The BBB disruption is characterized by the formation of pores, which increases free diffusion of small molecules. The pore-mediated BBB disruption has the most pronounced effect for molecules such as sucrose or M6G, which have very low BBB permeability coefficients, and has a less pronounced effect for molecules that have intermediate BBB permeability coefficients, such as morphine and urea. Thus, the BBB permeability for urea, sucrose, morphine, and M6G is nearly comparable using the dialysis fiber method, although these molecules have widely different BBB PS products. The artifactually high BBB permeability for low permeant molecules such as M6G or sucrose is caused by the injury associated with the implantation of a dialysis fiber in brain.

LAT1 large neutral amino acid transporter

Large neutral amino acids are transported across the BBB by a saturable large neutral amino acid carrier (Pardridge and Oldendorf, 1975a), which has recently been identified as the large neutral amino acid transporter type 1 isoform (LAT1) (Boado et al., 1999). The bovine BBB LAT1 cDNA was cloned from a size-fractionated cDNA library representing transcripts derived from freshly isolated bovine brain capillaries (Figure 3.13). The preparation of the size-fractionated BBB cDNA library was made possible by the isolation of >100 μg of polyA + mRNA purified from the total pool of freshly isolated capillaries obtained from >2000 g of bovine brain (Figure 3.13). This polyA + mRNA was then size-fractionated by sucrose density gradient ultracentrifugation prior to production of the individual size-fractionated cDNA libraries (Boado et al., 1999). A full-length cDNA encoding the bovine BBB LAT1 was isolated and used in Northern blotting analysis to show the LAT1 mRNA is 100-fold more abundant at the BBB than any other tissue, including rat brain (Boado et al., 1999). These Northern results suggest the following. First, the LAT1 gene, like the *Glut1* gene (Pardridge et al., 1990a), is only expressed in brain at the BBB with minimal expression in brain cells under normal conditions. Second, the LAT1 gene evolved specifically to execute the very specialized properties of the BBB large neutral amino acid transporter. As discussed below, the transport of amino acids through the BBB is mediated by a carrier with an affinity much higher than neutral amino acid carriers found in other tissues (Pardridge, 1977b). Accordingly, the K_m of BBB amino acid transport is in the 100 μmol/l range (Pardridge, 1977a), which means that the K_m approximates the plasma concentration of the amino acids, which is designated [S]. When the [S] approximates the K_m, then competition effects occur in the physiological range (Pardridge, 1977b). The low K_m of BBB amino acid transport is the reason why the brain is selectively impaired by selective hyperaminoacidemias such as

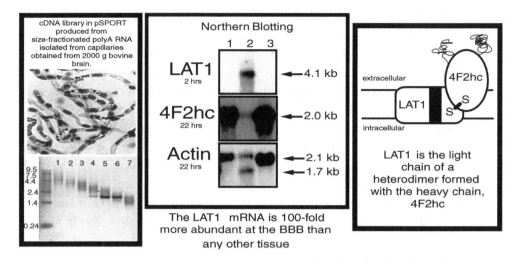

Figure 3.13   Molecular cloning of bovine blood–brain barrier large neutral amino acid transporter isoform 1 (LAT1). Left panel: PolyA+ mRNA was isolated from brain capillaries obtained from 2000 g of fresh bovine brain tissue and this was size-fractionated on a sucrose density ultracentrifugation for production of size-fractionated cDNA libraries. Middle panel: Northern blotting of polyA+ mRNA from rat brain (lane 1), bovine brain capillaries (lane 2), or C6 rat glioma cells (lane 3) using cDNAs to bovine LAT1, rat 4F2hc, or rat actin. Right panel: Scheme showing the heterodimer formed between the LAT1 and the 4F2hc inserted in the brain endothelial plasma membrane. From Boado et al. (1999) with permission. Copyright (1999) National Academy of Sciences, USA.

phenylketonuria, whereas other organs are not generally affected by hyperamino-acidemias. The K_m in peripheral tissues is in the 1–10 mmol/l range, which is 10- to 100-fold higher than the plasma concentration of amino acids in blood, which eliminates transport competition effects (Pardridge, 1983a).

The LAT1 protein is the light chain of a heterodimer formed with the heavy chain, 4F2hc (Kanai et al., 1998), as shown in Figure 3.13. The LAT1/4F2hc hetero-dimer is formed by a disulfide linkage, and the carbohydrate moieties of this trans-membrane heterodimer are linked to the heavy chain (Figure 3.13). Cloning of the BBB LAT1 cDNA allowed for prediction of the primary amino acid sequence of the BBB LAT protein and this is shown in Figure 3.14. This two-dimensional model of the LAT1 protein is based on hydropathy analysis (Kanai et al., 1998; Pineda et al., 1999), and predicts a single cysteine residue projecting in an extracellular direction and contained within a loop connecting the third and fourth transmembrane regions (Figure 3.14). This cysteine residue is believed to form the heterodimer with the 4F2hc (Mastroberardino et al., 1998). Cell culture studies indicate that the

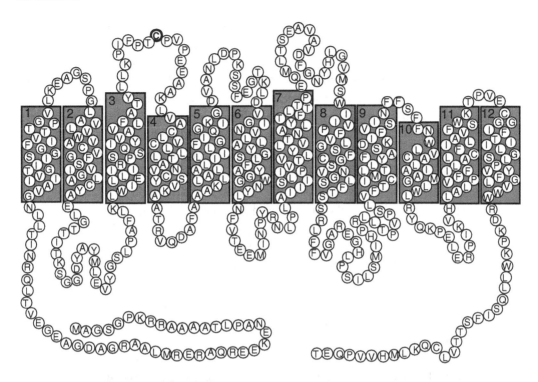

Figure 3.14   Predicted secondary structure of bovine blood–brain barrier (BBB) large neutral amino acid transporter isoform 1 (LAT1), which is comprised of 12 transmembrane regions and a cytoplasmic projecting amino terminus and carboxyl terminus. A single cysteine (C) residue that projects into the extracellular space is in the extracellular loop connecting the third and fourth transmembrane region. The structure is deduced from the cDNA sequence reported previously by Boado et al. (1999). Copyright (1999) National Academy of Sciences, USA.

LAT1 protein does not transport amino acids until it is inserted in the membrane as the heterodimer with the 4F2hc (Nakamura et al., 1999). Since this heterodimer is formed by the disulfide linkage, BBB neutral amino acid transport should be sensitive to sulfhydryl reagents. The sulfhydryl sensitivity was observed as the intracarotid arterial infusion of mercury ions selectively impairs BBB neutral amino acid transport, relative to BBB glucose transport (Pardridge, 1976). Since alkylating agents conjugate sulfhydryl residues (Golden and Shelly, 1987), it is also predicted that the intracarotid arterial perfusion of alkylating agents would result in a disruption of the LAT1/4F2hc heterodimer and thereby inhibit BBB neutral amino acid transport. Melphalan, which is phenylalanine mustard, and DL-2-amino-7-bis[(2-chloroethyl)amino]-1,2,3,4-tetrahydro-2-naphthoic acid (DL-NAM) are alkylating agents which inhibit BBB neutral amino acid transport at lower concentrations (Cornford et al., 1992; Takada et al., 1992). The DL-NAM has a very high affinity for the LAT1, and a peculiar property of BBB transport of DL-NAM is the very low V_{max} of BBB transport (Takada et al., 1992). The V_{max} is proportional to (a) the local membrane concentration of the LAT1, and (b) the rate at which amino acids shuttle through the stereospecific LAT1 carrier pore. If the DL-NAM alkylates the LAT1/4F2hc heterodimer at relatively low concentrations, owing to the high affinity of this drug for the carrier, this alkylation could disrupt the disulfide bond forming the heterodimer and this could lead to a reduced V_{max}. At higher concentrations, these alkylating agents conjugate numerous sulfhydryl agents on the brain capillary endothelial membrane, and this leads to BBB disruption. This was shown in the case of melphalan (Cornford et al., 1992). A saturation analysis of melphalan transport through the BBB revealed an unexpectedly high component of nonsaturable transport, as reflected in the high constant of nonsaturable transport, the K_D, which has units of μl/min per g. The high melphalan K_D was due to the disruption of the BBB caused by the administration of high concentrations of this alkylating agent.

Alkylating agents such as DL-NAM or melphalan are drugs that gain access to brain via the BBB LAT1 because these drugs have structures mimicking neutral amino acids. Other examples of neutral amino acid drugs include L-DOPA, used for Parkinson's disease, α-methyldopa, used for the treatment of hypertension, α-methyl-p-tyrosine, and gabapentin, a δ-aminobutyric acid (GABA) agonist that has a neutral amino acid-like structure and is used for the treatment of epilepsy. These drugs must compete with circulating neutral amino acids for BBB transport via LAT1. The affinity of the BBB LAT1 for neutral amino acids is extremely high compared to the affinity of other large neutral amino acid transporters in peripheral tissues. This is represented by a very low K_m of BBB large neutral amino acid transport (Table 3.1). Because the K_m of BBB neutral amino acid transport is approximately equal to the plasma concentrations of the amino acids, saturation effects for BBB transport normally occur in the physiological range (Pardridge, 1977a). Therefore, when hyperaminoacidemia is induced following a protein meal, the BBB transport of L-DOPA is diminished and this causes the "on-off" effect of L-DOPA therapy for Parkinson's disease (Mena and Cotzias, 1975; Nutt et al., 1984). Similarly, the brain uptake of α-methyldopa is inhibited by hyperaminoacidemia (Markovitz and Fernstrom, 1977). Conversely, hypoaminoacidemia, such as that induced by insulin secretion following a carbohydrate meal, would be expected to cause an increased brain uptake of neutral amino acid drugs such as L-DOPA or melphalan.

MCT1 monocarboxylic acid transporter

The BBB has a monocarboxylic acid transporter (MCT) that is responsible for brain uptake of circulating lactate, pyruvate, and ketone bodies (Oldendorf, 1973).

The BBB MCT is induced in states of ketosis such as the neonatal period or fasting (Cremer et al., 1979). The brain combustion of ketone bodies is rate-limited by the BBB MCT transporter (Hawkins et al., 1986). Like the *Glut* or LAT gene families, there are multiple isoforms within the MCT family of monocarboxylic acid transporters. The MCT1 isoform is selectively expressed at the BBB whereas the MCT2 isoform is expressed in astrocytes in brain (Gerhart et al., 1999). Polymerase chain reaction (PCR) techniques were first used to demonstrate expression of the MCT1 gene at the BBB (Takanaga et al., 1995). Subsequent electron microscopic immunogold analysis showed the immunoreactive MCT1 was upregulated 15-fold in capillaries of the 14-day-old rat brain as compared to adult rat brain (Leino et al., 1999). It is difficult to detect immunoreactive MCT1 at the BBB in adult brain (Leino et al., 1999). The inability to detect immunoreactive MCT1 protein or the MCT1 mRNA in capillaries of adult brain is indicative of a low expression of this gene that normally occurs at the BBB in adult brain (Pellerin et al., 1998). The consequence of this relatively low expression of BBB MCT1 in adult brain is the rapid build-up of lactic acid in cerebral anoxia (Pardridge and Oldendorf, 1977). In contrast, when the myocardium is subjected to anoxia, there is little build-up of lactic acid in heart owing to the very high permeability of lactic acid across myocardial capillaries. In the brain, there is relatively low vascular permeability to lactic acid, owing to the low gene expression of BBB MCT1 in the adult brain, and this may account for the selective vulnerability of the brain to a lactic acid build-up in brief periods of anoxia.

The BBB MCT1 is a portal of entry to the brain for monocarboxylic acid drugs. Butyric acid crosses the BBB on the MCT and this is cross-competed by probenecid, which has a K_i of 1.5 mmol/l (Pardridge et al., 1975). At high concentrations, monocarboxylic acid drugs such as penicillin or acetylsalicylic acid are neurotoxic, and these drugs may gain access to the brain via the BBB MCT. At lower concentrations, however, the brain uptake of monocarboxylic acid drugs may not be appreciable, despite the presence of the MCT on the BBB, because these drugs are rapidly effluxed back to blood via BBB carrier-mediated active efflux systems, as discussed below.

Adenosine transporter

The V_{max} of the BBB adenosine transporter is even lower than that of the BBB lactate carrier (Table 3.1). Since an adenosine carrier is expressed at the BBB in vivo (Cornford and Oldendorf, 1975), it is puzzling that the intracarotid arterial infusion of adenosine has no vasodilator effect in brain similar to that found in other organs (Berne et al., 1983). The absence of CNS pharmacologic effects of adenosine following intracarotid arterial infusion arises from an enzymatic barrier to the circulating adenosine (Pardridge et al., 1994c). More than 90% of adenosine is

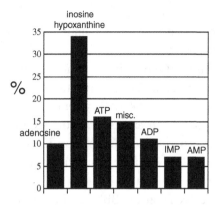

More than 90% of adenosine is metabolized following a 15-s internal carotid artery perfusion of [³H]-adenosine in the rat; brain metabolism was terminated by microwave irradiation of the head

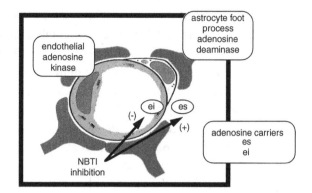

THE ENZYMATIC BARRIER TO CIRCULATING ADENOSINE EXPLAINS WHY INTRACAROTID INFUSED ADENOSINE HAS NO PHARMACOLOGIC EFFECT IN BRAIN.

Figure 3.15 Adenosine is transported by the blood–brain barrier adenosine carrier but is instantly metabolized at the brain microvasculature. Left: The percentage of brain radioactivity in various adenosine metabolites following a 15-s internal carotid artery perfusion of [³H] adenosine. ATP, adenosine triphosphate; ADP, adenosine diphosphate; IMP, inosine monophosphate; AMP, adenosine monophosphate. Right: Scheme showing differential expression of adenosine transporters on the luminal and abluminal membrane of the capillary endothelium and the relationship between these transporters, and the enzymatic barrier to adenosine formed by adenosine deaminase, localized in astrocyte foot processes. NBTI, S-4-nitrobenzyl-(6-thioinosine). The chromotagraphy data are from Pardridge et al. (1994c).

metabolized following a 15-s internal carotid artery perfusion of [³H]adenosine in the rat. In these studies, brain metabolism was instantly terminated by microwave radiation of the head and the principal metabolite was inosine and hypoxanthine (Figure 3.15). BBB transport of adenosine is insensitive to S-4-nitrobenzyl-(6-thioinosine) (NBTI) following intracarotid arterial infusion (Pardridge et al., 1994c). These studies suggest that the NBTI-sensitive adenosine transporter (designated es, and also known as ENT1) is not present on the luminal side of the BBB. However, high-affinity NBTI receptors are present in isolated brain capillaries (Kalaria and Harik, 1988). These observations suggest that the 'es' adenosine carrier is present on the abluminal side of the BBB, as depicted in Figure 3.15. Conversely, the in vivo evidence suggests that the NBTI-insensitive adenosine isoform (designated ei, or ENT2) is selectively expressed on the luminal membrane of the BBB (Figure 3.15).

The enzymatic barrier to circulating adenosine is distal to the BBB adenosine transporter at the endothelial cell plasma membrane, and may either be located in the endothelial cell cytoplasm or the astrocyte foot process. Adenosine deaminase, which converts adenosine to inosine, is localized at astrocyte foot processes with minimal localization at capillary endothelial cells in brain (Yamamoto et al., 1987). Since the principal metabolite formed during the intracarotid arterial infusion of adenosine is inosine (Pardridge et al., 1994c), the adenosine deaminase on astrocyte foot processes may be responsible for the enzymatic barrier to circulating adenosine. The activity of adenosine deaminase in rabbit brain capillaries was comparable to that of other adenosine metabolizing enzymes such as adenosine kinase, suggesting that adenosine deaminase could also be in the brain microvascular endothelium (Mistry and Drummond, 1986). However, as discussed below for p-glycoprotein, isolated brain capillaries are studded with remnants of astrocyte foot processes. Therefore, isolated brain capillary preparations contain enzymes that are purely of astrocyte foot process origin.

The BBB adenosine carrier, like the BBB *Glut1*, LAT1, or MCT1 carrier, is a portal of entry for drugs to the brain if the drug has a structure mimicking that of the endogenous nutrient. If the BBB adenosine carrier is to be targeted, then adenosine analogs that are resistant to adenosine deaminase must be developed to circumvent the BBB enzymatic barrier.

Choline transporter

There is a specific choline transporter at the BBB (Table 3.1), which also transports other drugs with quaternary ammonium derivatives such as hemicholinium and deanol (Cornford et al., 1978). Studies with rat serum suggest that there are compounds in plasma that compete for the BBB choline carrier other than choline itself (Cornford et al., 1978; Wecker and Trommer, 1984). Moreover, other studies suggest that there is a source of choline in the blood other than the free choline (Schuberth and Jenden, 1975), and that this source explains the net negative extraction of choline across the brain as determined by arterial–venous difference measurements (Aquilonius et al., 1975). The leading candidate for the alternative choline source is circulating lysolecithin, which is bound to high-affinity binding sites on albumin. However, no measurable transport of lysolecithin could be experimentally recorded using the BUI technique (Pardridge et al., 1979). It is also possible that there is no net extraction, i.e., net output, of choline by the brain. When arterial–venous differences are recorded by venous sampling techniques, it is possible to reverse the venous flow in the head if venous blood is sampled under negative pressure (Hertz and Bolwig, 1976). If there is not actual net export of choline from brain to blood, there may not be a need to posit an alternative source of circulating choline, since circulating lecithin or lysolecithin does not undergo significant transport across the BBB (Pardridge et al., 1979). Nevertheless, there is evidence that substrates in plasma, other than choline, compete with choline for entry into brain (Cornford et al., 1978; Wecker and Trommer, 1984). Carnitine is a possible candidate since this nutrient has a quaternary ammonium group, but competition studies indicated carnitine has a weak affinity for the BBB choline transporter (Cornford et al., 1978). The water-soluble vitamin thiamine has a quaternary ammonium group and competes for BBB choline transport (Kang et al., 1990), but the concentration of thiamine in the blood is insufficient to account for the competition effects observed with rat serum. That is, the affinity of thiamine for the choline carrier is not particularly high (Greenwood and Pratt, 1983), and the K_m of the choline carrier for thiamine is much higher than the plasma concentration, which means competition effects will not occur under physiologic conditions. These considerations illustrate that the affinity of the choline carrier for quaternary ammonium drugs is relatively low. As discussed above for lipid-mediated transport, the conversion of amino moieties on drugs to quaternary ammonium groups is one strategy for blocking BBB drug transport. This conversion could have paradoxical effects, if the lipid mediation of the drug was blocked, but the carrier mediation of the drug via the BBB choline carrier was enhanced.

Vitamin transport

There is evidence for a number of low-capacity (low V_{max}) vitamin carriers in the BBB. Some of these carriers may have evolved specifically to transport a given vitamin. Alternatively, CMT of vitamins through the BBB may occur because the vitamin has affinity for one of the endogenous nutrient carriers. As discussed above, thiamine may have some affinity for the BBB choline carrier (Kang et al., 1990). Although ascorbic acid (vitamin C) does not undergo transport across the BBB (Spector, 1981), the reduced form of vitamin C, dehydroascorbic acid, rapidly enters brain from blood, because this form of vitamin C is a substrate for the BBB *Glut1* glucose transporter (Agus et al., 1997). The dehydroascorbic acid is reduced in brain and thereby trapped in brain tissue in the form of ascorbic acid.

Methyltetrahydrofolic acid (MTFA) is a monocarboxylic acid, and is transported across the BBB by a saturable carrier-mediated system that is equally inhibited by 10 μmol/l concentrations of either MTFA or folic acid (Wu and Pardridge, 1999a). The folates are transported across biological membranes by either the folate receptor (FR) or the reduced folate carrier (RFC) (Zhao et al., 1997). The RFC has a preferential affinity for MTFA rather than folic acid, whereas the FR has an equal affinity for either MTFA or folic acid. The observation that both MTFA and folic acid compete for MTFA transport across the BBB suggests that the FR may be expressed at the BBB in vivo (Wu and Pardridge, 1999a). Western blotting studies show that the FR is expressed in brain only at the choroid plexus (Weitman et al.,

1994), but a selective expression of the FR at the BBB would not be detected in Western blotting studies of whole brain extracts.

The water-soluble vitamin, biotin, is also transported across the BBB via a saturable transport system (Spector et al., 1986), and the BBB PS product for biotin, 10.8 ± 1.0 μl/min per g (Kang et al., 1995b), is 10-fold greater than the BBB PS product for MTFA, 1.1 ± 0.3 μl/min per g (Wu and Pardridge, 1999a). Given the appreciable permeability of the BBB for biotin, one strategy for enhancing drug transport across the BBB is to biotinylate drugs such that these would have an affinity for the BBB biotin carrier. However, biotinylation of drugs does not cause BBB transport (Bickel et al., 1993a). This observation reinforces the idea that if the BBB CMT systems are to be used as portals of entry to the brain for drugs, then the drug must be converted to a structure that mimics the endogenous nutrient or vitamin. Conversely, when the drug is conjugated to the endogenous nutrient or vitamin, the affinity for the BBB CMT system is lost. The exception to this rule may be the folate transport system if, in fact, BBB transport of folate is mediated by the folate receptor. That is, folate transport across the BBB may be an RMT system, reviewed in Chapter 4, not a CMT system. Receptors, which operate on the order of minutes, are more tolerant of structural changes on the endogenous ligand than are carriers, which operate on the order of milliseconds.

Thyroid hormone transporter

There is a specific carrier at the BBB for thyroid hormones (Pardridge, 1979) and this carrier has a higher affinity for triiodothyronine (T_3) as compared to thyroxine (T_4). The BBB T_3 carrier is stereospecific with a 10-fold higher affinity for L-T_3 as compared to D-T_3 (Terasaki and Pardridge, 1987). A significant proportion of thyroid hormone action in the body may be mediated by thyroid hormone effects that take place within the brain. The intracerebroventricular injection of T_3 has a greater elevation of the heart rate in hypothyroidism than does intravenously injected T_3 (Goldman et al., 1985). The BBB T_3 carrier may be the site of the stereospecific action of thyroid hormone in the body. The oral administration of L-T_3 has a much greater pharmacologic effect than the oral administration of D-T_3. However, thyroid hormone binding to plasma proteins or thyroid hormone binding to the nuclear receptor is not stereospecific. These observations suggest that the principal locus of the stereospecificity of the thyroid hormonal action is the BBB T_3 carrier (Terasaki and Pardridge, 1987).

Summary of CMT

The BBB carrier-mediated transport systems listed in Table 3.1 are all portals of entry for brain drug-targeting systems. However, for the optimal use of these systems for brain drug targeting, it is preferable to convert the drug structure into a nutrient-mimetic structure, rather than coupling the drug to the nutrient and forming a conjugate of drug and nutrient. As illustrated in the case of morphine and M6G (Figure 3.12), the addition of a carbohydrate moiety to morphine does not mediate transport of the drug across the BBB via the *Glut1* glucose carrier (Wu et al., 1997a). The second principle with respect to drug targeting via the BBB CMT systems is that it is necessary to optimize the use of enzymatic BBB mechanisms. For example, L-DOPA is an effective precursor for dopamine in brain because once this neutral amino acid is transported across the BBB on LAT1, the drug is immediately decarboxylated by aromatic amino acid decarboxylase, which is abundant in the perivascular compartment (Wade and Katzman, 1975). Similarly, the adenosine deaminase in the astrocyte foot process rapidly inactivates adenosine once it is transported across the BBB (Yamamoto et al., 1987; Pardridge et al., 1994c). Much of these enzymatic barrier systems may reside in the astrocyte foot process or pericyte compartments. Although many BBB functions are generally ascribed to the endothelial cell, the pericyte and astrocyte foot process are two other cells that form the brain microvasculature (Pardridge, 1999a). The pericyte shares the basement membrane with the endothelial cell, and more than 99% of the surface of the capillary is invested by astrocyte foot processes. The intimate relationships between the brain capillary endothelial cell and the astrocyte foot process are illustrated in the case of p-glycoprotein, as discussed below.

Carrier-mediated efflux

p-Glycoprotein

p-Glycoprotein is a 170 kDa cell surface protein that is a product of the multidrug resistance (MDR) gene, which is a member of the ATP-binding cassette (ABC) gene family (Gao et al., 1998). p-Glycoprotein is responsible for an ATP-dependent active efflux of drugs from the cellular compartment to the extracellular space (Kartner et al., 1985). Certain drugs may induce p-glycoprotein expression in cancer cells and induce resistance to chemotherapeutic agents by virtue of the active efflux of the drug from the cancer cell. Immunoreactive p-glycoprotein was found at the brain microvasculature in either brain tissue sections (Cordon-Cardo et al., 1989) or in isolated brain capillaries (Jette et al., 1993). These observations gave rise to the idea that p-glycoprotein was responsible for active efflux of drug across the brain capillary endothelium and it is hypothesized that p-glycoprotein is expressed at the luminal membrane of the capillary endothelium in brain. However, there are several lines of evidence that argue against the selective expression of p-glycoprotein at the endothelial plasma membrane, particularly for the human brain. The systemic administration of p-glycoprotein inhibitors such as cyclosporin A or verapamil resulted in the increased uptake in peripheral tissues of a p-glycoprotein substrate, vinblastine, but there was no parallel increase in brain uptake of vinblastine (Arboix et al., 1997). Second, the intravenous injection in primates of radiolabeled MRK16, a monoclonal antibody to human p-glycoprotein, resulted in no binding to the brain microvasculature in vivo (Pardridge et al., 1997). There should have been binding observed because the MRK16 MAb binds an epitope of p-glycoprotein that projects into the extracellular space (Georges et al., 1993), and this should have been freely accessible to circulating MRK16, if p-glycoprotein is expressed at the luminal membrane of the brain capillary endothelium. For example, the intravenous injection of MAbs that target the BBB insulin receptor or TfR, which are expressed at the luminal membrane of the capillary endothelium in brain, are rapidly taken up by brain (Chapter 5). Third, the pattern of immunostaining of brain sections with p-glycoprotein antibodies was similar to that observed with antibodies directed against glial fibrillary acidic protein (GFAP), which is a marker of astrocyte cell bodies and astrocyte foot processes (Pardridge et al., 1997).

The close, indeed intimate, association of astrocyte foot processes and the capillary endothelium is shown in Figure 3.16. Confocal microscopy was used in conjunction with antibodies both to the *Glut1* glucose transporter, a brain capillary endothelial marker, and to GFAP, an astrocyte foot process marker, to show the dual staining of these two antigens at the brain microvasculature (Figure 3.16A). The elaborate architecture of the astrocyte foot process at the brain microvasculature is shown in the various panels of Figure 3.16. Kacem et al. (1998) propose that the astrocyte foot processes form a rosette-like structure at the microvasculature, which is seen in confocal microscopy (panels D, E, and F of Figure 3.16). The astrocyte cell bodies send foot processes to endothelial cells and this is shown in Figure 3.16C (Blumcke et al., 1995).

The detection of immunoreactive GFAP at astrocyte foot processes decorating the brain microvasculature is highly dependent on the technique that is used, both with respect to the fixation of the brain tissue and to the origin of the anti-GFAP antibody (Kacem et al., 1998). Some GFAP antibodies will only detect immunoreactive GFAP in astrocyte cell bodies and other GFAP antibodies will only detect astrocyte foot processes (Kacem et al., 1998). When isolated capillaries are prepared, there are remnants of astrocyte foot processes that remain adhered to the basement membrane of the isolated brain capillary. This was first shown by White et al. (1981) and subsequently demonstrated conclusively with confocal microscopy which showed colocalization of GFAP and the muscarinic acetylcholine receptor at astrocyte foot processes in preparations of isolated brain capillaries (Moro et al., 1995).

Similar to the colocalization of GFAP and the muscarinic acetylcholine receptor

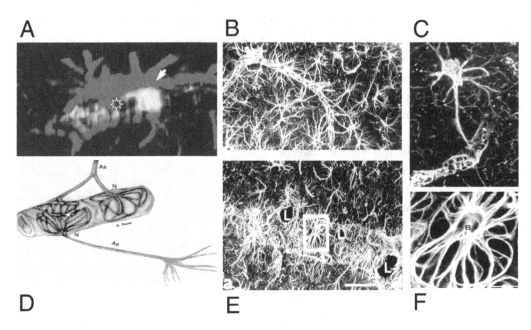

Figure 3.16   Confocal fluorescent microscopy of immunoactive glial fibrillary acidic protein (GFAP) in rat brain. A capillary dual-labeled with antibodies to GFAP and the *Glut1* glucose transporter shows the endothelial staining and the intimal relationship with the astrocyte foot process. Panel A: arrow shows endothelial *Glut1* glucose transporter. Panels B, E, and F are serial confocal scans reconstructed to show the three-dimensional relationship of immunoreactive GFAP bearing astrocyte foot processes with the brain microvasculature. The astrocyte foot processes form a rosette-like structure at the abluminal membrane of the capillary endothelium, as shown in panel D. Panel C shows an astrocyte cell body sending a projection to form a foot process on a neighboring capillary. Panel D: As, astrocyte; N, nucleus. Panel E: L, vessel lumen. Boxed area is magnified in panel F. Panel F: B, body of astrocyte. Panels A, B, D, E, and F are from Kacem et al. (1998) with permission and panel C is from Blumcke et al.: Relationship between astrocyte processes and "perioneuronal nets" in rat neocortex, Blumcke, I., Eggli, P. and Celio, M.R., *Glia*, copyright © (1995). Reprinted by permission of Wiley-Liss, Inc., a subsidiary of John Wiley & Sons, Inc.

in isolated brain capillaries, there is colocalization of GFAP and p-glycoprotein in this preparation (Golden and Pardridge, 1999). Isolated human brain capillaries were cytocentrifuged to a glass slide, and stained with antibodies to either the *Glut1* glucose transporter, an endothelial cell marker, or to GFAP, an astrocyte foot process marker. Using the MRK16 antibody to human p-glycoprotein, there is colocalization of immunoreactive p-glycoprotein at the human brain microvasculature with GFAP, not *Glut1*, as shown in Figure 3.17 (colour plate). The colocalization patterns of MRK16 and the anti-GFAP antibody are identical and overlap completely, whereas there is no overlap of MRK16 and *Glut1* (Figure 3.17).

These results suggest that brain microvascular p-glycoprotein, at least in the human brain, is localized to the astrocyte foot process (Golden and Pardridge, 1999). The presence of p-glycoprotein in brain astrocytes has been demonstrated for human brain (Tishler et al., 1995). In rat brain, astrocytic p-glycoprotein is increased after excitotoxic brain damage (Zhang et al., 1999a); these last findings are consistent with the observation that p-glycoprotein is expressed in C6 rat glial cells (Henderson and Strauss, 1991).

The finding that p-glycoprotein is expressed at astrocyte foot processes attached to human brain capillaries was not supported by studies with human brain microvessels that were prepared by an enzymatic homogenization technique (Seetharaman et al., 1998). In this study, there was no colocalization of immunoreactive p-glycoprotein and GFAP. However, when capillaries are isolated by an enzymatic homogenization technique, the basement membrane is dissolved and the astrocyte foot process remnants are separated from the endothelial cells in the subsequent Percoll density centrifugation (Pardridge et al., 1986). With this methodology, one would not expect to colocalize p-glycoprotein and GFAP in human brain capillaries, since the astrocyte foot processes are removed from the brain capillary preparation.

Three-cell model of BBB drug transport

The expression of p-glycoprotein at the astrocyte foot process is still consistent with a pivotal role played by this efflux system in regulating brain uptake of drugs. Moreover, the placement of p-glycoprotein at the astrocyte foot process leads to a three-cell model of how drug movement across the cerebral microvasculature is regulated (Pardridge, 1999a). The endothelium and the astrocyte foot process are separated by a distance of only 20 nm (Paulson and Newman, 1987), and this space is filled by capillary basement membrane. All drugs that enter brain must traverse the tiny compartment that exists between the endothelial abluminal membrane and the astrocyte foot process. Morever, a third cell, the brain capillary pericyte, which shares the basement membrane with the endothelium, is anatomically positioned to work in concert with the endothelium and the astrocyte foot process to regulate the flux of drugs across the brain microvasculature (Figure 3.18). Several ectoenzymes are expressed on the pericyte plasma membrane (Risau et al., 1992; Kunz et al., 1994). Therefore, pericyte ectoenzymes, astrocyte foot process p-glycoprotein, and endothelial active efflux systems at the endothelial abluminal membrane may all work in concert to prevent the brain uptake of xenobiotics. The inhibition of any one of these three systems would cause the brain/plasma drug concentration ratio to be increased. Indeed, the brain/plasma concentration ratio of a number of drugs is increased in the p-glycoprotein knockout mouse (Schinkel et al., 1995). However, the brain/plasma drug ratio is a function of several

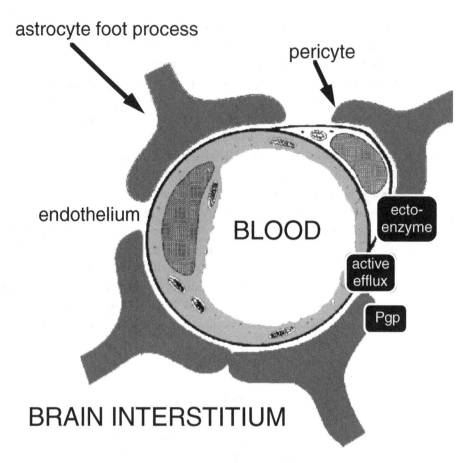

Figure 3.18   Three-cell model of the brain microvasculature showing the intimate relationship of active efflux systems within the brain capillary endothelial membrane, ectoenzymes in the pericyte plasma membrane, and p-glycoprotein (Pgp) in the plasma membrane of astrocyte foot processes. From Pardridge (1999a) with permission. © 1999 The Alfred Benzon Foundation, DK-2900 Hellerup, Denmark.

parameters, only one of which is the permeability of the BBB on the endothelial luminal membrane. The brain/plasma drug ratio is a function of (a) influx into brain, (b) efflux from brain to blood, (c) binding to cytosolic proteins in brain cells, and (d) metabolism of the drug by brain cells. The interaction of these multiple factors in the regulation of solute uptake by brain is discussed further below in the context of a physiologic model of plasma protein-mediated transport.

Endothelial active efflux systems

None of the three drugs that form the triple therapy of acquired immune deficiency syndrome (AIDS) – AZT, 3TC, or protease inhibitors – cross the BBB. The human immunodeficiency virus (HIV) protease inhibitors are all substrates for p-glycoprotein (Lee et al., 1998). Drugs such as AZT and 3TC are not substrates for p-glycoprotein (Lucia et al., 1995). Nevertheless, these drugs have a BBB penetration that is log orders less than that expected on the basis of the lipid-solubility of these drugs (Figure 3.3). This is because drugs such as AZT, 3TC, or dideoxyinosine (DDI) are all substrates for a probenecid-sensitive active efflux system at the brain microvasculature (Galinsky et al., 1990; Dykstra et al., 1993; Takasawa et al., 1997). These active efflux systems are similar to that expressed in kidney, which accounts for active renal secretion of AZT by a process that is inhibited by p-aminohippuric acid (PAH) (Griffiths et al., 1991). Initially, it was concluded that AZT readily penetrated the CNS and this was based on findings that AZT was transported into human cerebrospinal fluid (CSF) (Klecker et al., 1987). However, the AZT transport into CSF occurs because there is no active efflux of AZT at the choroid plexus, which forms the blood–CSF barrier (Chapter 2). Conversely, there is no significant transport of AZT into brain parenchyma (Ahmed et al., 1991), because there is active efflux of AZT at the BBB (Takasawa et al., 1997). To date, the system responsible for the active efflux of drugs such as AZT or 3TC at the BBB is not known.

There are probably numerous active efflux systems at the brain microvasculature that remain to be identified (Deguchi et al., 1995). Bile acids such as taurocholate undergo efflux from brain to blood at the BBB via a process that is sensitive to probenecid, but not PAH (Kitazawa et al., 1998). However, the BBB active efflux systems for bile acids, estrone sulfate, or other organic acids has not been clarified at the molecular level. Recent studies show that organic anion transporting polypeptide type 2 (oatp2) is selectively expressed in brain at the BBB (Gao et al., 1999; Li et al., 2001). oatp2 transports thyroid hormones, bile acids, and estrone sulfate. Although estrone is rapidly transported across the BBB by lipid mediation, estrone sulfate is not transported across the BBB (Steingold et al., 1986), and this may be due to active efflux of this molecule by BBB oatp2. Similarly, there is evidence that the permeability of the BBB for T_3 on the brain side of the barrier is greater than the permeability on the blood side (Pardridge, 1979). This asymmetry of BBB T_3 transport may be secondary to active efflux of T_3 via BBB transporters such as oatp2. At the present time, the ultrastructural localization of oatp2 in brain capillary endothelium has not been clarified. Given the availability of antibodies to immunoreactive oatp2, it would be useful to perform electron microscopic immunogold studies of oatp2 expression at the BBB similar to that done for the *Glut1* glucose transporter (Figure 3.11). Presumably, active efflux transport systems at the BBB are selectively localized on the endothelial abluminal membrane.

Codrugs and BBB active efflux systems

Novel BBB active efflux systems may be identified in a BBB genomics program that clones novel genes selectively expressed at the BBB and such strategies are discussed in more detail in Chapter 10. Such a "BBB genomics" program led to the finding of selective expression of oatp2 at the BBB, as reviewed in Chapter 10. Novel efflux systems at the BBB would be important new targets for enhancing brain uptake of drugs such as AZT or 3TC with the use of "codrug" therapy. In this approach, a codrug is administered along with the AZT or 3TC and the codrug inhibits the BBB active efflux system, which increases penetration of circulating AZT or 3TC into brain for the treatment of cerebral AIDS. Such a codrug approach would be analogous to the use of aromatic amino acid decarboxylase (AAAD) inhibitors in conjunction with L-DOPA therapy. These inhibitors, which do not cross the BBB (Clark, 1973), inhibit the peripheral degradation of L-DOPA by AAAD. Since the inhibitors do not cross the BBB, AAAD in the CNS is not inhibited by the codrugs. The codrug strategy is little used in present-day CNS drug therapy. However, the discovery of novel BBB active efflux systems could provide the molecular basis for future codrug discovery.

Plasma protein-mediated transport

Enhanced dissociation mechanism

Tryptophan and many drugs are bound by plasma proteins such as albumin, α_1-acid glycoprotein (AAG), or lipoproteins. A widely held view is that only the drug that is free in vitro, as determined by equilibrium dialysis or a comparable method, is available for transport across the BBB in vivo (Pardridge, 1998b). However, when the free drug hypothesis is subjected to direct empiric testing in vivo, it is found that the plasma protein-bound drug is operationally available for transport across the BBB in vivo. This occurs by a process of enhanced dissociation at the brain capillary endothelial interface. The enhanced dissociation results in transport of the drug into brain from the circulating plasma protein-bound pool without a parallel BBB transport of the plasma protein per se. This process is characterized by an increase in the dissociation constant (K_D) governing the ligand–plasma protein-binding reaction in vivo in the brain capillary, as compared to the K_D that occurs in vitro in a test tube (Table 3.2). The expansion of the K_D in vivo arises from conformational changes about the ligand-binding site on the plasma protein. This conformational change results in an increase in the dissociation rate of the ligand from the binding site in vivo in the brain capillary relative to the dissociation rate that occurs in vitro (Pardridge, 1998b). The in vivo K_D, designated K_D^a, can be measured with the KRC equation for a plasma protein with a single drug-binding site as follows:

$$E = 1 - e^{-f \cdot PS/F}$$
$$f = K_D^a / (K_D^a + A_F)$$

where E = the extraction of unidirectional influx, F = cerebral blood flow, f = bioavailable fraction, and A_F = the concentration of unoccupied plasma protein-

Table 3.2 Comparison of plasma protein binding of hormones and drugs in vitro and in vivo within the brain microvasculature

Plasma protein	Ligand	K_D(μmol/l) (in vitro)	$K_D{}^a$(μmol/l) (in vivo)
Bovine albumin	Testosterone	53 ± 1	2520 ± 710
	Tryptophan	130 ± 30	1670 ± 110
	Corticosterone	260 ± 10	1330 ± 90
	Dihydrotestosterone	53 ± 6	830 ± 140
	Estradiol	23 ± 1	710 ± 100
	T_3	4.7 ± 0.1	46 ± 4
	Propranolol	290 ± 30	220 ± 40
	Bupivacaine	141 ± 10	211 ± 107
	Imipramine	221 ± 21	1675 ± 600
hAAG	Propranolol	3.1 ± 0.2	19 ± 4
	Bupivacaine	6.5 ± 0.5	17 ± 4
	Isradipine	6.9 ± 0.9	35 ± 2
	Darodipine	2.5 ± 0.5	55 ± 7
	Imipramine	4.9 ± 0.3	90 ± 9
Human albumin	L-663,581	125 ± 16	675 ± 18
	L-364,718	8.2 ± 0.8	266 ± 38
	Diazepam	6.3 ± 0.1	157 ± 36
hVLDL	Cyclosporin	1.9 ± 0.5	1.8 ± 0.4 [a]
hLDL	Cyclosporin	0.81 ± 0.08	1.6 ± 0.4 [a]
hHDL	Cyclosporin	0.45 ± 0.10	0.44 ± 0.11[a]
HSA	Isradipine	63 ± 8	221 ± 7
	Darodipine	94 ± 5	203 ± 14

Notes:

hAAG, human α_1-acid glycoprotein; hVLDL, human very low density lipoprotein; hLDL, human low density lipoprotein; hHDL, human high density lipoprotein; HSA, human serum albumin; T_3, triiodothyronine.

[a] Units are grams per liter.

From Pardridge (1998b) with permission.

binding sites (Pardridge, 1998b). The in vivo $K_D{}^a$ will equal the K_D measured in vitro if there is no enhanced dissociation of the ligand from the plasma protein-binding site in vivo in the brain capillary compartment (Table 3.2).

The drug-binding sites on albumin are shown in the three-dimensional structure of albumin (Carter and He, 1994). The structure of human serum albumin (HSA) has been determined by X-ray diffraction (Figure 3.19). Free fatty acids and

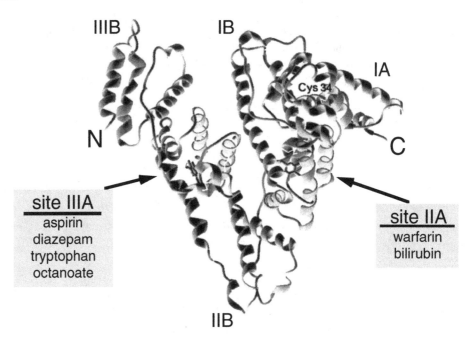

Figure 3.19   Three-dimensional structure of human serum albumin predicted from X-ray diffraction. The amino (N) and carboxyl (C) termini are indicated. The six different drug-binding sites in the albumin molecule are designated IA, IB, IIA, IIB, IIIA, and IIIB. The main drug-binding sites on albumin are IIA and IIIA. From Carter and He (1994) with permission.

tryptophan bind to subdomain IIIA, and bilirubin and warfarin bind to subdomain IIA. The three-dimensional structure of proteins that is determined with X-ray diffraction yields a static image of relatively rigid protein molecules. However, the original three-dimensional model of albumin formulated by Brown (1977) envisions "springs" comprising the ligand-binding sites. These springs reflect the constant random fluctuations of molecular motion that allows for sudden conformational transitions. These conformational changes can either be selective at specific binding sites on the albumin molecule or can be of a global nature throughout the entire molecule. Albumin should not be considered to be in a static state, but is a "kicking and screaming stochastic" molecule (Peters, 1985). Kragh-Hansen (1981) noted the flexible nature of the albumin molecule and classified the conformational changes as being either of large amplitude, similar to a "breathing" molecule, or small amplitude with conformational changes that have a half-time in the order of nanoseconds.

The flexibility of the albumin molecule is reduced by either acid pH or by binding of cationic drugs (Kragh-Hansen, 1981). The latter finding is of interest since the binding of lipophilic amines, such as propranolol or bupivacaine, to albumin is not associated with enhanced drug dissociation in vivo in the brain capillary (Pardridge, 1998b). The absence of enhanced dissociation of certain lipophilic amines from albumin is demonstrated by the equality between the in vivo K_D^a and the in vitro K_D, as shown in Table 3.2. Conversely, the binding of lipophilic amine drugs to AAG is characterized by marked enhanced dissociation at the brain capillary in vivo, and this is shown by the increased K_D^a in vivo in the brain capillary as compared to the in vitro K_D value (Table 3.2). The increase in the K_D^a in vivo is mediated by the collision of the albumin molecule with the endothelial glycocalyx. This collision triggers the conformational changes about the binding site on the plasma protein (Horie et al., 1988; Reed and Burrington, 1989).

In summary, plasma protein-mediated transport into brain, and in peripheral tissues, is a widely observed phenomenon. Transport of plasma protein-bound drug that is restricted to only the free fraction measured in vitro is the exception, not the rule. These findings indicate that drug targeting to the brain cannot be predicted on the basis of in vitro measurements of plasma protein binding of drugs. Rather, in vivo methodology such as the BUI method or the internal carotid artery perfusion method (Chapter 4) should be used to determine the extent to which plasma protein binding restricts BBB transport of a given drug or ligand in vivo. Using the in vivo methods enables the measurement of the dissociation constant governing the drug/protein binding reaction in vivo within the brain capillary compartment. When this is done, the typical finding is that the in vivo K_D^a is much higher than the in vitro K_D (Table 3.2), consistent with the enhanced dissociation mechanism.

Physiologic model of brain uptake of drugs

A method that is often used to measure BBB permeability of a given drug is the determination of the brain/plasma ratio, which is equivalent to an organ volume of distribution (V_D). The organ V_D is actually a complex function of many parameters, only one of which is BBB permeability. A physiologic model of the distribution in brain of a drug that is bound by both plasma proteins and brain cytosolic proteins is shown in Figure 3.20 (Pardridge and Landaw, 1985). The influx of the drug through the BBB is a function of the on and off rates of drug binding to albumin (K_7, K_8, Figure 3.20), drug binding to plasma globulins such as AAG (K_1, K_2, Figure 3.20), and to BBB permeability on the endothelial luminal membrane (K_3, Figure 3.20). The efflux of drug from brain to blood is a function of the BBB permeability on the endothelial abluminal membrane (K_4, Figure 3.20), the on and off rates of drug binding to cytosolic proteins in brain cells (K_5, K_6, Figure 3.20), and brain metabolism of the drug (K_{met}, Figure 3.20). The brain/plasma drug ratio is determined by all of these factors.

The pool of drug available for transport through the BBB, which is L_F in Figure

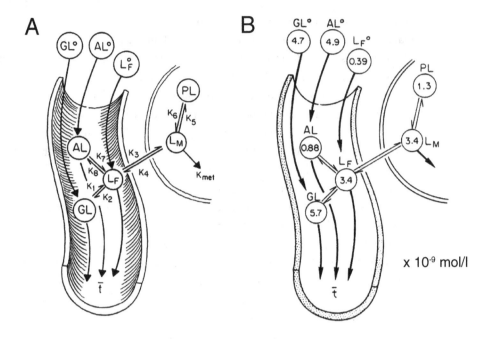

Figure 3.20 (A) Physiological model of drug transport through the brain capillary wall and into brain cells. Pools of globulin-bound, albumin-bound, and free drug in the systemic circulation are denoted as GL^0, AL^0, and L_F^0, respectively; pools of globulin-bound, albumin-bound, and plasma bioavailable drug in the brain capillary are denoted as GL, AL, and L_F, respectively. Pools of free and cytoplasmic-bound drug in brain cells are denoted as L_M and PL, respectively; $\bar{t}$ is the mean capillary transit time in brain. (B) Predicted steady-state concentrations of testosterone in the various pools of the brain capillary and in brain cells. The pool size concentrations are nmol/l, and the concentration of free cytosolic testosterone in brain cells (L_M) is predicted to approximate the concentration of albumin-bound testosterone in the circulation (AL^0), but is more than 10-fold greater than the concentration of free hormone (L_F^0) measured in vitro by equilibrium dialysis. From Pardridge (1998b) with permission.

3.20, is much larger than the pool of drug that is free, as measured by in vitro methods, which is L_F^0 in Figure 3.20. This is due to the enhanced dissociation of drug from the plasma protein-bound pool within the brain capillary (Table 3.2). The pool of drug that is free inside brain cells (L_M in Figure 3.20) cannot be experimentally measured. However, this pool is driven solely by the pool of "bioavailable" drug in the brain capillary compartment (L_F), and this can be experimentally measured with the BUI technique, as reviewed elsewhere (Pardridge, 1998b). The brain concentration of drug is the sum of the free pool (L_M) and the protein-bound pool

(PL in Figure 3.20). The PL pool is a function of the cytosolic-binding proteins in brain cells. However, the concentration of free drug inside brain cells, L_M, which drives the formation of the drug–receptor complex, is independent of the activity of brain cytosolic binding systems (Pardridge, 1998b). The L_M pool is proportional to the pool of bioavailable drug in the brain capillary, L_F, as well as rates of organ metabolism of drug, as reflected in the K_{met} parameter (Figure 3.20).

In summary, many drugs are avidly bound by plasma proteins. Measurement of this binding by in vitro techniques such as equilibrium dialysis or ultrafiltration can give a false picture of drug transport at the BBB interface in vivo, because many drugs undergo enhanced dissociation at the BBB in vivo (Table 3.2). Also, measurement of the brain/plasma drug concentration ratio gives a false picture of BBB permeability. This is because the brain/plasma drug concentration ratio is a complex function of several parameters regulating drug influx and efflux between the plasma and brain compartments (Figure 3.20).

4

Receptor-mediated transcytosis of peptides

- Introduction
- Receptor-mediated transcytosis
- Absorptive-mediated transcytosis
- Neuropeptide transport at the blood–brain barrier
- Summary

Introduction

Receptor-mediated transcytosis (RMT) systems exist at the blood–brain barrier (BBB) in parallel with the carrier-mediated transport (CMT) systems reviewed in Chapter 3. The CMT systems mediate the BBB transport of small molecule nutrients, vitamins, and hormones and operate on the order of milliseconds. In contrast, the RMT systems mediate the BBB transport of circulating peptides and plasma proteins such as transferrin (Tf), and operate on the order of minutes. The CMT systems are stereospecific pores formed by transmembrane regions of the transporter protein that traverse the luminal or abluminal endothelial plasma membranes. In contrast, BBB receptors have relatively small transmembrane regions and large extracellular projecting portions that form the ligand-binding site. The receptor–ligand complex is endocytosed into the endothelial cell, packaged within an endosomal system, and traverses the endothelial cytoplasm for exocytosis in a matter of minutes. The distance that must be traversed in the process of transcytosis through the BBB is only 200–300 nm. This short distance may be the reason why BBB transcytosis is relatively rapid and occurs within minutes. There are numerous peptide receptor systems expressed at the BBB, and many of these mediate the RMT of the circulating peptide through the BBB (Figure 4.1).

The capillary endothelial barrier of the vertebrate brain is unique with respect to other endothelial barriers in peripheral tissues. The capillaries perfusing organs other than brain or spinal cord are porous and contain both transcellular and paracellular pathways for peptide transport through the endothelial barrier. The transcellular pathway is the extensive pinocytosis that occurs across the endothelium in peripheral tissues, and the paracellular pathways are the interendothelial junctional spaces that are open in peripheral capillaries because these lack epithelial-like tight

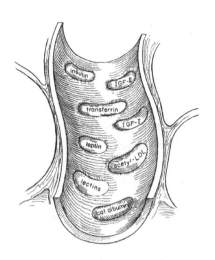

OBSERVATION:

PEPTIDE RECEPTORS ARE PRESENT ON THE BRAIN CAPILLARY ENDOTHELIUM, AND SOME OF THESE MEDIATE PEPTIDE TRANSCYTOSIS THROUGH THE BBB.

CHIMERIC PEPTIDE HYPOTHESIS:

DRUG DELIVERY TO THE BRAIN MAY BE ACHIEVED BY ATTACHMENT OF THE DRUG TO PEPTIDE OR PROTEIN "VECTORS," WHICH ARE TRANSPORTED INTO BRAIN FROM BLOOD BY ABSORPTIVE- OR RECEPTOR-MEDIATED TRANSCYTOSIS THROUGH THE BBB.

Figure 4.1   Blood–barrier peptide receptors and chimeric peptide hypothesis. IGF, insulin-like growth factor; LDL, low density lipoprotein. From Pardridge (1997) with permission.

junctions. Because of the availability of these pathways for free solute diffusion across endothelial barriers in peripheral tissues, circulating peptides such as insulin or Tf readily gain access to the interstitial space of peripheral tissues without the intervention of RMT systems at the endothelial barrier. For example, the transport of insulin across the endothelial barrier in peripheral tissues is not saturable (Steil et al., 1996). Similarly, the microvasculature of brain is selectively immunostained by antibodies to the Tf receptor (TfR), whereas the endothelial barrier in most peripheral tissues does not contain significant amounts of immunoreactive TfR (Jefferies et al., 1984).

Chimeric peptide hypothesis

The observation that peptide receptors are present on the brain capillary endothelium and some of these mediate peptide transcytosis through the BBB gave rise to the chimeric peptide hypothesis (Pardridge, 1986). It was hypothesized that drug delivery to the brain may be achieved by attachment of the drug to peptide or protein "vectors," which are transported into brain from blood by receptor- or absorptive-mediated transcytosis through the BBB (Figure 4.1). These vectors may be endogenous peptides or plasma proteins which are ligands for the receptor- or absorptive-mediated transcytosis systems at the BBB. Alternatively, the vectors may be peptidomimetic monoclonal antibodies (MAbs) that bind exofacial epitopes on the specific endogenous BBB receptors and "piggy-back" across the BBB via the peptide RMT system (Pardridge et al., 1991). This process occurs without significant inhibition of transport of the endogenous ligand (Skarlatos et al., 1995), and this is possible if the binding site for the peptidomimetic MAb is removed from the binding site for the endogenous ligand on the receptor.

Peptidomimetic monoclonal antibodies

The concept of peptidomimetic MAbs dates back many years when it was shown that certain MAbs to peptide receptors may have agonist-like properties (Shechter et al., 1982; Zick et al., 1984; Heffetz et al., 1989; Soos et al., 1989). Binding of the peptide receptor-specific MAb to the receptor triggers conformational changes within the receptor that are subsequently followed by peptide-like signal transduction phenomena. Similarly, certain MAbs may be "endocytosing MAbs" and undergo receptor-mediated endocytosis into the cell by virtue of MAb binding to an exofacial epitope on the peptide receptor. Similar events occur at the BBB. The OX26 MAb, which is a murine antibody to the rat TfR (Jefferies et al., 1985), binds the BBB TfR in rats and, like circulating Tf, undergoes RMT through the BBB subsequent to its binding to the endogenous BBB TfR (Chapter 5). The OX26 MAb and circulating Tf undergo binding and transport through the BBB at comparable rates, as determined by internal carotid artery perfusion studies (Skarlatos et al., 1995), as discussed below and in Chapter 5. There is no competition between the OX26 MAb and Tf for the BBB TfR (Skarlatos et al., 1995), because the MAb and the Tf bind to different binding sites on the TfR. For this reason, the MAb binding site is unsaturated in vivo, whereas the Tf binding site on the TfR is fully saturated by the high concentration (25 μmol/l) of circulating Tf in the plasma. At very high doses of the MAb there can be competition for Tf binding sites (Ueda et al., 1993), but no competition occurs at the pharmacologic doses of the MAb (Skarlatos et al., 1995).

Drug/vector conjugates

A chimeric peptide is formed when a peptide or peptidomimetic MAb is conjugated to a drug that is normally not transported through the BBB (Pardridge, 1986). The formation of the vector/drug conjugate must be accomplished in such a way that the bifunctionality of the conjugate is retained. That is, the drug must be biologically active in the form of the conjugate and the peptide or peptidomimetic MAb must still bind the BBB and trigger RMT in the form of the drug/vector conjugate. Therefore, an important component in the formation of chimeric peptides is the strategy by which the drug and vector are linked and these linker strategies are discussed in Chapter 6. The discovery and genetic engineering of BBB transport vectors are discussed in Chapter 5. The applications of chimeric peptides with protein-based drugs are discussed in Chapter 7 and the applications with antisense-based therapeutics are discussed in Chapter 8. The extension of the chimeric peptide hypothesis to gene targeting to the brain is discussed in Chapter 9, and the discovery of BBB-specific targets with a BBB genomics program is described in Chapter 10.

Peptide-mediated signal transduction phenomena at the blood–brain barrier

It is possible that many peptide receptors on the BBB do not mediate the transcytosis of the circulating peptide through the brain capillary endothelial barrier. Instead, the binding of a circulating peptide to its cognate receptor on the luminal surface of the endothelium may trigger signal transduction phenomena within the brain capillary endothelial cytoplasm to mediate the biological response of the peptide (Pardridge, 1983b). Similarly, there may be peptide receptors selectively expressed on the abluminal membrane of the capillary endothelium, and these may function to trigger signal transduction phenomena within the endothelial cytoplasm by virtue of secretion of the neuropeptide from the brain compartment. Many vasoactive peptides trigger signal transduction phenomena at the BBB without undergoing transcytosis through the endothelial barrier. Atrial natriuretic peptide (ANP) increases the formation of cyclic guanosine monophosphate (GMP) in brain capillary endothelial cells grown in primary tissue culture (Vigne and Frelin, 1992). Whether a similar phenomenon occurs in vivo is at present not known, but the intracarotid arterial perfusion of dibutyryl cyclic GMP results in increased endothelial pinocytosis (Joo et al., 1983). The application of substance P to isolated brain capillaries mediates the translocation of protein kinase C from the endothelial cytoplasm to the plasma membrane of the brain capillary (Catalan et al., 1989). The addition of parathyroid hormone (PTH) increases the formation of cyclic adenosine monophosphate (AMP) in isolated brain capillaries (Huang and Rorstad, 1984). There is evidence for receptors for vasoactive peptides such as angiotensin II (Speth and Harik, 1985), ANP (Chabrier et al., 1987), and bradykinin (Homayoun and Harik, 1991) in isolated brain capillary preparations. These receptors may trigger signal transduction within the endothelial cytoplasm following peptide binding at either the brain or blood interface of the capillary endothelium. These signal transduction phenomena may alter intracellular calcium and the stabilization of endothelial tight junctions and lead to BBB disruption, as discussed in Chapter 2.

Receptor-mediated transcytosis

Receptor-mediated transcytosis in peripheral tissues

RMT occurs in epithelial barriers (Cardone et al., 1996), and the trancytosis across capillary endothelial barriers in peripheral tissues was described many years ago

(Simionescu, 1979). The RMT of peptides is prominent in the intestinal barrier, particularly in the postnatal period. Certain trophic factors, such as nerve growth factor (NGF), present in the maternal milk gain access to the general circulation of the suckling infant by virtue of RMT of the NGF across the intestinal epithelial barrier (Siminoski et al., 1986). Similarly, passive immunity in the young is acquired by the RMT of immunoglobulin G (IgG) molecules in the gut lumen. The RMT of the luminal IgG across the intestinal epithelial barrier decreases as the individual is weaned from the suckling period (Hobbs and Jackson, 1987).

The pathway of RMT through an epithelial or endothelial barrier involves several sequential steps (Broadwell et al., 1996). First, there is binding of the circulating peptide or peptidomimetic MAb to the cognate receptor on the luminal membrane of the brain capillary endothelium and this is followed by endocytosis of the receptor–ligand complex. The endocytosis may occur within either smooth or clatharin-coated pits (Goldfine, 1987). Following entry into the preendosomal compartment immediately distal to the plasma membrane, the peptide is triaged into one of at least three different pathways: (a) transcytosis to the abluminal membrane for exocytosis, (b) movement into the endothelial lysosomal compartment, or (c) retroendocytosis whereby the peptide returns to the luminal membrane of the capillary endothelium for exocytosis back to the blood compartment. As discussed below, the retroendocytosis model has been proposed for Tf/receptor interactions at the BBB (Bradbury, 1997). The intraendothelial triaging to these various pathways may or may not involve movement through the trans-Golgi network (TGN). In cultured cells, the role of the TGN may be either prominent or minimal depending on the ligand and cell type (Pesonen et al., 1984; Vogel et al., 1995). The exocytosis of the ligand at the abluminal membrane at the capillary endothelium may or may not involve the cognate receptor. The receptor–ligand complex may move across the endothelial barrier and participate in exocytosis where the receptor can also mediate endocytosis on the abluminal membrane of the capillary endothelium. Alternatively, there may be dissociation of the receptor–ligand complex within the endothelial compartment followed by return of the receptor to the luminal endothelial membrane in parallel with exocytosis of the peptide at the abluminal membrane of the capillary endothelium. For example, in cultured cells, the receptor for epidermal growth factor (EGF) participates in only endocytosis, not exocytosis (Brandli et al., 1991). Conversely, as discussed below, there is evidence for expression of the TfR at both luminal and abluminal membranes of the brain capillary endothelium (Huwyler and Pardridge, 1998), which suggests that the BBB TfR moves back and forth between the luminal and abluminal membranes.

Protein phosphorylation and dephosphorylation at the blood–brain barrier

Protein phosphorylation plays a crucial role in RMT (Casanova et al., 1990), particularly exocytosis (Almers, 1990). If RMT was a prominent pathway at the BBB, then protein phosphorylation and dephosphorylation at the brain capillary endothelium should be active so that the exocytosis arm of the RMT pathway could be regulated. Protein phosphatases appear to play a crucial role in exocytosis, which is inhibited with inhibition of protein phosphatases (Davidson et al., 1992). In addition, protein-dependent phosphatases also play a role in regulation of endocytosis (Lai et al., 1999). Protein phosphorylation at the BBB may involve the interaction of cyclic AMP and A-kinases, cyclic GMP and G-kinases, calcium and protein kinase C, or calcium/calmodulin kinases. There are approximately 100 protein phosphorylation pathways specific to the brain and these involve alternate cycles of protein phosphorylation and dephosphorylation (Nestler et al., 1984).

Protein phosphorylation at the brain synapse is a site of one of the most active areas of protein phosphorylation in the body (Nestler et al., 1984). In order to investigate protein phosphorylation and dephosphorylation at the BBB, these pathways were compared in isolated bovine brain capillaries and capillary-depleted brain synaptosomal preparations, as shown in Figure 4.2. The level of protein phosphorylation in isolated brain capillaries is as high as the activity of protein phosphorylation in brain synaptosomes (Pardridge et al., 1985b), and the activity of protein dephosphorylation in brain capillaries exceeds the phosphatase activity in brain synaptosomes (Figure 4.2). The dephosphorylation pathway for the 80 kDa phosphoprotein doublet in brain capillaries is extremely rapid and is nearly complete within 5 s of incubation at 0 °C. This level of activity is typical of peptide–receptor interactions. For example, the protein phosphorylation of the EGF receptor is complete within 30 s at 0 °C (Soderquist and Carpenter, 1983). The rapidity of the protein phosphorylation or dephosphorylation is indicative of the biological significance of these pathways in vivo (Nestler et al., 1984).

In the brain capillary a prominent protein that is phosphorylated is an 80 kDa doublet that electrophoretically runs nearly parallel to a protein of comparable molecular weight in the synaptosomal membrane (Figure 4.2). An 80 kDa synaptosomal phosphoprotein is synapsin I (Nestler et al., 1984), but it is unknown whether synapsin I is also expressed at the BBB in vivo. The 80 kDa doublet in the isolated bovine brain capillary preparation is largely dephosphorylated within 5 s of incubation at 0 °C and is completely dephosphorylated within 2 min of incubation at 0° C (Figure 4.2, left panel). Conversely, there is no dephosphorylation of the synaptosomal 80 kDa protein (Figure 4.2). Another major phosphoprotein in the brain capillary preparation is a triplet in the 50–55 kDa molecular weight range and these proteins are not present in the synaptosomal preparation (Figure 4.2).

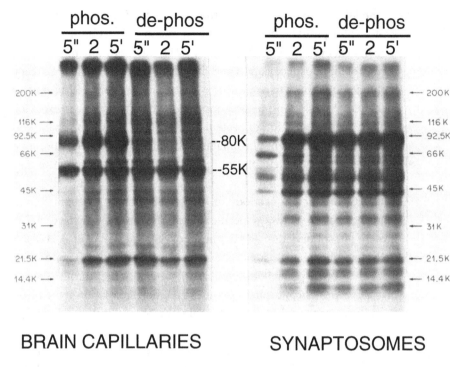

Figure 4.2   Autoradiograms of bovine brain capillary plasma membranes (left) and bovine brain
capillary-depleted synaptosomal membranes (right) after 0.08–5 min phosphorylation
and dephosphorylation assays at 0 °C. The migration of molecular weight standards is
shown on the left and right margins. SDS-PAGE was done with 6–20% gradient gels. The
phosphorylation assays were initiated by adding [^{32}P]γ-ATP to the membrane preparation
and the assay was terminated by the addition of SDS sample buffer. The
dephosphorylation assay was executed by extending the phosphorylation assay for a
period of 5 min. At the end of the phosphorylation period, 1 mmol/l unlabeled ATP and
7.5 mmol/l EDTA were added to the assay solution, and the assay was continued for
0.08–5 min prior to the addition of the SDS sample buffer. From Pardridge et al. (1985b)
with permission.

Thus, there are differences in the pattern of protein phosphorylation and dephosphorylation in the BBB membranes versus the brain synaptosomal membranes,
and this tissue-specific pattern of protein phosphorylation at the BBB likely has
important functional significance for the regulation of transport across the BBB in
vivo.

The identities of these prominent protein kinases and phosphatases at the BBB
are at present not known. Catalan et al. (1996) have provided evidence that an
80 kDa phosphoprotein in brain capillaries is myristoylated alanine-rich C kinase

bovine brain capillaries

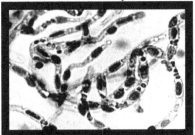

ISOLATED HUMAN AND ANIMAL BRAIN CAPILLARIES:
AN IN VITRO MODEL SYSTEM OF THE BLOOD-BRAIN BARRIER

bovine brain capillaries

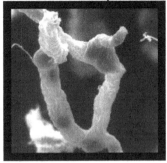

human brain capillaries

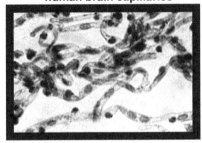

Figure 4.3   Isolated bovine brain capillaries are shown at the light microscopic level (top left panel) and with scanning electron microscopy (right panel). Autopsy human brain capillaries are shown at the light microscopic level (bottom left panel).

substrate (MARCKS) and Weber et al. (1987) isolated a 56 kDa phosphatase from porcine brain capillaries. Calcineurin is a phosphatase of the type 2B category, and plays a role in calcium-dependent endocytosis (Lai et al., 1999). Whether calcineurin is expressed in the BBB in vivo is at present not known. In summary, there is extensive protein phosphorylation and dephosphorylation at the BBB and these pathways are as active as – and in some cases more than – similar pathways in brain synaptosomal preparations (Figure 4.2). These observations suggest that extensive signal transduction pathways take place on a second-to-second basis in the brain capillary endothelium and many of these pathways may regulate the RMT of peptides through the endothelial barrier in brain in vivo. The initial triggering of the signal transduction pathways or the RMT is binding of the peptide to the brain capillary endothelial peptide receptor.

Endogenous blood–brain barrier peptide receptors

The isolated brain capillary model

The biochemical characterization of BBB peptide receptors may be performed with the isolated animal or human brain capillary preparation (Figure 4.3). Capillaries were initially purified from fresh animal brain or from human autopsy brain

(Siakotos et al., 1969; Brendel et al., 1974; Goldstein et al., 1975; Joo, 1985). In the latter case, an intact preparation of purified human brain capillaries can be obtained from brain that is removed up to 40 h after death (Pardridge et al., 1985a). When capillaries were isolated from rabbit brain, there was no change in the parameters of amino acid uptake into the capillaries following isolation of the microvessels at either 0 or 40 h postmortem (Choi and Pardridge, 1986). Scanning electron microscopy shows the capillary is visibly free of contiguous brain tissue (Figure 4.3). However, as discussed in Chapter 3, the isolated brain capillary contains remnants of astrocyte foot processes that remain studded to the basement membrane surface of the capillary. It is the basement membrane "straightjacket" that enables the purification of isolated microvessels from homogenates of the brain tissue.

The isolated brain capillary preparation should be viewed as an intact membrane preparation and not as a metabolically viable cellular compartment. Whether capillaries are isolated with either mechanical or enzymatic homogenization techniques, these capillaries are metabolically impaired and have a 90% reduction in cellular concentrations of adenosine triphosphate (ATP), even when capillaries are immediately isolated from fresh brain (Lasbennes and Gayet, 1983). This is an unusual property of the brain capillary since it is possible to isolate cells from other organs with enzymatic homogenization techniques and these cells maintain normal levels of ATP. However, the distinctive property of the brain capillary is that these cells are metabolically impaired and have seriously low levels of ATP following homogenization from fresh brain using either mechanical or enzymatic homogenization techniques. The isolated brain capillary preparation has been used as an intact membrane preparation for the study of animal or human BBB receptors and transporters. The activation of brain capillary adenyl cyclase is also possible using the isolated brain capillary preparation (Huang and Rorstad, 1984). In addition, BBB CMT can be studied with this model (Choi and Pardridge, 1986). The pattern of amino acid competition for BBB LAT1 in the human brain capillary preparation is identical to what is observed when BBB LAT1 RNA is injected into frog oocytes and neutral amino acid competition studies are performed in the RNA-injected oocytes (Hargreaves and Pardridge, 1988; Boado et al., 1999).

The isolated brain capillary preparation has been used to investigate the kinetics of endogenous peptide binding to its cognate receptor and the binding constants for a number of human BBB peptide receptors are shown in Table 4.1. The affinity of the BBB peptide receptor is high, as represented by dissociation constants (K_D) in the low nmol/l range. The maximal binding capacities for the BBB peptide receptors is in the range of 0.1–0.3 pmol/mg protein (Table 4.1). For comparison purposes, this receptor density is 1000-fold less than the B_{max} of D-glucose inhibitable cytochalasin B binding to isolated brain capillaries (Dwyer and Pardridge, 1993),

Table 4.1 Peptide-binding parameters for isolated human brain capillary receptors

Peptide	K_D (nmol/l)	B_{max} (pmol/mg$_p$)
Leptin	5.1 ± 2.8	0.34 ± 0.16
IGF-2	1.1 ± 0.1	0.21 ± 0.01
IGF-1	2.1 ± 0.4	0.17 ± 0.02
Insulin	1.2 ± 0.5	0.17 ± 0.08
Transferrin	5.6 ± 1.4	0.10 ± 0.02

Notes:

IGF, insulin-like growth factor.

From Golden et al. (1997) with permission.

which reflects the density of the *Glut1* glucose transporter at the BBB (Chapter 3). The B_{max} of BBB peptide receptors is approximately 50-fold lower than the B_{max} of glucose transporter binding sites in brain synaptosomal membranes (Pardridge et al., 1990a). The lower B_{max} of BBB peptide receptor systems parallels the much lower concentration of circulating peptides in the blood relative to circulating nutrients such as glucose. Despite the fact that the B_{max} of BBB peptide receptors is 2–3 log orders lower than the B_{max} of BBB CMT systems such as the glucose transporter, the existence of the BBB peptide receptors is readily detected with immunocytochemistry and receptor-specific antibodies. As discussed below, these illuminate the brain microvasculature in immunocytochemical detection of BBB peptide receptor systems.

Blood–brain barrier insulin receptor

The presence of saturable binding sites for radiolabeled circulating insulin was demonstrated more than 20 years ago by emulsion autoradiography studies (Van Houten and Posner, 1979). Subsequently, the isolated brain capillary preparation was used to quantify the kinetics of insulin binding to the BBB and these studies showed the K_D of insulin binding to the BBB was identical to the K_D of insulin binding to the insulin receptor in peripheral tissues (Frank and Pardridge, 1981). Affinity cross-linking studies were performed to determine the molecular weight of the BBB insulin-binding site (Figure 4.4). In these studies, isolated human brain capillaries (Figure 4.4A) were incubated with [^{125}I]insulin, which was then affinity cross-linked to the brain capillaries in the presence of either low (6 ng/ml) or high (10 μg/ml) insulin concentrations (lanes 1 and 2, respectively, Figure 4.4B). These studies showed that the only saturable binding site for insulin at the human BBB had a molecular weight of 130 kDa (Pardridge et al., 1985a), which is identical to the molecular weight of the α subunit of the insulin receptor. The transport of

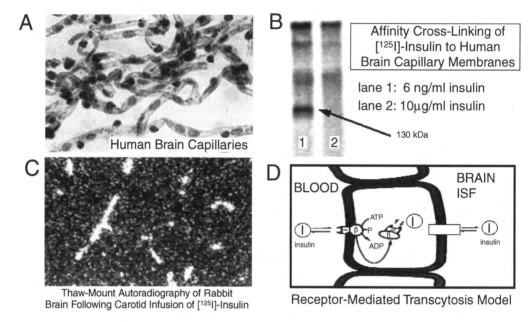

Figure 4.4   Human blood–brain barrier (BBB) insulin receptor and brain capillary transport of circulating insulin. (A) Human brain capillaries. (B) Film autoradiogram following SDS-PAGE of [[125I]insulin affinity cross-linked to human brain capillary membranes in the presence of either 6 ng/ml insulin (lane 1), or 10 μg/ml insulin (lane 2). A specific 130 kDa saturable binding site for insulin is shown. (C) Darkfield emulsion autoradiography of rabbit brain following a 10-min carotid arterial infusion of [125I]insulin. Insulin within the brain capillary compartment is shown as well as insulin diffusely spread throughout brain parenchyma. (D) Model for receptor-mediated transcytosis of insulin through the BBB in vivo. ISF, interstitial fluid; ATP, adenosine triphosphate; ADP, adenosine diphosphate; P, phosphate. From Pardridge et al. (1985a) and reprinted from *Brain Res.*, **420**, Duffy, K.R. and Pardridge, W.M. Blood–brain barrier transcytosis of insulin in developing rabbits, 32–8, copyright (1987), with permission from Elsevier Science.

insulin into brain was demonstrated with thaw mount autoradiography of rabbit brain following the intracarotid arterial infusion of [125I]-labeled insulin (Duffy and Pardridge, 1987). As shown in Figure 4.4C, the brain capillaries are revealed in this darkfield micrograph of rabbit brain following a 10-min carotid artery infusion of [125I]insulin. However, silver grains are also found throughout the brain parenchyma, indicating that the circulating insulin rapidly diffuses in brain following transport through the BBB. Most of the silver grains seen in the capillary compartment represent radiolabeled insulin confined to the capillary volume, since this brain preparation was not saline-perfused subsequent to the carotid artery perfusion of the [125I]insulin. Reverse-phase high performance liquid chromatography (HPLC) of ethanol extracts of brain demonstrated that the metabolism and conversion of the insulin infused into the carotid artery to [^{125}I]tyrosine were not significant. Therefore, the silver grains in brain parenchyma reflected the transport of unmetabolized insulin into brain (Duffy and Pardridge, 1987).

The transport of radiolabeled insulin into brain parenchyma in the rabbit was completely saturated by the inclusion of high concentrations of unlabeled insulin in the carotid artery perfusate (Duffy and Pardridge, 1987). Since the only saturable binding site for insulin at the BBB has a molecular weight identical to that of the insulin receptor (Pardridge et al., 1985a), the model of insulin transport through the BBB is RMT (Figure 4.4D). Transcytosis was inferred because there is no paracellular pathway for insulin transport through the BBB, owing to the presence of the epithelial-like tight junctions in the brain capillary endothelium. At this point, the term transcytosis is used provisionally as this model would require confirmation with ultrastructural studies using electron microscopy. The electron microscopic confirmation of the BBB RMT model is discussed below in the case of the BBB TfR (Bickel et al., 1994a).

The BBB insulin receptor enables the brain uptake of circulating insulin. There is indirect evidence that suggests that the brain takes up circulating insulin and this corroborates the direct demonstration of RMT through the BBB shown in Figure 4.4. Insulin is a neuromodulator substance in the central nervous system (CNS) and regulates the formation of nascent synapses in developing neurons (Puro and Agardh, 1984). There is also insulin receptor widely distributed throughout the CNS (Zhao et al., 1999), and insulin concentrations are readily measurable in the brain (Baskin et al., 1983a). However, there is no insulin mRNA in brain (Giddings et al., 1985), indicating the brain is not a site of insulin synthesis. In earlier work it was suggested that insulin was made in the brain and this hypothesis was put forward on the basis of the observation that the concentration of insulin in the brain exceeded the concentration of insulin in blood (Havrankova and Roth, 1979). However, this high brain insulin concentration was subsequently shown to be an artifact due to errors in brain extraction of insulin. When brain insulin is properly extracted, the concentration of insulin in the brain is less than the concentration of insulin in plasma and the brain/plasma ratio or volume of distribution in rat brain is approximately 0.2 ml/g (Frank et al., 1986). There was also initial confusion about the molecular weight of the brain insulin receptor. Some studies found a molecular weight of approximately 130 kDa (Haskell et al., 1985), such as that shown in Figure 4.4B, while other studies showed a slightly lower molecular weight of approximately 120 kDa (Hendricks et al., 1984). These discrepancies were subsequently resolved by studies showing there are two populations of insulin receptor in the brain that arise from a single insulin receptor gene (Zahniser et al., 1984). These two populations are characterized by differences in glycosylation of the α subunit, accounting for the slightly lower molecular weight of the insulin receptor found in brain synaptosomal membranes as compared to the molecular weight of the insulin receptor found in brain capillaries.

The activity of the BBB insulin receptor is regulated under pathophysiologic conditions and is upregulated in development (Frank et al., 1985), and is downregulated in streptozotocin (STZ)-induced diabetes mellitus (Frank et al., 1986). In STZ diabetes, the brain/plasma insulin ratio in the rat decreases from 0.092 ± 0.024 to 0.029 ± 0.001 (Frank et al., 1986). This decrease in the brain volume of distribution of insulin in STZ diabetes suggests there is a downregulation of the BBB insulin receptor, since the only source of brain insulin is from the circulation via the BBB transport system. This downregulation was demonstrated, as the activity of the BBB insulin receptor in capillaries isolated from rats subjected to STZ diabetes is decreased compared to control rat brain capillaries (Frank et al., 1986). In the developing rabbit brain, the brain/plasma ratio increases to 0.67 ± 0.09 ml/g in newborn rabbit brain, which is increased threefold compared to the brain/plasma ratio of insulin in adult rabbit brain, 0.22 ± 0.08 ml/g (Frank et al., 1985). This suggests that the BBB insulin receptor activity is increased in developing brain and this was confirmed. The B_{max} of insulin binding to capillaries obtained from suckling rabbit brain was increased relative to the B_{max} of insulin binding to capillaries obtained from adult rabbit brain (Frank et al., 1985). The higher brain/plasma ratio of insulin in adult rabbit brain, relative to adult rat brain, suggests the BBB insulin RMT system is more active in rabbits than in rats, and rabbits may be a preferred model system for studying BBB RMT of insulin in vivo.

Blood–brain barrier transferrin receptor

The BBB TfR can be detected immunocytochemically with antibodies to the TfR, as discussed in Chapter 5. When immunocytochemistry is performed with such antibodies using a panel of tissues, the brain vasculature is immunostained whereas the microvasculature in peripheral tissues is not visualized (Jefferies et al., 1984). These studies indicated that the TfR is selectively expressed at the vasculature in brain compared to peripheral tissues. Subsequently, the saturable binding of radiolabeled Tf to human brain capillaries was demonstrated using the isolated human brain capillary preparation (Table 4.1). An MAb was used in immunocytochemistry to demonstrate continuous immunostaining of the capillary preparation, indicating that the microvascular TfR was of endothelial origin (Pardridge et al., 1987a). These studies of isolated brain capillaries show that the affinity of the BBB TfR was high with a K_D in the low nmol/l range (Table 4.1), and that the BBB TfR mediates the endocytosis of radiolabeled Tf (Pardridge et al., 1987a).

The RMT of Tf through the BBB in vivo was demonstrated by Fishman et al. (1987) with arterial perfusions of radiolabeled Tf in the rat. However, the RMT of Tf through the BBB in vivo was subsequently stated to be "controversial" (Begley,

1996), and the RMT model for Tf was called into question on the basis of three observations. First, when [125I]transferrin and 59Fe are coadministered, the brain uptake of the 59Fe is much greater than the brain uptake of the [125I]Tf when brain uptake is measured over days, even weeks (Morris et al., 1992). This observation gave rise to the "retroendocytosis" model of BBB Tf transport (Bradbury, 1997), which posits that the circulating Tf–iron (Fe) complex is endocytosed into the brain capillary endothelial cytoplasm subsequent to binding to the BBB TfR on the luminal endothelial membrane. The Tf–Fe complex is hypothesized to separate within the brain capillary endothelial endosomal system. It is further hypothesized that the apotransferrin is exported back to blood, and that the iron is exported to brain interstitium via undefined pathways across the abluminal membrane. In the retroendocytosis model, it is also necessary to explain how the Fe is taken up by brain cells in the absence of Tf. In fact, the principal observation supporting the retroendocytosis model is also compatible with the model of Tf RMT through the BBB. In the RMT model, the Tf–Fe complex is transcytosed through the BBB and is then endocytosed into brain cells. The dissociation of Fe and Tf takes place within brain cells wherein brain cell ferritin can absorb the iron. The apotransferrin may then either be degraded in brain cells with the release of the [125I] radioactivity back to blood, or undergo exocytosis back to blood. In the case of either the RMT model or the retroendocytosis model, the brain radioactivity of 59Fe would be sequestered relative to the brain radioactivity of the [125I].

The second observation used to support the retroendocytosis model is the finding of Roberts et al. (1993) that the intracarotid artery perfusion of a conjugate of Tf and horseradish peroxidase (HRP) results in peroxidase activity within the endothelial cytoplasm, but not in compartments in brain distal to the endothelial cytoplasm. However, Broadwell et al. (1996) subsequently demonstrated that conjugates of HRP and Tf are transcytosed through the endothelial cytoplasm and HRP activity is found in compartments in brain distal to the endothelial space. Moreover, as shown in Figure 4.5, both biochemical and morphologic evidence demonstrated the transcytosis of radiolabeled Tf through the endothelial compartment in brain in vivo. In the physiologic studies, the internal carotid artery perfusion (ICAP) and the capillary depletion techniques were used (Figure 4.5A). In the morphologic approach, thaw mount autoradiography was used (Figure 4.5B). Following ICAP of radiolabeled Tf, the brain volume of distribution rapidly reached 50–60 μl/g within a 5-min perfusion (Figure 4.5A). The capillary depletion technique was used to show that more than 80% of the brain radioactivity had distributed to the postvascular supernatant compartment and less than 20% was confined to the vascular pellet (Figure 4.5A). These ICAP/capillary depletion studies confirmed the initial observations of Fishman et al. (1987). The thaw mount autoradiography showed that the circulating Tf readily distributes

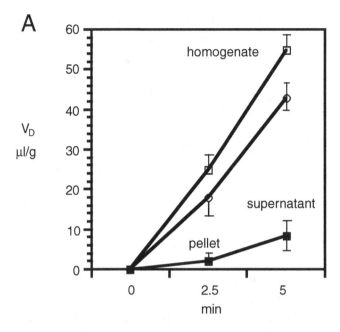

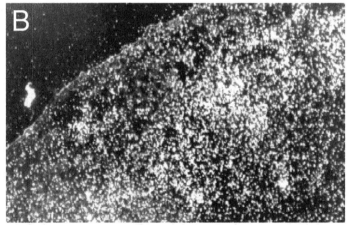

Figure 4.5   (A) Brain volume distribution (V_D) of [^{125}I]rat holotransferrin in the homogenate, postvascular supernatant, and vascular compartments after 5 or 10 min internal carotid artery perfusion in the anesthetized rat. Data are mean ± SE ($n = 3$ rats). The internal carotid artery perfusions were performed at a flow rate of 3.7 ml/min to prevent admixture with circulating rat plasma. (B) Darkfield micrograph of emulsion autoradiogram of rat brain following a 5-min internal carotid perfusion of [^{125}I]rat holotransferrin in physiologic saline at a rate of 3.7 ml/min. Unlike the autoradiography studies shown in Figure 4.4C, the brain was postperfused in these experiments with saline for 30 s at 3.7 ml/min prior to decapitation of the animal. This study shows extensive and rapid distribution of blood-borne transferrin throughout brain parenchyma. Reprinted from *Brain Res.*, **683**, Skarlatos, S., Yoshikawa, T. and Pardridge, W.M., Transport of [^{125}I]transferrin through the blood–brain barrier in vivo, 164–71, copyright (1995), with permission from Elsevier Science.

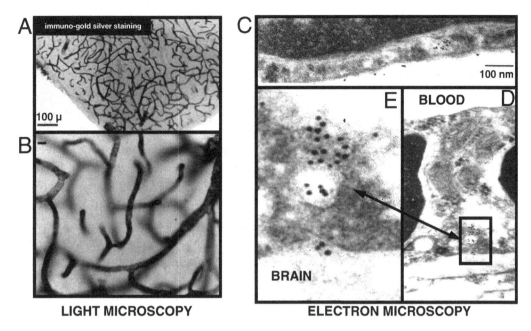

LIGHT MICROSCOPY   **ELECTRON MICROSCOPY**

Figure 4.6   Transcytosis of 5 nm gold monoclonal antibody (MAb) conjugate through the blood–brain barrier in vivo. (A) Silver-enhanced vibratome section of rat brain hemisphere perfused with a conjugate of 5 nm gold and the OX26 MAb. The coronal section is at the level of the frontal cortex. (B) Higher magnification of the same section as in (A). Silver deposits line the vascular wall. (C) Electron micrograph of a brain capillary endothelial cell after perfusion with the OX26–gold conjugate. Clusters of intracellular gold particles trapped in endosomal structures are seen within the endothelial cytoplasm. (D) A transverse section through the brain capillary endothelial cell shows an endosomal cluster of gold–OX26 conjugates moving toward the abluminal membrane. (E) Higher magnification shows the gold–OX26 MAb conjugate within the endosomal structure and demonstrates exocytosis of the conjugate into the brain interstitial space. (Reproduced, with permission, from Bickel, U., Kang, Y.-S., Yoshikawa, T. and Pardridge, W.M. In vivo demonstration of subcellular localization of anti-transferrin receptor monoclonal antibody against βA4 protein: a potential probe for Alzheimer's disease. *J. Histochem. Cytochem.* **42**: 1493–7, 1994.)

throughout brain parenchyma (Figure 4.5B), similar to the RMT of radiolabeled insulin (Figure 4.4C).

Transcytosis through the endothelial compartment mediated by the BBB TfR was directly confirmed with ultrastructural studies using immunogold electron microscopy (Figure 4.6). In these investigations, a conjugate of 5 nm gold and the OX26 MAb was prepared and infused in the internal carotid artery for a 10-min period in anesthetized rats (Bickel et al., 1994a). The brain capillary compartment was subsequently cleared with a postperfusion saline wash and the brain was fixed in situ with carotid artery perfusion of glutaraldehyde. At the light microscopic level, the detection of the OX26 MAb/gold conjugate in brain was made with immunogold silver staining (Figure 4.6A, B). These light microscopic studies of fixed sections showed staining of the microvasculature throughout the brain, indicating that the BBB TfR is widely distributed in brain. The capillaries shown in panels A and B of Figure 4.6 contain the OX26 MAb/gold conjugate within the endothelial cytoplasmic compartment, because the brain capillary lumen was flushed with a postperfusion saline wash. When these sections were examined ultrastructurally, OX26 MAb/gold conjugate was seen decorating the luminal membrane of the brain capillary endothelium, as shown in Figure 4.6C. MAb/gold conjugate was also found in the endothelial cytoplasmic compartment, but this cytoplasmic MAb/gold conjugate was uniformly confined to endosomal-like structures with a diameter of 80–100 nm (Figure 4.6). The endosomal structures were observed to move across the endothelial cytoplasm from the direction of blood to brain (Figure 4.6D), and at high magnification, the MAb/gold conjugate is seen to exocytose from the endothelial compartment into brain interstitial space (Figure 4.6E).

One of the factors that makes it difficult to demonstrate transcytosis across the BBB with morphologic techniques is the dilution that the tracer undergoes following exocytosis into brain interstitium. The volume of the brain interstitium is about 200 μl/g, whereas the volume of the brain capillary endothelial compartment is <1 μl/g. Therefore, the tracer is diluted >200-fold as soon as the molecule is exocytosed from the endothelial cell. Uptake into brain cells will dilute the tracer even further. This dilution phenomenon explains why the capillary compartment is visualized so well, while the brain is not visualized, at the light microscopic level (Figure 4.6A, B). Conversely, the use of radioisotopic techniques makes the demonstration of RMT through the BBB in vivo straightforward, as shown in Figure 4.5.

The third observation used to buttress the validity of the retroendocytosis model was the absence of immunoreactive TfR on the abluminal membrane of the capillary endothelium using preembedding immunolabeling methods (Roberts et al., 1993). However, Vorbrodt (1989) has shown that receptors on the abluminal endothelial membrane cannot be detected with preembedding immunolabeling procedures. This is because only the luminal membrane is exposed when tissue sections are incubated with the labeling antibody in a preembedding method. When the receptor systems on the abluminal membrane are to be detected, it is necessary to perform postembedding immunolabeling procedures. However, this requires aldehyde fixation of the tissue for subsequent ultrastructural studies, and this will denature the abluminal TfR and abort immunodetection of the abluminal TfR.

These technical limitations pertaining to electron microscopic detection of abluminal receptor can be set aside by taking advantage of confocal fluorescent microscopy and the ability to resolve the luminal and abluminal membranes of the capillary endothelium with this technology using isolated brain capillaries (Figure 4.7, colour plate). Fluorescein-labeled immunoliposomes, conjugated with either the OX26 MAb (Figure 4.7B) or the mouse IgG_{2a} isotype control (Figure 4.7A), were incubated with freshly isolated rat brain capillaries that were cytocentrifuged to a glass slide without fixation prior to examination with confocal microscopy (Huwyler and Pardridge, 1998). Incubation with the OX26 immunoliposomes resulted in staining of both the luminal and abluminal membranes of the brain capillary endothelium (panels B and C of Figure 4.7). In contrast, no immunostaining was noted when immunoliposomes were prepared with the mouse IgG_{2a} isotype control (Figure 4.7A). A computer-aided reconstruction of the consecutive optical sections through the brain capillary showed that the luminal and abluminal membranes could be separated with confocal microscopy and that immunoreactive TfR was found on both membranes (Figure 4.7C). Rat brain capillaries were also incubated with unconjugated OX26 MAb and the binding of the OX26 MAb to the isolated rat brain capillary preparation was detected with a fluorescein-labeled secondary antibody yielding the green color shown in panels E and F of Figure 4.7. These capillaries were also colabeled with phosphatidyl ethanolamine (PE) conjugated with rhodamine to yield the red color in panels D and F of Figure 4.7. This colabeling allowed for the demonstration of endocytosis of the OX26 MAb into the rat brain endothelial compartment, as revealed by the punctate staining pattern that was separated from the membrane staining revealed by the rhodamine-PE. This indicated that the OX26 MAb had moved into the endothelial compartment subsequent to receptor binding (Huwyler and Pardridge, 1998).

In summary, the BBB TfR has been characterized with a radioreceptor assay using human brain capillaries (Table 4.1), and the BBB TfR is shown to mediate the RMT of either Tf (Figure 4.5) or a Tf peptidomimetic MAb (Figure 4.6) through the endothelial cytoplasm in vivo. The RMT of circulating Tf–Fe complexes enables the brain uptake of circulating iron as well as the brain uptake of other heavy metals that are also bound to circulating Tf such as gallium, aluminum, or manganese (Aschner and Aschner, 1990; Pullen et al., 1990; Roskams and Connor, 1990).

Blood–brain barrier insulin-like growth factor receptor

The insulin-like growth factors (IGF), IGF1 or IGF2, bind specific type 1 or type 2 IGF receptors, respectively. The type 2 IGF receptor also binds mannose-6-phosphate (M6P). Studies with isolated bovine brain capillaries demonstrated that both the type 1 and type 2 IGF receptors are present on animal brain capillaries (Frank et al., 1986). However, subsequent studies with human brain capillaries showed that the human BBB IGF receptor is a variant IGF receptor also found in human placenta (Steele-Perkins et al., 1988), and which binds both IGF1 and IGF2 with high affinity (Duffy et al., 1988). In these experiments, isolated human brain

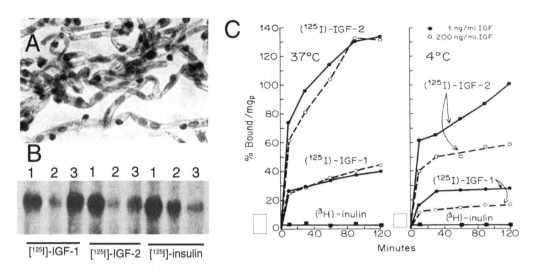

Figure 4.8 (A) Isolated human brain capillaries. (B) Affinity cross-linking of [^{125}I]insulin-like growth factor-1 (IGF1), [^{125}I]IGF2, or [^{125}I]insulin to isolated human brain capillaries using disuccinimidylsuberate (DSS). Capillaries were incubated with labeled hormone in the presence of no additive (lane 1), 250 ng/ml IGF mixture (lane 2), or 400 ng/ml porcine insulin (lane 3). The molecular weight of the insulin binding site is 133 kDa, and the molecular weight of the IGF binding site is 141 kDa. Both IGF1 and IGF2 bind to a receptor of identical molecular weight whereas the molecular weight of the insulin receptor is slightly lower. (C) Time course of [^{125}I]IGF1 and [^{125}I]IGF2 binding to isolated human brain capillaries in the presence of either 1 ng/ml IGF (closed circles) or 200 ng/ml (open circles) at either 37 °C (left) or 4 °C (right). The uptake of [^{3}H]inulin, an extracellular space marker, was not significantly different at either temperature and the values observed at 37 °C are shown in the figure (closed squares). There is no significant difference between the uptake at the IGFs in the presence of 1 or 200 ng/ml IGF at 37 °C. However, nonspecific binding was about half that of the total binding at 4 °C. From Duffy et al. (1988) with permission.

capillaries (Figure 4.8A) were used along with either [^{125}I]IGF1 or [^{125}I]IGF2 and either affinity cross-linking studies (Figure 4.8B) or radioreceptor assays (Figure 4.8C). Both radiolabeled IGF1 and IGF2 avidly bound to human brain capillaries and this binding was so rapid that endocytosis into the capillary compartment was rate-limiting. Since endocytosis is nonsaturable, the binding of IGF1 or IGF2 to human brain capillaries was not saturable at 37 °C (Figure 4.8C, left panel). When the incubations were repeated at 4 °C, the cold temperatures inhibited endocytosis to a greater extent than membrane binding and the saturability of IGF1 or IGF2 to the human brain capillary plasma membrane could then be demonstrated (Duffy et al., 1988). The dissociation constant of IGF1 or IGF2 binding to the human BBB was in the low nmol/l range (Table 4.1).

The molecular weight of the IGF1 or IGF2 receptor at the human BBB was 141 kDa (Figure 4.8B). Affinity cross-linking of IGF1, IGF2, or insulin to human brain capillaries is shown in Figure 4.8B. Lane 1 represents binding of the peptide in tracer concentration; lane 2 represents binding in the presence of 250 ng/ml IGF1/IGF2, and lane 3 represents binding in the presence of 400 ng/ml insulin. Binding of IGF1 or IGF2 to human brain capillary was not inhibited by high concentrations of insulin, but was inhibited by high concentrations of IGF1 or IGF2. The molecular weight of the IGF1 or IGF2 binding site was 141 kDa, which is comparable to the molecular weight of the α subunit of the variant IGF receptor found in human placenta, which has a high affinity for both IGF1 and IGF2 (Steele-Perkins et al., 1988).

The IGF2 receptor on animal brain capillaries is the type 2 receptor (Frank et al., 1986), which also binds M6P (Braulke et al., 1990). This suggests that certain lysosomal enzymes that have M6P moieties could be taken up from blood by brain via the BBB type 2 IGF receptor. There is evidence that a lysosomal enzyme such as β-glucuronidase is taken up from blood by brain in the mouse (Birkenmeier et al., 1991). If BBB transport of certain M6P-bearing enzymes does take place, then the mechanism of this uptake may be RMT via the BBB type 2 IGF receptor. However, the type 2 IGF receptor is apparently absent at the human BBB (Duffy et al., 1988), as IGF transport is mediated by the variant IGF receptor (Figure 4.8). This means that lysosomal enzymes or other ligands of the M6P receptor may not be taken up by the human brain from blood.

The IGFs are avidly bound by a series of IGF-binding proteins in the plasma and >99.9% of circulating IGF1 or IGF2 is plasma protein-bound and <0.1% is free in the circulation (Clemmons, 1990). Because of the avid binding of the IGFs to specific binding proteins, there is no increase in the IGF1 concentration in cerebrospinal fluid (CSF) following peripheral administration of the peptide (Hodgkinson et al., 1991). In the absence of the binding proteins, the RMT of IGF1 or IGF2 across the BBB can be demonstrated by ICAP of the radiolabeled peptides (Reinhardt and Bondy, 1994). However, because most complexes of the IGFs and the binding proteins do not interact with the IGF receptors, the transport of IGF1 or IGF2 from blood to brain is minimal in vivo. This explains why the concentrations of IGF1 in rat brain and rat CSF are very low (Merrill and Edwards, 1990), despite the presence of a specific IGF receptor on the BBB (Frank et al., 1986; Duffy et al., 1988). In contrast, IGF2 is measurable in both rat brain and CSF (Haselbacher et al., 1984). The high level of IGF2 in rat brain or CSF does not necessarily mean that the IGF2-binding protein complex is transported through the BBB via the brain capillary IGF2 receptor. Instead, the high brain IGF2 arises from the de novo synthesis of IGF2 in brain. The concentration of the IGF2 mRNA in adult rat brain is highest among any organs of the body including liver (Ueno et al., 1988). However, subsequent in situ hybridization experiments could not demonstrate IGF2 transcript in brain parenchyma, although IGF2 mRNA was readily detected in choroid plexus (Bondy et al., 1990). This observation gave rise to the hypothesis that the origin of IGF2 in brain parenchyma was the choroid plexus synthesis and secretion to CSF. However, as discussed in Chapter 10, it has recently been shown that the brain microvasculature is a rich source of IGF2 transcript in the brain. This suggests that the brain IGF2 actually originates from synthesis in the brain microvascular compartment with direct secretion to brain. In this regard, the BBB acts as an "endocrine organ," as discussed further in Chapter 10.

Blood–brain barrier leptin receptor

Leptin (OB) is a 16 kDa polypeptide secreted by adipocytes in response to a meal (Zhang et al., 1994). Circulating leptin is then taken up by brain to induce satiety. The existence of leptin was hypothesized following the parabiosis experiments (Coleman, 1978). This work showed that lean litter mates stopped eating when their circulation was surgically connected to obese mice. The ob/ob mice are shown in Figure 4.9A. The db/db obese mouse has a defect in the OB receptor (OBR) and consequently this mouse has a very high level of circulating OB. This high level of circulating OB was transferred to the lean litter mate and resulted in cessation of food consumption. The genes for both OB and the OBR were subsequently cloned and sequenced and the OBR was found to be a member of the class I cytokine receptor family (Zhang et al., 1994; Tartaglia, 1997). The OBR is expressed in tissues as both long and short forms, designated OBR_L and OBR_S, respectively. The short and long forms of the receptor arise from a common gene and are due to alternate RNA splicing at the carboxyl terminal exon (Tartaglia, 1997). This results in truncation of the cytoplasmic portion of the receptor, and the short form of the OBR has a reduced participation in signal transduction pathways. The long form of the OBR is predominant in the hypothalamus (Schwartz et al., 1996).

Like the situation for insulin (Giddings et al., 1985), the mRNA for OB is not detectable in brain (Masuzaki et al., 1995). Therefore, OB in the brain arises from the circulation via RMT on the BBB OBR (Figure 4.9). The immunoreactive OBR is detected in human or rat brain frozen sections with an OBR-specific antiserum (Boado et al., 1998a), and this shows selective staining of the brain microvasculature in brain (Figure 4.9B). The microvascular immunostaining is continuous, suggesting an endothelial origin of the OBR at the microvasculature (Figure 9B). The kinetics of binding of $[^{125}I]OB$ (leptin) to human brain capillaries is shown in Figure 4.9C and indicates that leptin is bound to a high-affinity OBR in human brain capillaries (Golden et al., 1997). This binding was not cross-competed with either insulin or IGF. Polymerase chain reaction (PCR) studies with cDNA derived from polyA+ RNA isolated from rat brain capillaries and primers that amplify

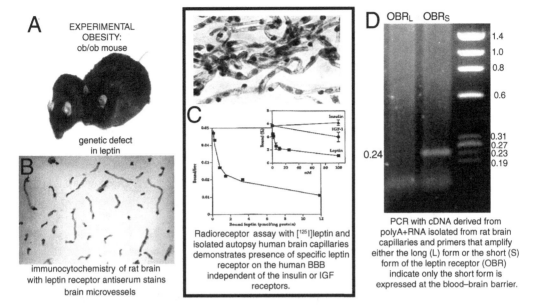

A EXPERIMENTAL OBESITY: ob/ob mouse

genetic defect in leptin

B

immunocytochemistry of rat brain with leptin receptor antiserum stains brain microvessels

C

Radioreceptor assay with [^{125}I]leptin and isolated autopsy human brain capillaries demonstrates presence of specific leptin receptor on the human BBB independent of the insulin or IGF receptors.

D OBR$_L$ OBR$_S$

0.24

1.4
1.0
0.8
0.6
0.31
0.27
0.23
0.19

PCR with cDNA derived from polyA+RNA isolated from rat brain capillaries and primers that amplify either the long (L) form or the short (S) form of the leptin receptor (OBR) indicate only the short form is expressed at the blood–brain barrier.

Figure 4.9   Human and rodent blood–brain barrier (BBB) leptin receptor (OBR): system for delivery of leptin from blood to brain. (A) Mouse models for experimental obesity. (B) Immunocytochemistry of frozen section of rat brain with an OBR antiserum that reacts to all isoforms. (C) Isolated human brain capillaries were used to show saturable binding of [^{125}I]leptin to the BBB OBR using standard radioreceptor analyses. No cross-competition with insulin-like growth factor-1 (IGF1) or insulin is observed. (D) Polymerase chain reaction (PCR) analysis shows the predominant OBR isoform at the BBB is the short form. From Golden et al. (1997) with permission and Boado et al. (1998a) with permission.

either the OBR$_L$ or OBR$_S$ indicated that the short form of the OBR was the variant predominantly expressed at the BBB (Boado et al., 1998a). This suggests the short form may act as a transport system at cellular barriers such as the BBB or choroid plexus, whereas the long form may mediate signal transduction in brain and in particular in the hypothalamus. Much of leptin's biological effect in the body may in fact be regulated via the CNS. For example, when leptin is administered intravenously, the alteration in hepatic glucose output caused by leptin is mediated via the brain (Liu et al., 1998).

The immunostaining of the microvasculature with an antibody to the OBR (Figure 4.9B) demonstrates that immunocytochemistry is the preferred method for detecting the presence of peptide receptors in brain. Oftentimes the existence of peptide receptors in the brain is determined with film autoradiography which has a resolution that is insufficient to resolve capillaries. Consequently, when the OBR in brain was initially detected with film autoradiography, it was only found at the

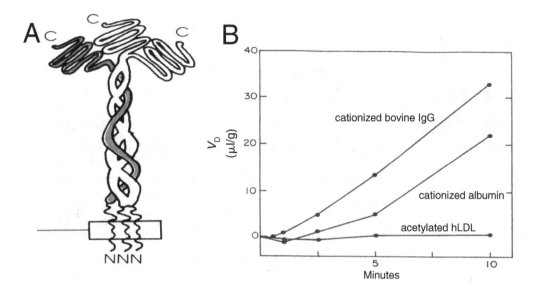

Figure 4.10   (A) Type I scavenger receptor. (B) Postvascular volume of distribution (V_D) of radiolabeled cationized bovine IgG, cationized bovine albumin, or acetylated human low density lipoprotein (hLDL). Internal carotid artery perfusions were performed for up to 10 min in the anesthetized rat and capillary depletion analysis was used to determine the postvascular supernatant V_D. Reprinted from *Adv. Drug. Del. Rev.*, **10**, Bickel, U., Yoshikawa, T. and Pardridge, W.M., Delivery of peptides and proteins through the blood–brain barrier, 205–45, copyright (1993), with permission from Elsevier Science.

choroid plexus and not at the brain microvasculature (Lynn et al., 1996). This mistake of missing brain microvascular receptors or gene products with film autoradiography is made many times. The problem is that film autoradiography lacks the resolution to detect brain microvessels which have a diameter of only approximately 5 μm. If peptide receptors or gene products are to be detected in brain, it is best to perform this with either emulsion autoradiography or immunocytochemistry, which has a much higher resolution than film autoradiography.

Blood–brain barrier lipoprotein receptors

Many of the lipoprotein receptors belong to the low density lipoprotein (LDL) receptor gene family, and include the LDL receptor, the LDL-related protein (LRP), and gp330/megalin (Stockinger et al., 1998). In addition, there are scavenger receptors (SR) and various SR isoforms are found either on macrophages or on both macrophages and endothelial cells (Figure 4.10A). The SR isoform on endothelial cells also binds unmodified LDL with high affinity and saturation studies of radiolabeled LDL binding to membranes could represent the underlying expression of either the LDL receptor or the SR (Rigotti et al., 1995).

There is evidence for an LDL receptor on brain capillaries (Meresse et al., 1989). Initial studies with isolated brain capillaries demonstrated that binding of radiolabeled LDL to brain capillaries was nonsaturable. This suggests that the endocytosis of LDL at the isolated brain capillary preparation is rate-limiting, compared to membrane binding, similar to the case of IGF binding to human brain microvessels (Figure 4.8C). Saturable binding of LDL could be demonstrated, however, when partially purified brain capillary plasma membrane preparations were used (Meresse et al., 1989). There was also evidence for transcytosis of LDL through an in vitro BBB model comprised of cultured brain capillary endothelial cells (Dehouck et al., 1997). Whether there is transcytosis of LDL or high density lipoprotein (HDL) through the BBB in vivo is at present not known, but would be of importance to the pathogenesis of brain vascular atherosclerosis.

LDL binding to brain capillaries may be mediated by the type II scavenger receptor, which binds the LDL with high affinity (Rigotti et al., 1995). The ligands for the scavenger receptor are modified forms of LDL such as acetylated LDL. Uptake of LDL by the BBB SR would be expected to mediate only the endocytosis of the LDL into the brain capillary endothelial compartment, and not transcytosis through the endothelium. The lack of transcytosis of the acetylated LDL via the BBB SR was demonstrated with ICAP experiments, as shown in Figure 4.10B. Whereas radiolabeled forms of cationized bovine immunoglobulin (IgG) or cationized bovine albumin were transcytosed through the BBB via absorptive-mediated transcytosis (see below), the ICAP experiments demonstrated the absence of transcytosis of acetylated human LDL (hLDL), as shown in Figure 4.10B. The brain volumes of distribution (V_D) shown in Figure 4.10B are for the postvascular supernatant. In contrast, the brain V_D for radiolabeled acetylated LDL in the total brain homogenate was several-fold above the brain plasma volume marker, but this was completely sequestered within the vascular pellet, as determined with the capillary depletion technique (Triguero et al., 1990). These studies demonstrate that the BBB SR is responsible for the receptor-mediated endocytosis of circulating lipoproteins into the capillary endothelial compartment and not the RMT of these ligands through the BBB in vivo.

Absorptive-mediated transcytosis

Lectins

Lectins are glycoproteins, typically of plant origin, that bind specific carbohydrate residues present on membrane proteins. Nag (1985) has demonstrated that a variety of different lectins bind the brain endothelial plasma membranes, including wheat germ agglutinin (WGA). WGA is a homodimer comprised of two 18 kDa subunits and binding of WGA to cells causes agglutination due to a lectin-induced cross-linking of membrane-bound receptors (Grant and Peters, 1984). This cross-linking can deplete membrane proteins, which can then lead to lipid transitions and result in a significant alteration in membrane fluidity and permeability.

WGA undergoes absorptive-mediated transcytosis through the BBB. Broadwell et al. (1988) injected a conjugate of HRP and WGA intravenously, and used electron microscopy to demonstrate movement of this conjugate through the endothelial cytoplasm. HRP activity was found in pericytes, indicating there was transcytosis of the conjugate through the endothelial compartment in vivo. Several hours were required for the WGA–HRP conjugate to move through the endothelial cytoplasm (Broadwell et al., 1988). In contrast, ligands that utilize the RMT pathway at the BBB move through the endothelial cytoplasm within minutes, as shown in the case of insulin (Figure 4.4) or transferrin (Figures 4.5 and 4.6).

Cationic proteins

Cationic proteins with a net positive charge undergo absorptive-mediated endocytosis into cells, in general, and absorptive-mediated transcytosis through the BBB in vivo. Such proteins include those that are naturally cationic or proteins that have been cationized by the addition of amino groups to the surface of the protein.

Cationized albumin

The cationization of proteins enhances cellular uptake of the protein by triggering absorptive-mediated endocytosis into cells (Basu et al., 1976; Bergmann et al., 1984). Proteins are typically cationized by conjugating bifunctional amino groups to surface carboxyl residues via amide linkages. Cationization involves the conversion of a carboxyl moiety of a surface glutamate or aspartate residue into an extended primary amino group and this results in a significant increase in the isoelectric point (pI) of the protein. The cationization of proteins is a pH-controlled reaction and cationization is enhanced with decreasing pH (Lambert et al., 1983), owing to protonation of the surface carboxyl groups. If the cationization reaction is too vigorous, then there can be extensive intermolecular cross-linking and aggregation of the protein. BBB transport of cationized human serum albumin (HSA) is shown in Figure 4.11. The pI of the HSA was increased from approximately 5.2, in the case of native HSA, to approximately 8.1, for the cationized HSA (Figure 4.11A). The cationized HSA was then conjugated to a neutral light avidin (NLA) and the cationized HSA (cHSA)–NLA conjugate was radiolabeled by attachment to [^{3}H]biotin, which was bound by the NLA moiety with high affinity (Kang and Pardridge, 1994a). The [^{3}H]biotin conjugated to the cHSA/NLA was injected intravenously into anesthetized rats, and brain uptake and plasma and brain stability studies were performed (Figure 4.11B,C). The biotin/cHSA/NLA conjugate was stable in blood for periods as long as 6 and 24 h (top panel, Figure 4.11B). However, the conjugate was selectively degraded in brain and approximately 50% of the brain radioactivity migrated with the intact conjugate, and approximately 50% migrated

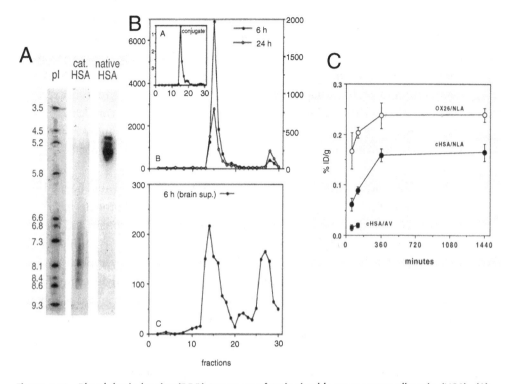

Figure 4.11   Blood–brain barrier (BBB) transport of cationized human serum albumin (HSA). (A) Isoelectric focusing of cationized (cat.) HSA, native HSA, and isoelectric standards (pI). (B) Elution through a gel filtration high performance liquid chromatography (HPLC) column of [³H]biotin bound to the purified cationized HSA (cHSA)/neutral light avidin (NLA) conjugate before injection into rats is shown in the inset. The elution of the plasma obtained 6 and 24 h after a single intravenous injection of [³H]biotin bound to the cHSA/NLA conjugate is shown in the top panel. The elution of rat brain obtained 6 h after a single intravenous injection of [³H]biotin bound to the cHSA/NLA conjugate is shown in the bottom panel. (C) The percentage of injected dose (ID) per gram brain of [³H]biotin bound to either cHSA/NLA or cHSA/AV for up to 24 h after administration is shown, in comparison with the brain uptake of [³H]biotin bound to OX26/NLA. Mean ± SE (n = 3 rats per point). AV, avidin. From Kang and Pardridge (1994a) with permission.

with low molecular weight biotin (bottom panel, Figure 4.11B). These gel filtration metabolism studies indicate the conjugate is stable in blood and the uptake of brain radioactivity reflects the intact conjugate. The studies also demonstrate the conjugate is degraded in brain following absorptive-mediated transcytosis through the BBB (Kang and Pardridge, 1994a). The extent to which the cHSA/NLA conjugate crosses the BBB was compared to BBB transport of (a) a conjugate of the OX26 MAb and NLA, which is designated OX26/NLA, and (b) a conjugate of avidin and cHSA, which is designated OX26/AV, as shown in Figure 4.11C. The brain uptake of the [³H]biotin bound to the cHSA/AV was very low and this was due to the reduced plasma area under the concentration curve (AUC) of this conjugate (Kang and Pardridge, 1994b). As discussed in more detail in Chapter 6, avidin, a cationic protein, is rapidly removed from blood by absorptive-mediated endocytosis in peripheral tissues, particularly liver (Kang et al., 1995b). In contrast, the NLA is a neutral form of avidin (Chapter 6) and NLA conjugates of BBB transport vectors have optimized pharmacokinetic parameters, relative to avidin conjugates (Kang and Pardridge, 1994b). The brain uptake of the OX26/NLA conjugate is approximately 50% higher than the brain uptake of the cHSA/NLA conjugate (Figure 4.11C).

The cHSA studies demonstrate that cationized forms of HSA could be used as a BBB transport vector (Kang and Pardridge, 1994a). Cationized proteins have been shown to be toxic due largely to the immunogenicity of these proteins and the formation of immune complexes that are deposited in the kidney (Gauthier et al., 1982; Muckerheide et al., 1987). However, this toxicity may only apply to cationization of heterologous proteins, which have a preexisting underlying immunogenicity. The immunogenicity of the heterologous protein is increased following cationization, probably owing to increased uptake by antigen-presenting cells. Conversely, if the protein to be cationized is homologous (i.e., same species), and lacks an underlying immunogenicity, then there is no enhanced immunogenicity of the protein following cationization (Pardridge et al., 1990b). This was demonstrated in the case of cationized rat serum albumin (RSA). The cationized and native RSAs were administered daily at a dose of 1 mg/kg subcutaneously to groups of rats for 4- and 8-week periods. These doses resulted in no toxicity, as the animals treated with the cationized RSA had normal weight gain, normal tissue histology, and normal serum chemistry. The animals exhibited low-titer antibody responses to the cationized RSA as shown by radioimmunoassay, and this antibody response was comparable to the low-titer antibody reaction observed in the animals receiving native RSA (Pardridge et al., 1990b).

Cationized immunoglobulin G

Antibody molecules such as IgG could be used for the diagnosis and treatment of brain diseases, should these proteins be made transportable through the BBB in vivo. Cationization of IgG is one option available for increasing brain uptake of circulating antibodies. Similar to cationization of HSA, IgG molecules were cationized by conversion of surface carboxyl groups to extended primary amino groups, shown in Figure 4.12A. The structure of the IgG was unchanged following cationization (Triguero et al., 1989), as sodium dodecylsulfate polyacrylamide gel electrophoresis (SDS-PAGE) showed there was no change in the size of the heavy chain or the light chain of the IgG following cationization (Figure 4.12B). The pI of a mixture of bovine IgG molecules ranged from 5–7.5, and this was uniformly

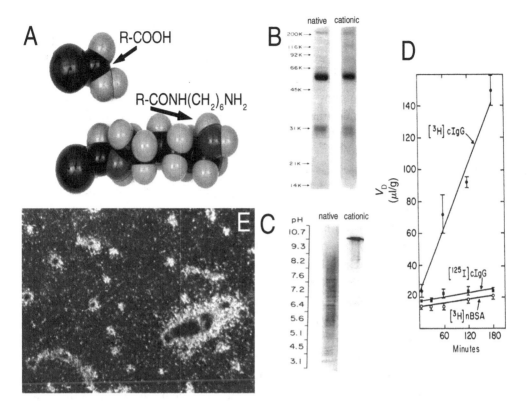

Figure 4.12   Transport of cationized immunoglobulin G (IgG) through the blood–brain barrier. (A) Atomic model of surface carboxyl groups (R-COOH) and carboxyl groups converted to an extended primary amine group [R-CONH(CH$_2$)$_6$NH$_2$]. (B) SDS-PAGE of either native or cationized bovine IgG. (C) Isoelectric focusing of either native or cationized bovine IgG. (D) Brain volume distribution (V_D) of [^{3}H]cationized IgG (cIgG), [^{125}I]cIgG, or [^{3}H] native bovine serum albumin (nBSA). Isotopes were injected intravenously in anesthetized rats and brain uptake was measured for the next 3 h. (E) Darkfield micrograph of emulsion autoradiography of rat brain following a 10-min carotid arterial perfusion of [^{125}I]cationized bovine IgG. The brain was not saline-cleared following the 10-min carotid artery perfusion of the labeled protein. From Triguero et al. (1989, 1991) with permission.

increased to a range of 9.5–10 following cationization, as determined by isoelectric focusing (Figure 4.12C). The cationized IgG (cIgG) was then radiolabeled with [^{3}H] and injected into anesthetized rats (Triguero et al., 1991). Brain uptake was measured over a period of 3 h and these studies showed a progressive increase in the brain volume of distribution (V_D) of the [^{3}H]cIgG compared to a plasma volume marker, [^{3}H]-native BSA (nBSA), as shown in Figure 4.12D. The radiolabeled cIgG underwent absorptive-mediated transcytosis through the BBB and this was demonstrated by emulsion autoradiography of rat brain following ICAP of the radiolabeled IgG (Figure 4.12E). These autoradiography studies revealed radiolab-eled cIgG entrapped in the brain capillary compartment. In these experiments, the brain was not saline-cleared following the perfusion of the radiolabeled cIgG, which accounts for the dense labeling of the microvasculature (Figure 4.12E). The emulsion autoradiography studies also show abundant silver grains in brain paren-chyma, indicating rapid transcytosis of cationized IgG through the BBB within a 10-min carotid artery infusion period (Figure 4.12E).

Cationized IgG and serum binding

A significant problem encountered with cIgG or cationized MAb is the binding of constituents in serum to the cIgG, and this binding neutralizes the cationic charge on the protein, and eliminates the enhanced uptake into brain and other organs (Triguero et al., 1991). A property of this phenomenon is that it is sensitive to the method by which the cIgG is radiolabeled, and also varies amongst different MAbs. If the cationized bovine IgG is labeled with [^{125}I] via oxidative iodination, and then injected into rats, there is so significant increase in brain uptake of the [^{125}I]cIgG, as shown in Figure 4.12D. However, when the same form of cIgG is radiolabeled with [^{3}H]sodium borohydride, there is a significant and time-dependent increase in brain uptake of the [^{3}H]cIgG (Figure 4.12D). This serum inhibition phenome-non could also be demonstrated with isolated brain capillaries (Triguero et al., 1991). When rat serum was added to isolated bovine brain capillaries incubated with the [^{3}H]cIgG, there was no inhibition of the binding and uptake of the cIgG to the brain capillary in vitro caused by the rat serum. However, there was nearly complete inhibition of binding and uptake of the cIgG to the brain capillary prep-aration caused by rat serum when the cIgG was radiolabeled with [^{125}I]. This binding by serum components is specific to the type of IgG or MAb that is under investigation. For example, the AMY33 MAb, which is a mouse IgG1 and is directed against the Aβ-amyloidotic peptide of Alzheimer's disease, was cationized and radiolabeled with either [^{125}I] or [^{111}In] (Bickel et al., 1994b). The cationized AMY33 that was radiolabeled with [^{125}I] had enhanced clearance from plasma in vivo, with no demonstrable inhibition by serum components (Bickel et al., 1995b). On the other hand, the cationized AMY33 that was radiolabeled with [^{111}In] dem-onstrated pronounced serum inhibition such that the plasma clearance of the cationized MAb, radiolabeled with [^{111}In], was no different from the plasma clear-ance of the native MAb (Bickel et al., 1995b). If the labeled cIgG is subject to the serum inhibition phenomenon, then further in vivo studies with the cIgG are pre-cluded, since the increase in tissue uptake is neutralized. Further studies are needed to determine the nature of the serum inhibition and to develop strategies for elim-inating this inhibition.

In working with cationized MAbs, it is important to perform a pharmacokinetic analysis of the radiolabeled protein early in the drug development process. The

Table 4.2 Monoclonal antibodies (MAbs) that have been cationized with retention of biological activity

MAb	Target	Purpose
MAb 111	rev	AIDS therapy
AMY 33	Aβ	Brain amyloid imaging
D146	ras	Cancer therapy
Humanized 4D5	p185^{HER2}	Cancer imaging

Notes:
AIDS, acquired immune deficiency syndrome.
From Bickel et al. (1994b); Pardridge et al. (1994a, 1995c, 1998a) with permission.

plasma pharmacokinetics will demonstrate whether there is serum neutralization of the cationic MAb. If serum inhibition is present, then the plasma clearance of the cationized antibody is not substantially increased relative to the plasma clearance of the native MAb. The serum inhibition is not observed with all cationized antibodies.

Cationized monoclonal antibodies

MAbs directed against specific receptors or proteins in brain are potentially new agents for the diagnosis or treatment of brain diseases. However, native MAbs do not cross cell membranes, and it is necessary physically to inject the antibody into the cytoplasm of cultured cells to obtain a biological response (Lane and Nigg, 1996). Cationized MAbs are potential new therapeutic agents, because these agents can traverse the BBB via absorptive-mediated transcytosis. Cationized MAbs may be particularly useful for brain imaging, because the cationized MAb is removed from blood very rapidly, and this reduces the plasma concentration of the radio-labeled MAb, which will reduce the "noise" of the imaging signal. The specific MAbs that have been cationized and investigated are shown in Table 4.2. The potential applications of these agents include the treatment of cerebral acquired immune deficiency syndrome (AIDS) or brain cancer, or the diagnosis of Alzheimer's disease or brain cancer. Because cationization increases the immunogenicity of heterologous proteins (Muckerheide et al., 1987), cationized mouse MAbs cannot be administered to humans. However, murine MAbs can be converted to human proteins by genetic engineering, as discussed in Chapter 5. Humanized MAbs may be ideal candidates for IgG cationization because these agents may have minimal immunogenicity in humans.

The humanized 4D5 MAb directed against the p185^{HER2} oncogenic protein was cationized and initial studies were performed, as shown in Figure 4.13. The immunoreactive p185^{HER2} was expressed on the plasma membrane in human tumor cells,

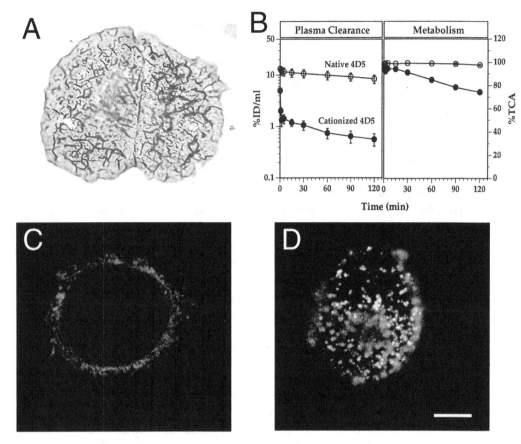

Figure 4.13   (A) Immunocytochemistry demonstrating localization of the p185^{HER2} protein to the plasma membrane and to the tubular network of the endoplasmic reticulum in SK-BR3 human breast cancer cells in tissue culture. Immune staining was done with the humanized 4D5 monoclonal antibody (MAb) to p185^{HER2}. (B) Left: Plasma concentration expressed as percentage of injected dose (ID)/ml of plasma after the intravenous injection in rats of [^{125}I]-labeled native humanized 4D5 antibody or [^{125}I]-cationized humanized 4D5 antibody. Data are mean ± SE (n = 3 rats per point). Right: The percentage of plasma radioactivity that is precipitable by trichloroacetic acid (TCA) is shown for the native or cationized 4D5 antibody. (C, D) Confocal microscopy of SK-BR3 cells incubated with either fluorescein-labeled native humanized 4D5 antibody (C) or fluoresceinated cationized humanized 4D5 antibody (D). Cells were incubated for 60 min at 4 °C with fluoresceinated antibody and then incubated at 37 °C for 90 min prior to confocal microscopy. The magnification bar in (D) is 8 μm. From Pardridge et al. (1998a) with permission.

but was also largely confined to the intracellular endoplasmic reticulum, as shown by the immunocytochemistry studies in Figure 4.13A. The native 4D5 MAb cannot access the intracellular target because antibodies are not taken up by cells in the absence of specific transport mechanisms. This is demonstrated by confocal microscopy (Pardridge et al., 1998a). In these studies, the native humanized 4D5 MAb was directly conjugated with fluorescein and added to p185^{HER2}-bearing tumor cells. However, even after prolonged incubations, the native MAb was confined to the plasma membrane (Figure 4.13C). Conversely, the cationized, humanized MAb readily distributed into the cytoplasmic compartment (Figure 4.13D). Both the native and the humanized MAb were labeled with ^{125}I, and a pharmacokinetic analysis in rats was performed (Figure 4.13B). These studies showed the cationized, humanized MAb was rapidly removed from the plasma compartment, indicating no inhibition of the cationic moiety by serum substituents (Pardridge et al., 1998a).

In summary, cationized humanized MAbs are potential new agents for the diagnosis and treatment of disorders of the brain or other organs. Owing to the rapid removal from plasma (Figure 4.13B), cationized MAbs may be particularly suited as diagnostic agents. However, the rapid removal from plasma results in a greatly reduced plasma AUC. In this respect, cationization of proteins is analogous to lipidization of small molecules. Both processes increase cellular uptake, in general, and this results in a reduced plasma AUC. Since the brain uptake (percentage of injected dose per gram brain: %ID/g) is directly proportional to the plasma AUC (Chapter 3), any modification that reduces the plasma AUC will tend to offset the increase in BBB PS product. Nevertheless, cationization of MAbs is a novel way of increasing the cellular uptake of the MAb. The alternative is to transfect the cell with a gene encoding the MAb (Marasco et al., 1993), to produce an "intrabody," but this changes the problem of antibody targeting to the cell to gene targeting to the cell, and the latter can be more difficult than the former. However, gene targeting to the brain is feasible, as discussed in Chapter 9.

Protamine

Protamine is a 7 kDa arginine-rich, cationic protein that is produced in spermatozoa to complex DNA. Both protamine and polyarginine, to a much greater extent than polylysine, cause BBB disruption following ICAP of the polypeptide (Westergren and Johansson, 1993). These observations correlate with other studies showing that the intravenous injection of protamine increases albumin flux across capillary beds in general (Vehaskari et al., 1984). An unexplained finding was that the brain interstitial concentration of the small molecule, glutamic acid, was not increased following the intracarotid arterial infusion of protamine (Westergren et

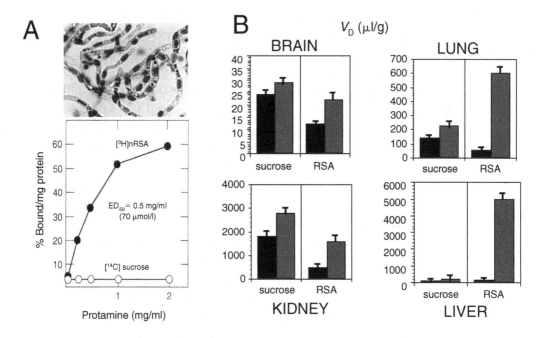

Figure 4.14   (A) In vitro: Bovine brain capillaries are shown in the top panel. The bottom panel shows
the percentage binding per mg protein of either [^{3}H]-native rat serum albumin (nRSA) or
[^{14}C]sucrose in the presence of varying concentrations of unlabeled protamine.
Incubations were performed at 37 °C for 30 min. (B) In vivo: Organ volume distribution
(V_D) for either [^{14}C]sucrose or [^{3}H]-native RSA measured 5 min after the intravenous
injection of 1.5 mg/kg salmon protamine (sigma grade 4, histone-free), using the external
organ technique. Mean $\pm$ SE ($n = 3$ rats per point). From Pardridge et al. (1993) with
permission.

al., 1994). This suggested that the BBB was selectively disrupted to large molecules
such as albumin, but not to small molecules such as glutamic acid.

The mechanism of protamine interaction with the BBB was initially investigated
in vitro with isolated brain capillaries (Figure 4.14A). In the absence of protamine,
the binding of [^{3}H]-native RSA by isolated bovine brain capillaries was minimal
and not significantly different from the binding of [^{14}C]sucrose, as shown in Figure
4.14A. However, with increasing concentrations of protamine, ranging from 0 to
2 mg/ml, there was a selective and progressive increase in the binding of [^{3}H]RSA,
with a 50% effective dose of 0.5 mg/ml (70 μmol/l) protamine (Pardridge et al.,
1993). In contrast, the protamine did not increase the brain capillary uptake of the
sucrose (Figure 4.14A). The protamine-mediated uptake of the [^{3}H]RSA by the
brain capillary was competitively inhibited by either γ-globulin or native bovine

serum albumin. This suggested that the protamine was forming a complex with the native RSA and was actually carrying the native RSA into the brain capillary cytoplasm in a vectorial mechanism. That is, protamine is normally rapidly bound and endocytosed by the brain capillaries in an absorptive-mediated endocytosis process. Whereas native RSA has no interaction with the brain capillary, the RSA–protamine complex may be taken up by the endothelium by attachment to the protamine binding sites. The high-affinity binding of albumin to protamine was demonstrated with equilibrium dialysis, which showed the binding dissociation constant (K_D) was 6–9 μmol/l. Therefore, at the concentrations used in these studies (Figure 4.14 A), protamine and native RSA were forming a complex and this could account for the selective increase in uptake of the RSA relative to sucrose (Figure 4.14 A). In contrast to protamine, an anionic substance such as dextran sulfate resulted in comparable increase in brain capillary uptake of either the [^{3}H]-native RSA or the [^{14}C]sucrose (Pardridge et al., 1993). This indicated that the anionic dextran sulfate was causing some kind of disruption of the brain capillary endothelial membrane and increasing the uptake of all solutes in the medium, including both low and high molecular weight substances. This correlates with other studies showing that the intracarotid arterial infusion of heparin sulfate results in BBB disruption (Nagy et al., 1983).

The selective effect of protamine on capillary transport of serum proteins, as opposed to small molecules such as sucrose, was confirmed in vivo with the intravenous injection/external organ technique (Pardridge et al., 1983). The organ volume of distribution (V_D) of [^{3}H]-native RSA was measured in brain, kidney, lung, and liver at 5 min after intravenous injection of [^{3}H]-native RSA and [^{14}C]sucrose, and either 0 or 1.5 mg/kg type IV salmon protamine base. These results are shown in Figure 4.14B. There is a selective increase in the organ uptake of the albumin, relative to sucrose, caused by the coinjection of the protamine. These studies were consistent with the hypothesis that protamine undergoes absorptive-mediated transcytosis through the capillary barrier in brain, as well as other tissues, and that protamine can act as a vector by binding albumin, and that the protamine–albumin complex also crosses the brain capillary barrier. At higher concentrations, protamine causes actual BBB disruption with increased pinocytosis across the brain capillary endothelium (Vorbrodt et al., 1995).

Other naturally cationic proteins

Proteins that are naturally cationic, like protamine, have a preponderance of arginine and lysine residues, relative to glutamate and aspartate residues. Several naturally cationic proteins undergo absorptive-mediated transport through the BBB, and these include histone (Pardridge et al., 1989a), an adrenocorticotropic hormone (ACTH) analog (Shimura et al., 1991), the soluble extracellular domain of the lymphocyte CD4 receptor (Pardridge et al., 1992), and the cationic "import peptides" discussed below. The cationic proteins bind the anionic sites on the brain capillary endothelium, and this binding triggers the absorptive-mediated endocytosis and transcytosis. The anionic sites on the luminal membrane of the brain capillary endothelium are mainly sialic acid residues, and the anionic charges on the abluminal membrane are primarily heparan sulfate (Vorbrodt, 1989).

Import peptides

The rev and tat proteins are produced by the human immunodeficiency virus (HIV) and these proteins are critical to viral replication. Both proteins are highly cationic, and tat has been used to mediate the cellular uptake of tat–protein conjugates (Fawell et al., 1994). The part of the tat protein that mediates cell uptake is a highly cationic, arginine-rich sequence between residues 37 and 58 (Chen et al., 1995), and a synthetic peptide encompassing amino acid residues 48–60, GRKKR-RQRRRPPQC, is actively taken up by cells (Vivés et al., 1997). The fusion of part of this sequence, YGRKKRRQRRR, to the amino terminus of β-galactosidase results in increased uptake of the fusion protein by many organs in vivo, including the brain (Schwarze et al., 1999).

Tat, rev, histone, and protamine are all cationic proteins that bind either DNA or RNA. Other cationic peptides are derived from the third helix of the Antennapedia protein, which is a homeoprotein that belongs to a family of DNA binding proteins first identified in *Drosophila*. These peptides include a lysine/arginine-rich sequence of RQILIWFQNRRMKWK (Derossi et al., 1994), or an arginine-rich sequence of RRWRRWWRRWWRRWRR (Williams et al., 1997). These import peptides are said to enter cells by nonendocytosis mechansisms, but confocal microscopy uniformly demonstrates the inclusion of the peptides in intracellular endosomal vesicles (Allinquant et al., 1995; Williams et al., 1997).

Cationic import peptides have been used to enhance doxorubicin transport across the BBB in vivo, and these peptides include an arginine-rich 18-mer called SynB1, and a lysine/arginine-rich 16-mer, called D-penetratin (Rousselle et al., 2000). Doxurubicin was conjugated to the amino terminus of either peptide, and the BBB transport of the drug/cationic peptide conjugate was greatly increased compared to the unconjugated doxorubicin following ICAP in the absence of serum. However, only marginal increases in brain uptake of the conjugate were observed following intravenous administration. The reduced activity of the vector following intravenous administration was due in part to extensive plasma protein binding of the proteins, which is on the order of 96–99.5% (Rousselle et al., 2000). This inhibition of BBB transport caused by plasma protein binding is similar to the effects of plasma protein binding on the BBB transport of phosphorothioate oligodeoxynucleotides, as discussed in Chapter 8.

There are two problems associated with the use of highly cationic proteins as BBB drug-targeting systems. First, the cationic proteins are widely taken up by peripheral tissues and are rapidly removed from the blood stream (Pardridge et al., 1989a). Therefore, based on the "pharmacokinetic rule" (Chapter 3), these proteins have a reduced plasma AUC and a proportionate reduction in the brain %ID/g. The cationization of proteins is analogous to the lipidization of small molecules. Similarly, the attachment of a cationic carrier has the same effect as attachment of a lipid carrier. Both modifications result in an increase in the BBB permeability–surface area (PS) product and a parallel decrease in the plasma AUC, which tends to have offsetting effects on the brain %ID/g. Because the plasma AUC is reduced, the brain %ID/g is not increased in proportion to the increase in BBB PS product. Second, cationic proteins can be toxic to cells. Histone causes nonspecific increases in BBB permeability (Pardridge et al., 1989a). The tat protein induces apoptosis of hippocampal neurons (Kruman et al., 1998).

Neuropeptide transport at the blood–brain barrier

Introduction

There are conflicting statements in the literature as to whether neuropeptides cross the BBB. Various claims have been made on the basis of interpretation of studies involving the intravenous injection of peptides that are radiolabeled with [^{125}I]iodine on peptide tyrosine residues. Even within the same review, there are conflicting statements as to whether neuropeptides cross the BBB in pharmacologically significant amounts (Brownlees and Williams, 1993). The mechanism of neuropeptide transport through the BBB, if it occurs, is said to be either free diffusion owing to lipid-solubility of the peptide, or CMT of the peptide.

The central finding in support of neuropeptide transport through the BBB is the observation that the brain/plasma ratio or brain volume of distribution (V_D) of the labeled peptide exceeds that of a plasma volume (V_O) marker such as native albumin. However, when brain uptake is measured from radioactivity determinations, the brain V_D can exceed the brain V_O simply due to the brain uptake of labeled peptide metabolites that are generated by the peripheral metabolism and degradation of the labeled peptide (Pardridge, 1983b). In this setting, the radiolabeled peptide is rapidly taken up by peripheral tissues, degraded, and radiolabeled metabolites, such as iodotyrosine or iodide, are released to the circulation. These metabolites, particularly iodotyrosine are taken up by the brain by CMT systems such as large neutral amino acid transporter type 1 (LAT1) at the BBB (Chapter 3), and essentially all of the radioactivity arising in the brain is due to the brain uptake of the metabolite, not the original neuropeptide. As discussed below, it can be shown that when the peripheral metabolism or release of the radiolabeled metabolites is blocked, the brain V_D of the labeled peptide decreases to the V_O value, because the artifact, i.e., the brain uptake of radiolabeled metabolites, has been removed from the experimental setting.

Mechanisms of neuropeptide transport through the blood–brain barrier

Free diffusion

Small oligopeptides may traverse the BBB by lipid mediation owing to the lipid-solubility of the peptide (Banks et al., 1991). However, as reviewed in Chapter 3, once a small molecule forms at least 8–10 hydrogen bonds in solvent water, the transport through the BBB in pharmacologically significant amounts is minimal. Owing to the extensive hydrogen bonding of the amide group, which forms the basic structure of an oligopeptide, there is extensive hydrogen bonding between the neuropeptide and solvent water. Even an oligopeptide as small as two amino acids will form eight hydrogen bonds with water and a tripeptide will form >10 hydrogen bonds with water. These considerations pertain to naturally occurring peptides that do not have an artificial blockade of the hydrogen bond forming functional groups on the amide structures. For example, a dipeptide that is cyclized to form a diketopiperazine will have a substantial increase in lipid-solubility owing to the reduced hydrogen bonding associated with the formation of the cyclic structure.

Another approach towards the reduction in hydrogen bonding of peptides is the synthesis of artificial peptides that are acetylated at the amino terminus and N-methylated at internal amide bonds, because these modifications eliminate hydrogen bonding. Such structural changes of di- and tri-peptides of phenylalanine can increase the lipid-solubility of the peptide (Chikhale et al., 1995), and in this setting, free diffusion of the synthetic oligopeptide through the BBB is possible. However, this situation is not representative of most peptides, which form numerous hydrogen bonds with solvent water. For example, octreotide is a cyclic octapeptide, but this peptide still forms enough hydrogen bonds effectively to eliminate free diffusion across a monolayer of brain capillary endothelial cells (Jaehde et al., 1994). Ermisch et al. (1993) have concluded that the free diffusion of peptides through the BBB is without physiologic significance.

Carrier-mediated transport of peptides at the blood–brain barrier

The existence of a series of peptide transport systems (PTS), designated PTS-1 through PTS-4, have been proposed to mediate the brain uptake of a wide variety of neuropeptides (Banks and Kastin, 1990). However, there has been no biochemical characterization of these putative peptide transport systems. Affinity cross-linking experiments using radiolabeled ligand and SDS-PAGE have not been performed to determine the molecular weight of the putative PTS at the BBB, similar to that performed for BBB RMT systems (Figures 4.4 and 4.8). Moreover, despite the molecular cloning of a wide variety of CMT systems, there has been no cloning of PTS specific for the neuropeptides that have been proposed to undergo CMT through the BBB. Recently, an oligopeptide transporter (OPT) type 1, OPT-1, has been cloned from yeast and the K_m of OPT-1 for leucine enkephalin is 0.35 mmol/l (Hauser et al., 2000). There has been no demonstration that peptide transporters such as OPT-1 are expressed in mammalian systems, much less at the BBB. If OPT-1 was expressed at the BBB to mediate the transport of leucine enkephalin, then the V_{max} of this system would have to be high, given the very low affinity (high K_m) of OPT-1 for leucine enkephalin. Other studies have proposed that synthetic enkephalin analogs such as [D-penicillamine^{2,5}] enkephalin (DPDPE) cross the BBB by as yet unknown mechanisms (Williams et al., 1996). DPDPE is a weak substrate for organic anion transporting polypeptide type 2 (oatp2) (Kakyo et al., 1999) and, as reviewed in Chapter 10, oatp2 is selectively expressed at the BBB (Li et al., 2001). However, the principal substrate for oatp2 is estrone sulfate (Noe et al., 1997), and estrone sulfate does not cross the BBB (Steingold et al., 1986). This suggests that oatp2 is an active efflux system that is preferentially involved in movement of substrate from brain to blood, rather than from blood to brain.

Artifacts in brain neuropeptide uptake caused by peripheral metabolism of the peptide

Enkephalin

Early studies reported a moderate brain uptake index (BUI) for radiolabeled enkephalin (Kastin et al., 1976). However, subsequent studies showed that the BUI of labeled enkephalin could be blocked by the coadministration of unlabeled tyrosine (Zlokovic et al., 1985). The peptide is labeled at the amino terminal tyrosine, and aminopeptidases on the endothelial glycocalyx remove the amino terminal tyrosine residue, enabling the labeled tyrosine to undergo CMT through the BBB on LAT1 (Chapter 3). This can be demonstrated with isolated brain capillaries, as shown in Figure 4.15A. When radiolabeled leucine enkephalin is added to the capillaries there is a time-dependent increase in the brain uptake of the neuropeptide (Pardridge and Mietus, 1981). However, this uptake is blocked completely to the background level by the inclusion of 5 mmol/l L-tyrosine in the incubation medium (Figure 4.15B). Parallel chromatographic studies showed that the leucine enkephalin was progressively converted to free tyrosine during the incubation with the bovine brain capillaries (Figure 4.15C), owing to the action of capillary aminopeptidase. Therefore, there is no actual binding or uptake of the leucine

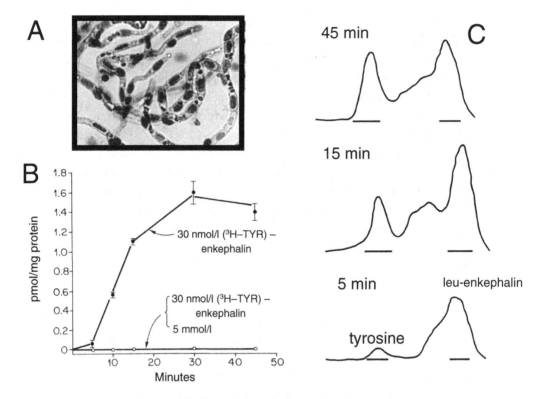

Figure 4.15   (A) Bovine brain capillaries. (B) Time course of uptake of [³H]leucine enkephalin in isolated bovine brain capillaries incubated in the presence of either 0 or 5 mmol/l unlabeled tyrosine. Mean ± SE (*n* = 3–4). (C) Radioscans of thin-layer chromatograms of medium radioactivity obtained following incubation of brain capillaries with [tyrosyl-³H]leucine enkephalin for 5, 15, or 45 min. The migration of tyrosine or leucine enkephalin standards in the chromatography is shown by the horizontal bars. From Pardridge and Mietus (1981) with permission.

enkephalin, per se, by the brain capillary, but there is active uptake of the radiolabeled tyrosine metabolite.

Leptin

The intravenous injection of [^{125}I]leptin in rats is followed by the appearance of radioactivity in the brain and this has been interpreted as evidence for saturable transport of leptin across the BBB (Banks et al., 1996). Owing to the presence of the OBR on the BBB (Golden et al., 1997), there may in fact be RMT of leptin through the BBB in vivo. However, the measurement of brain radioactivity following the intravenous injection of radiolabeled leptin is not interpretable owing to the extensive metabolism of this neuropeptide in the periphery following intravenous administration in the rat (Golden et al., 1997). The radioactive iodotyrosine is released following the degradation of the leptin in the periphery and this will then undergo CMT through the BBB in vivo and lead to measurable brain radioactivity. In an attempt to block artifactual uptake of tyrosine by brain, Banks et al. (1996) have administered unlabeled tyrosine in the leptin injection studies. However, the dose of tyrosine used in these investigations, 0.4 mg/kg, is >100-fold lower than the dose necessary to cause significant increases in plasma tyrosine such that the BBB LAT1 is inhibited (Tyfield and Holton, 1976). No competition effects for brain uptake of radiolabeled tyrosine are caused by a systemic administration of a dose of unlabeled tyrosine as low as 0.4 mg/kg.

Brain-derived neurotrophic factor (BDNF)

Neurotrophic factors such as nerve growth factor (NGF) or BDNF have been radio-labeled with [^{125}I] and injected intravenously for brain uptake studies (Poduslo and Curran, 1996; Pan et al., 1998). These neurotrophic factors are said to cross the BBB. However, the neurotrophic factors are highly cationic proteins that are rapidly taken up by peripheral tissues such as liver and rapidly converted to radiolabeled metabolites (Pardridge et al., 1994b). When this peripheral metabolism is inhibited by protein pegylation (Chapter 6), there is a decrease in the peripheral metabolism of the neurotrophic factor and a parallel decrease in the brain volume of distribution (V_D), as shown in Figure 4.16. The brain "uptake" of the radiolabeled BDNF decreases to zero in proportion to the inhibition of peripheral metabolism of peptide (Sakane and Pardridge, 1997). The decrease in peripheral metabolism of the BDNF is caused by progressive pegylation of the BDNF with polyethylene glycol (PEG) ranging from 2 to 5 kDa in molecular weight, designated PEG^{2000} and PEG^{5000} (Figure 4.16). The inhibition of peripheral degradation of the pegylated BDNF is reflected in the progressive increase in the plasma AUC caused by converting BDNF to BDNF-PEG^{2000} or BDNF-PEG^{5000} (Figure 4.16). The brain V_D of native BDNF is in excess of 150 μl/g (Figure 4.16) and this would lead to the calculation of a significant BBB PS product. However, the brain V_D decreases to a level that is not significantly different from the brain plasma volume (V_O) with progressive pegylation of the neurotrophic factor (Figure 4.16). This study indicates that if the peripheral metabolism of the neurotrophic factor is removed, there is no artifactual uptake of radiolabeled metabolites, and there is no recording of radioactivity in the brain above the plasma volume level. The loss of brain "uptake" of the BDNF following protein pegylation is not due to loss of biologic activity of the neurotrophic factor. As discussed in Chapter 6, the neurotrophic factor was pegylated on carboxyl residues, which allows for complete retention of the biologic activity of the BDNF (Sakane and Pardridge, 1997), despite the pegylation modification of the protein. The studies shown in Figure 4.16 demonstrate that it

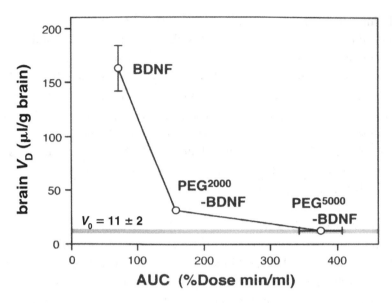

Figure 4.16 Artifactual brain uptake of a radiolabeled neuropeptide. The brain volume distribution (V_D) of [^{125}I]brain-derived neurotrophic factor (BDNF), [^{125}I]BDNF-PEG^{2000}, and [^{125}I]BDNF-PEG^{5000} is plotted vs the corresponding 60-min plasma area under the concentration curve (AUC). The brain uptake of radiolabeled BDNF decreases to zero in proportion to the inhibition of peripheral metabolism of the peptide, which is caused by progressive pegylation of the BDNF. The brain plasma volume (V_0) is shown by the horizontal line. Mean $\pm$ SE ($n = 3$ rats). From Sakane and Pardridge (1997) with permission.

is possible to increase markedly the plasma AUC of a peptide therapeutic without altering biologic activity, as discussed in Chapter 6.

Epidermal growth factor (EGF)

EGF does not cross the BBB and there is no EGF receptor on the BBB (Kurihara et al., 1999). However, if EGF is radiolabeled with [^{125}I] and injected intravenously, a significant level of brain radioactivity is observed, as shown in Figure 4.17B. In this case, the brain uptake is in excess of 0.03%ID/g brain in the rat (Kurihara et al., 1999), which is the level typically recorded for the brain uptake of neuropeptides that are proposed to cross the BBB. However, there is extensive metabolism of [^{125}I]EGF in peripheral tissues, as shown by the measurement of plasma radioactivity that is precipitable by trichloroacetic acid (TCA) (Figure 4.17A). This study shows that the plasma TCA is <80% at 15 min and <20% at 60 min after intravenous injection. Given this degree of peripheral metabolism of the [^{125}I]EGF, there will be substantial formation of [^{125}I]tyrosine released to blood. This problem of release of radiolabeled metabolites to the blood following peripheral metabolism

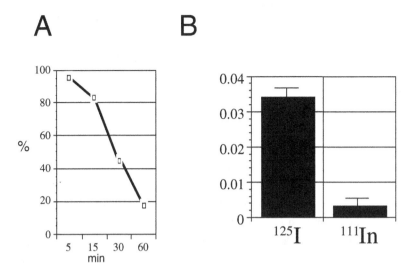

A   **B**

Figure 4.17   (A) The percentage of plasma trichloroacetic acid (TCA) precipitable radioactivity is plotted versus time following intravenous injection of [^{125}I]epidermal growth factor (EGF) in anesthetized rats. (B) Brain uptake (percentage of injected dose per gram brain: %ID/g) of either [^{125}I]EGF or [^{111}In]EGF at 60 min after intravenous injection of either isotope in anesthetized rats. Reproduced with permission from Kurihara et al. (1999). Copyright (1999) American Chemical Society.

can be eliminated by radiolabeling the peptide with indium-111 (Kurihara et al., 1999). When the EGF is radiolabeled with [^{111}In] that is chelated to a diethylene-triaminepentaacetic acid (DTPA) moiety, which is conjugated to lysine residues, the brain "uptake" of the [^{111}In]-labeled EGF is decreased 10-fold to a value no greater than a plasma volume marker, as shown in Figure 4.17B. Serum TCA measurements cannot be performed with peptides labeled with [^{111}In] because this would result in dissociation of the radionuclide from the DTPA chelator moiety. Therefore, serum gel filtration fast protein liquid chromatography (FPLC) measurements were performed, and this showed that there was no formation of low molecular weight radiolabeled metabolites in blood following the intravenous injection of EGF labeled with [^{111}In] (Kurihara et al., 1999). The rate of plasma clearance of [^{125}I]EGF and [^{111}In]EGF is identical, indicating that the method of radioiodination does not alter the uptake of EGF in peripheral tissues (Kurihara et al., 1999). Both forms of EGF are taken up equally rapidly and metabolized in peripheral tissues. However, the [^{111}In] stays sequestered in peripheral tissue and is not released to the general circulation (Press et al., 1996). Conversely, the radiolabeled metabolites containing [^{125}I] are rapidly released to the plasma compartment. The differential processing and exportation of these two radionuclides to the circulation explain the 10-fold difference in brain "uptake" of the [^{125}I]EGF following intravenous administration. EGF does not cross the BBB, and the apparent brain uptake of the radioactivity following intravenous injection of [^{125}I]EGF is strictly a function of the peripheral metabolism of the peptide and brain uptake of [^{125}I] metabolites (Kurihara et al., 1999).

Artifacts of brain uptake of neuropeptides secondary to vascular binding

Opioid peptides

The problem of peripheral metabolism of peptides can be eliminated using the ICAP technique. In this case, the radiolabeled peptide is perfused in saline buffer in the absence of serum proteins for various times followed by measurement of the brain volume of distribution (V_D). If the brain V_D exceeds the sucrose or plasma volume (V_O), then the peptide is said to cross the BBB. The brain V_D of a metabolically stable opioid peptide, [^{3}H]DALDA, was measured with the ICAP technique and the V_D values exceeded that of sucrose (Samii et al., 1994). However, the calculated BBB PS product for the [^{3}H]DALDA was many-fold greater than the PS product determined following intravenous injection. The artifactually high PS product following ICAP relative to the lower PS product after intravenous injection was not due to plasma protein binding (Samii et al., 1994). In addition, the BBB PS product measured following intravenous injection was reliable because there was no metabolic degradation of this metabolically stable neuropeptide. The artifactually high BBB PS product determined with the ICAP technique was subsequently demonstrated to be due to nonspecific vascular absorption of the opioid peptide during the ICAP. This was shown by a series of experiments in which the brain V_D of the [^{3}H]DALDA was measured after a postperfusion wash protocol involving the infusion of physiologic buffer containing 5% bovine serum albumin following the ICAP with the labeled opioid peptide. These experiments showed the apparent brain V_D of the [^{3}H]DALDA was reduced by the postperfusion wash, indicating the neuropeptide had not undergone transport through the BBB, but was nonspecifically absorbed to the vascular compartment during the ICAP procedure.

Aβ^{1-40} amyloid peptide

The Aβ^{1-40} amyloid peptide is a potential imaging agent for quantifying the deposition of amyloid in brain in Alzheimer's disease, as reviewed in Chapter 7. [^{125}I]Aβ^{1-40} is said to cross the BBB based on measurements of brain radioactivity after the intravenous injection of the peptide (Poduslo et al., 1999). However, like other neuropeptides, [^{125}I]Aβ^{1-40} is rapidly degraded in peripheral tissues, which confounds interpretation of brain uptake data. To circumvent this problem, the BBB transport of [^{125}I]Aβ^{1-40} has been measured by the ICAP method, and this shows that the brain V_D of Aβ^{1-40} exceeds the V_O for labeled sucrose (Saito et al.,

1995). When the capillary depletion technique was performed, however, the V_D of [^{125}I]Aβ^{1-40} in the postvascular supernatant was not significantly different from the V_O in that compartment for radiolabeled sucrose. These studies indicated that, although Aβ^{1-40} was sequestered by the capillary endothelium, there was no significant trans-BBB passage of this peptide (Saito et al., 1995).

Summary

Data on the brain uptake of a given neuropeptide should be interpreted with consideration to how the brain V_D is experimentally measured. If the radiolabeled neuropeptide was administered intravenously, it is likely that peripheral metabolism of the neuropeptide was responsible for the brain uptake of radiolabeled metabolites rather than the neuropeptide per se. If the radiolabeled neuropeptide was administered by ICAP, consideration should be made as to whether there is nonspecific vascular sequestration of the peptide, particularly if the peptide is radiolabeled by radioiodination, which enhances absorption to vascular surfaces. If the neuropeptide is believed to cross the BBB by free diffusion, then the 1-octanol/saline partition coefficient should be measured. If the neuropeptide crosses the BBB by free diffusion, then the log PS of the neuropeptide should fall on the lipid-solubility trendline when the log PS is plotted versus log P, as discussed in Chapter 3. If the neuropeptide is believed to cross the BBB by CMT, then parallel biochemical investigations should be performed using studies such as affinity cross-linking, which documents the molecular weight of the putative peptide transporter. Thus far, no mammalian oligopeptide transporters have been cloned or identified at the molecular level, and shown to be expressed at the BBB.

5

Vector discovery: genetically engineered Trojan horses for drug targeting

- Introduction
- Peptidomimetic monoclonal antibodies
- Genetically engineered vectors
- Brain-specific vectors
- Summary

Introduction

Brain drug-targeting vectors are peptides, modified plasma proteins, or peptidomimetic monoclonal antibodies (MAbs) that are ligands for blood–brain barrier (BBB) endogenous receptors (Pardridge, 1986; Kumagai et al., 1987). This property enables these molecules to act as "transportable peptides" and undergo receptor- or absorptive-mediated transcytosis through the BBB in vivo. Endogenous peptides or peptidomimetic MAbs undergo receptor-mediated transcytosis (RMT) through the BBB and lectins or cationized proteins such as cationized albumin are transported through the BBB via absorptive-mediated transcytosis. These transportable peptides may be used as molecular "Trojan horses" to ferry drugs across the BBB via the endogenous peptide receptor transport systems. A chimeric peptide is formed when a drug, that is normally not transported through the BBB, is conjugated to a BBB transport vector or "transportable peptide" using linker strategies outlined in Chapter 6. Endogenous peptides that are ligands for BBB RMT systems could be used as vectors, and these are discussed in Chapter 4. In addition, peptidomimetic MAbs can be used as BBB brain drug-targeting vectors provided these MAbs bind the endogenous BBB peptide receptors. This binding enables the MAb to act as a "transportable peptide" and to undergo RMT through the BBB in vivo. For example, either insulin (Fukuta et al., 1994) or an insulin receptor peptidomimetic MAb (Wu et al., 1997b) has been used to deliver chimeric peptides through the BBB. The ability of MAbs to mimic the action of an endogenous peptide was demonstrated in the 1980s (Beisiegel et al., 1981; Soos et al., 1989). Based on the property of MAbs to mimic an endogenous peptide, it was shown that drugs could be delivered to cells by conjugating the drug either to an

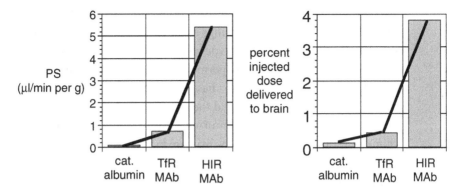

Figure 5.1   Evolution in brain vector discovery. Left: The blood–brain barrier permeability–surface area (PS) product is shown for three different brain drug-targeting vectors: cationized (cat.) albumin, peptidomimetic monoclonal antibody (MAb) to the transferrin receptor (TfR), and peptidomimetic MAb to the human insulin receptor (HIR). Right: The percentage of injected dose delivered to the brain for the three different vectors is shown.

endogenous peptide such as transferrin (Raso and Basala, 1984) or to a corresponding transferrin receptor (TfR) peptidomimetic MAb (Domingo and Trowbridge, 1985).

Evolution in brain drug vector discovery

Initially, insulin and then cationized albumin were used as vectors for brain drug targeting (Pardridge, 1986; Kumagai et al., 1987). Subsequently, anti-TfR peptidomimetic MAbs such as the OX26 murine MAb to the rat TfR was demonstrated to undergo transcytosis through the BBB via the endogenous BBB TfR (Friden et al., 1991; Pardridge et al., 1991). Jefferies et al. (1984) showed selective binding of the OX26 MAb to the brain microvasculature, which was consistent with selective expression of the TfR at the BBB. The BBB permeability–surface area (PS) product of the OX26 anti-TfR MAb is approximately three- to four-fold greater than that for cationized albumin (Figure 5.1). Since cationized albumin and the TfR MAb have approximately the same plasma area under the concentration curve (AUC), the percentage of injected dose delivered to the brain with the TfR MAb is approximately fourfold greater than that of cationized albumin (Figure 5.1). However, a human insulin receptor (HIR) peptidomimetic MAb has a nearly ninefold higher BBB PS product (Pardridge et al., 1995b), relative to that of TfR peptidomimetic MAbs (Friden et al., 1996). There is a corresponding ninefold increase in the brain uptake of the HIR MAb, relative to the TfR MAb. The brain uptake in primates of MAbs to the human TfR ranges from 0.2 to 0.3%ID/brain (Friden et al., 1996). The ratio of the brain uptake of the TfR MAb relative to a control immunoglobulin G

(IgG) was approximately 5. Conversely, the brain uptake of an HIR MAb in the primate is 3–4%ID/brain (Pardridge et al., 1995b), and the ratio in brain uptake of the HIR MAb relative to an isotype control IgG is about 40. This increased brain uptake is due to the higher BBB permeability to the HIR MAb (Figure 5.1). As discussed below, the HIR MAb has been genetically engineered to form a human/mouse chimeric MAb and the affinity of the chimeric MAb for the HIR is identical to that of the original murine MAb (Coloma et al., 2000). Similarly, the chimeric HIR MAb is taken up by primate brain to the same extent as the original murine HIR MAb. The avid uptake of the HIR MAb by the primate brain is put in context by considering the following. The brain uptake of the HIR MAb is ninefold greater than the brain uptake of a TfR MAb, and the brain uptake of a TfR MAb is >fivefold greater than the brain uptake of a neuroactive small molecule, morphine (Pardridge, 1997). Therefore, transportable peptides, that act as brain-targeting vectors, are taken up by brain at a level that is well within the range to cause in vivo central nervous system (CNS) pharmacologic effects.

Interpretation of the brain uptake (%ID/g)

The brain uptake of the HIR MAb in the primate is 3–4%ID/brain (Pardridge et al., 1995b). Since the brain of a rhesus monkey weighs approximately 100g, the %ID/g is approximately 0.04%ID/g in the primate. This level is 10-fold lower than the brain uptake of the OX26 anti-TfR MAb in the rat brain, which is 0.44%ID/g, as discussed below. The comparison of %ID/g in primates versus the %ID/g in rats would seem to contradict the statement that the brain uptake of the HIR MAb is nearly 10-fold greater than the brain uptake of the TfR MAb. However, it is erroneous to compare %ID/g amongst species of vastly different body weights. As discussed in Chapter 3, under considerations of the pharmacokinetic rule, the %ID/g $= (PS) \times (AUC)$. The plasma AUC is inversely related to the blood volume of the animal, which is fairly constant at 80 ml/kg between a 30-g mouse and a 70 000-g human. When an MAb is injected intravenously into an animal, it is instantly diluted in the blood volume. The blood volume in a 12-kg rhesus monkey is approximately 60-fold greater than the blood volume in a 200-g rat. Therefore, simply from dilutional effects caused by the increased body weight and increased blood volume, the plasma AUC of the same MAb in a primate is 60-fold lower than the plasma AUC in a rat. Given comparable BBB PS products in the two species, the %ID/g will be 60-fold lower in the primate compared to the rat. Drug dosing is based on kilogram body weight. Therefore, the absolute dose administered to the primate will be 60-fold greater than the dose administered to the rat on a total body weight basis, and the actual concentration of the drug in brain will be a function of the %ID/whole brain, not %ID/g brain. These considerations on the %ID/g relative to body weight of the animal are further discussed below in comparing brain uptake of TfR MAbs in rats and mice.

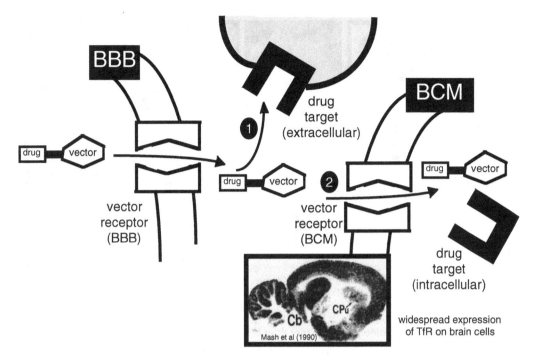

Figure 5.2   Transport of a chimeric peptide or vector/drug conjugate through the blood–brain barrier (BBB) and through the brain cell membrane (BCM). If the receptor of the drug is located in the synaptic cleft or other parts of the extracellular space, then the chimeric peptide need only undergo transport through one barrier, at the BBB. However, if the drug target is intracellular, then the chimeric peptide must undergo transport through two barriers, the BBB and the BCM. The film autoradiography study of Mash et al. (1990) shows widespread expression of the transferrin receptor (TfR) on brain cells. Therefore, transportable ligands that act as brain drug-targeting vectors and which target the TfR may enable transport through both barriers, the BBB, and the BCM. Cb, cerebellum; CPu, caudate putamen.

Membrane targeting in brain: one or two barriers

Brain drug targeting may be a one- or two-barrier targeting problem depending on the drug. The target for many protein-based therapeutics is a receptor positioned in the synaptic or extracellular space of brain, and these are discussed in Chapter 7. In this case, it is only necessary to target the drug through a single barrier, the BBB. Conversely, the targets for other drugs may be intracellular, such as for antisense-based therapeutics, as discussed in Chapter 8, or gene medicines, as discussed in Chapter 9. In this case, it is necessary to target the drug through two barriers in series: (a) the BBB and (b) the brain cell membrane (BCM), as depicted in Figure 5.2. One of the advantages of using ligands to either the TfR or the insulin

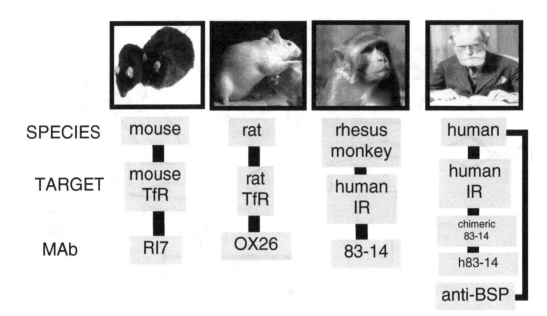

SPECIES	mouse	rat	rhesus monkey	human
TARGET	mouse TfR	rat TfR	human IR	human IR
				chimeric 83-14
				h83-14
MAb	RI7	OX26	83-14	
				anti-BSP

Figure 5.3   Species-specific blood–brain barrier drug-targeting vectors. Monoclonal antibodies (MAb) are species-specific with respect to the reactivity to either the transferrin receptor (TfR) or the insulin receptor (IR). BSP, brain capillary-specific protein.

receptor as brain drug-targeting vectors is that these receptors are expressed not only at the BBB, but are also widely expressed on the plasma membrane of cells throughout the brain (Mash et al., 1990; Zhao et al., 1999). The widespread distribution of the TfR on the BCM is demonstrated by the film autoradiography of rat brain in Figure 5.2. Therefore, conjugation of drugs to vectors that bind the TfR or insulin receptor enable drug transport through both the BBB and the BCM barriers in brain. The ability of the TfR MAb to circumvent both the BBB and the BCM barriers in brain enabled the development of both antisense drugs and gene medicines for the brain. These antisense agents or gene medicines are delivered to intracellular sites deep within brain cells, as discussed in Chapters 8 and 9, respectively.

Species-specificity of peptidomimetic MAbs

Brain drug targeting with peptidomimetic MAbs in different species requires the discovery of a panel of species-specific peptidomimetic MAbs, as outlined in Figure 5.3. The OX26 MAb is a murine antibody to the rat TfR (Jefferies et al., 1984), and this antibody is only effective in rats (Lee et al., 2000). As discussed below, the OX26 MAb does not recognize the murine TfR and is completely ineffective as a brain drug-targeting vector in the mouse. Similarly, the 83–14 HIR MAb, which is a mouse MAb to the human insulin receptor, does not bind to the mouse insulin receptor (Paccaud et al., 1992). The 83–14 HIR MAb does bind to the insulin receptor in Old World primates such as the rhesus monkey (Pardridge et al., 1995b). However, the 83–14 HIR MAb does not bind to the insulin receptor in New World primates such as the squirrel monkey and this vector cannot be used in that species (Pardridge et al., 1995b). The differential binding of the 83–14 HIR MAb to the insulin receptor in New World and Old World primates is consistent with the greater genetic similarity of Old World primates compared to humans in contrast to New World primates (Bourne, 1975). The murine 83–14 HIR MAb cannot be used in humans because this mouse protein would be highly immunogenic in humans. However, chimeric or humanized forms of the HIR MAb may be administered to humans (Figure 5.3), and preparation of the genetically engineered HIR MAbs is discussed below. The development of MAbs that bind brain capillary-specific proteins (BSP) is also discussed below and these agents are brain-specific drug-targeting vectors. A BSP is a protein that is expressed only at the BBB and not in other cells of the brain and not in other organs of the body (Pardridge, 1991). Although an anti-BSP MAb would be BBB-specific, and not deliver drug to peripheral tissues, the anti-BSP MAb would be ineffective in delivering drug across the brain cell membrane, as depicted in Figure 5.2.

Peptidomimetic monoclonal antibodies

HIR MAb in Old World primates and humans

HIR MAb binding to the human blood–brain barrier in vitro

Two different HIR MAbs were studied with respect to binding to isolated human brain capillaries and these MAbs are designated 83–14 and 83–7 (Soos et al., 1986). The 83–7 HIR MAb binds an epitope within amino acids 191–297 of the α subunit of the HIR, and the 83–14 MAb binds an epitope on the α subunit within amino acids 469–592 (Zhang and Roth, 1991), as shown in Figure 5.4A. Both MAbs equally immunoprecipitate the HIR and equally stimulate thymidine incorporation in cells (Soos et al., 1986). However, the unexpected observation was that the 83–14 binds human brain capillaries, used as an in vitro system of the human BBB, approximately 10-fold greater than binding observed for the 83–7 HIR MAb (Figure 5.4B). More than 70% of the 83–14 MAb that was bound to the human brain capillary was endocytosed based on acid wash studies (Figure 5.4B).

Both HIR MAbs yielded continuous immunostaining of microvessels in rhesus monkey brain (Pardridge et al., 1995b), as shown in Figure 5.4C. The continuous immunostaining indicates the immunoreactive insulin receptor at the brain micro-vasculature is of endothelial origin. The immunostaining of the microvasculature in brain with an HIR MAb is comparable to that observed with an antiserum to the

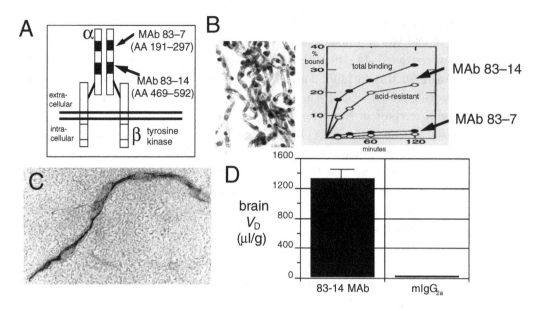

Figure 5.4   Brain targeting via a monoclonal antibody (MAb) to an extracellular epitope on the human insulin receptor. (A) Structure of the insulin receptor tetramer which is formed by two α subunits and two β subunits. The transmembrane region is in the β subunit, as is the intracellular tyrosine kinase domain. The entire α subunit projects into the extracellular space, which at the luminal membrane of the brain capillary endothelium is the plasma compartment. MAb 83–7 and 83–14 bind to amino acid (AA) epitopes on the α subunit. (B) Isolated human brain capillaries are used as an in vitro model system of the human BBB and standard radioreceptor methodology was used to demonstrate binding and endocytosis of [^{125}I]-labeled MAb 83–14 or MAb 83–7. Both antibodies bound to human brain capillaries and more than 70% of this binding was resistant to a mild acid wash, indicating the antibody was endocytosed. The binding of the 83–14 MAb was approximately 10-fold greater than the binding of the 83–7 MAb. (C) Immunoperoxidase immunocytochemistry of frozen sections of rhesus monkey brain immunolabeled with the 83–14 MAb. The continuous immunostaining is indicative of an endothelial origin of the insulin receptor in capillaries of rhesus monkey brain. (D) Brain volume of distribution (V_D) of [^{125}I]83–14 MAb or mouse immunoglobulin G (IgG) isotype control at 3 h after intravenous injection in anesthetized rhesus monkey. From Pardridge et al. (1995b) with permission.

leptin receptor, as shown in Figure 4.9B. Conversely, there was no specific immunostaining of the microvasculature in the brain of squirrel monkey (Pardridge et al., 1995b), which is a New World primate, because the HIR MAb is not active in New World primates such as squirrel monkeys.

The binding of the [^{125}I]83–14 MAb to human brain microvessels was equally inhibited by high concentrations (80 μg/ml) of either unlabeled 83–14 MAb or

83–7 MAb, but the binding was not inhibited by the corresponding isotype control antibodies, mouse IgG_{2a} and mouse IgG_1, respectively. High concentrations of insulin (0.5 µmol/l) caused minimal inhibition of binding of 83–14 MAb to human brain microvessels, indicating that insulin and the 83–14 MAb attach to different binding sites on the HIR. Scatchard analysis of the saturable binding of the 83–14 MAb to human brain microvessels indicated that binding was high affinity with a K_D of 0.45 ± 0.10 nmol/l with a maximum binding, B_{max} of 0.50 ± 0.11 pmol/mg protein. Therefore, the B_{max} of binding of the HIR MAb to human brain microvessels was comparable to the B_{max} of insulin binding to the human brain capillary (Table 4.1), which is consistent with binding of both insulin and the HIR MAb to the same insulin receptor on the human BBB. Although high concentrations of insulin have a minimal effect on 83–14 binding to human brain capillaries, it is possible that high concentrations of the 83–14 HIR MAb may inhibit insulin binding to the receptor. However, minimal inhibition of insulin binding to human brain capillaries was observed in the presence of 0.1–1.0 µg/ml concentrations of the 83–14 MAb (Pardridge et al., 1995b).

Brain drug targeting of the HIRMAb in rhesus monkeys

The 83–14 HIR MAb was radiolabeled with [^{125}I] and injected intravenously into anesthetized 7–8 kg rhesus monkeys. The pharmacokinetic parameters of plasma clearance and brain uptake of the [^{125}I] mouse 83–14 HIR MAb in the anesthetized rhesus monkey are shown in Table 5.1. These parameters are discussed below in the context of pharmacokinetic parameters for the chimeric HIR MAb. Capillary depletion analysis showed the murine 83–14 HIR MAb was transcytosed through the primate BBB in vivo. The uptake of the HIR MAb in gray matter of primate brain was approximately 2.5-fold greater than the brain uptake of the 83–14 MAb in white matter of primate brain (Pardridge et al., 1995b). This is consistent with the greater vascular density, and thus greater density of the insulin receptor, in gray matter relative to white matter (Lierse and Horstmann, 1959). This increased density of the insulin receptor in gray matter is visualized in brain scans of primate brain which show an increased brain uptake in gray matter relative to white matter tracks, as discussed below for the chimeric HIR MAb. The brain volume of distribution (V_D) of the 83–14 MAb exceeded 1200 µl/g brain at 3 h after intravenous injection, whereas the brain V_D of the mouse IgG_{2a} isotype control was 30 ± 2 µl/g (Figure 5.4D). Therefore, the brain V_D of the 83–14 HIR MAb was more than 40-fold greater than the V_D of the mouse IgG_{2a} isotype control (Pardridge et al., 1995b).

Table 5.1 Pharmacokinetic and brain uptake parameters of the human insulin receptor (HIR) monoclonal antibody (MAb) in the primate

Parameter (units)	HIR MAb	
	[^{111}In]-chimeric	[^{125}I]-murine
K_1/min	0.12 ± 0.01	0.27–0.29
K_2/min	0.0018 ± 0.0010	0.060–0.14
$t^1_{1/2}$ (min)	5.8 ± 0.6	1.9–2.4
$t^2_{1/2}$ (min)	380 ± 39	300–672
A_1 (%ID/ml)	0.15 ± 0.01	0.21–0.27
A_2 (%ID/ml)	0.10 ± 0.01	0.027–0.038
AUCl^∞_0 (%ID·min/ml)	55 ± 5	12.5–38.1
V_{SS} (ml/kg)	116 ± 11	367–406
Cl (ml/min per kg)	0.22 ± 0.08	0.39–1.00
MRT (h)	8.9 ± 0.9	6.8–15.9
Brain V_D (μl/g)	287 ± 3	1263–1329
BBB PS (μl/min per g)	1.7 ± 0.1	5.3–5.4
%ID/100 g brain	2.0 ± 0.1	2.5–3.8
V_D (sup)/V_D (capillary)	0.78 ± 0.08	0.60–0.80

Notes:

K, exponential rate constant; $t_{1/2}$, half-time; A, intercept; AUC, area under the plasma concentration curve; V_{SS}, systemic volume of distribution; Cl, systemic clearance; MRT, mean residence time; V_D, brain volume of distribution; BBB PS, blood–brain barrier permeability–surface area; %ID, percentage injected dose.

The chimeric data were measured over a 2-h period for one monkey and the data are mean of triplicate measurements from the same animal (Coloma et al., 2000). The murine data were measured over a 3-h period reported previously, and the range for two monkeys is shown. From Pardridge et al. (1995b) with permission.

TfR MAb in rats and mice

OX26 MAb in rats

The OX26 antibody is a murine MAb to the rat TfR and initial studies of Jefferies et al. (1984) showed selective immunostaining of the microvasculature in rat brain with the OX26 MAb. Conversely, the microvasculature was not immunostained in peripheral tissues with this antibody, which indicated a selective expression of the TfR on the endothelium comprising the capillaries perfusing brain. Subsequently, the TfR on the BBB was shown to mediate the transcytosis of transferrin through the BBB (Fishman et al., 1987; Pardridge et al., 1987a). Anti-TfR MAbs had previ-

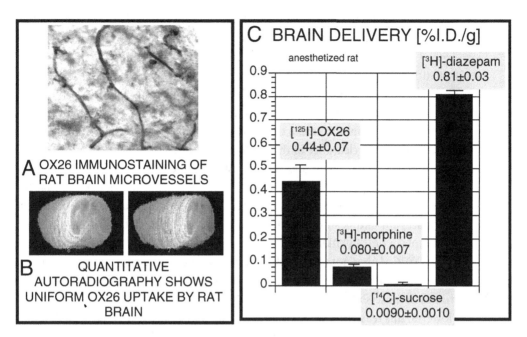

Figure 5.5   Brain delivery of a transferrin receptor monoclonal antibody (MAb). (A) Immunostaining of frozen sections of rat brain with the OX26 MAb shows continuous immunostaining, indicative of an endothelial origin of the blood–brain barrier (BBB) transferrin receptor. (B) Computerized reconstruction of serial coronal frozen sections of rat brain obtained 60 min after the intravenous injection of [^{125}I]OX26 MAb. (C) Brain uptake, expressed as percentage injected dose (ID) per gram brain, is shown for four different test substrates, all measured 30–60 min after intravenous injection in anesthetized rats. Data are mean ± SE ($n = 3$ rats).

ously been shown to deliver drugs to TfR-positive cells (Domingo and Trowbridge, 1985). Therefore, since the BBB TfR was shown to be a transcytosis system (Fishman et al., 1987; Pardridge et al., 1987a), the OX26 MAb was developed as a BBB drug-targeting vector (Friden et al., 1991; Pardridge et al., 1991).

The continuous immunostaining of microvessels in frozen sections of rat brain with the OX26 MAb is shown in Figure 5.5A. There is also background staining of the brain parenchyma owing to the expression of the TfR on brain cells, which is also shown by the autoradiography studies in Figure 5.2. The TfR is widely expressed on the BBB throughout the brain and this is demonstrated by the uniform distribution of brain uptake of the [^{125}I]OX26 MAb in rat brain. Film autoradiograms of serial sections of rat brain were reconstructed and the computerized three-dimensional images are shown in Figure 5.5B.

The brain uptake of the [^{125}I]OX26 MAb in the rat at 60 min after intravenous injection is $0.44 \pm 0.07\%ID/g$ and this level of brain uptake is more than fivefold greater than the brain uptake of morphine, a neuroactive small molecule (Figure 5.5C). Conversely, the brain uptake of a molecule that penetrates the BBB poorly is $0.0090 \pm 0.0010\%ID/g$, as observed for $[^{14}C]$sucrose (Figure 5.5C). Diazepam is a drug that represents the other end of the brain uptake spectrum, and the brain uptake of $[^3H]$diazepam is $0.81 \pm 0.03\%ID/g$ in the anesthetized rat (Figure 5.5C). Diazepam is a lipophilic amine that is 100% extracted across the BBB on a single pass and the brain clearance of this molecule is limited by cerebral blood flow. The brain uptakes of diazepam and sucrose establish the upper and lower bounds of brain uptake, respectively, as shown in Figure 5.5C. This analysis shows that the brain uptake of the OX26 MAb is intermediate between the brain uptake of sucrose and diazepam and is substantially in excess of the brain uptake of morphine. A brain uptake of $0.44\%ID/g$ indicates that approximately 99% of the injected dose of the OX26 MAb is not taken up by brain, since the rat brain weighs 1–2 g. On this basis, one could reject further uses of the OX26 MAb for brain drug-targeting studies because so little of the injected dose is actually taken up by the rat brain. However, this reasoning would lead to a comparable rejection of the drug development of diazepam! Although diazepam is 100% extracted on a single pass by brain, the brain uptake of diazepam in the anesthetized rat is only $0.8\%ID/g$ (Figure 5.5C), and this level of brain uptake is limited by the cardiac output to the brain. A brain uptake of approximately $1.0\%ID/g$ is a near maximal level of uptake for a drug in the anesthetized rat. Moreover, pharmacologically active concentrations of drugs can be delivered to the brain at relatively low systemic dosages, given a level of brain uptake of just $0.1\% ID/g$. For example, the brain concentration of a neuro-trophic factor can be increased from 1 to 5 ng/g or 500% by the peripheral administration of just 5 μg of drug, given a brain uptake of $0.1\%ID/g$ (Chapter 7).

RI7–217 and 8D3 TfR MAb in mice

The species-specificity of the OX26 MAb was demonstrated following the intravenous injection of $[^{125}I]$OX26 MAb in mice (Lee et al., 2000). These studies showed that the BBB PS product of the OX26 MAb in mice was negligible. The very low uptake of the OX26 MAb by mouse tissues explains the high plasma AUC of this antibody in mice (Figure 5.6B). Despite the very high plasma AUC for the OX26 MAb in mice, the brain uptake of this antibody was very low owing to the negligible PS product in this species. The BBB PS product, the plasma AUC, and the brain uptake of the OX26 MAb in mice are shown in Figure 5.6B.

Given the availability of transgenic mouse models, it would be advantageous to have a brain drug-targeting vector that is active in this species. Therefore, two different anti-TfR MAbs were evaluated as brain drug-targeting vectors in mice. These MAbs, the 8D3 MAb (Kissel et al., 1998), or the RI7–217 MAb (abbreviated

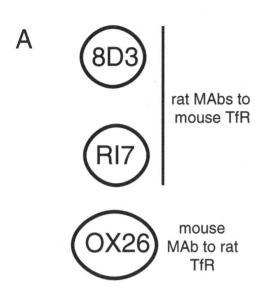

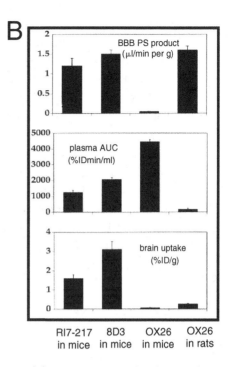

Figure 5.6   Brain drug targeting in the mouse. (A) The 8D3 and the RI7–217 monoclonal antibodies (MAbs) are rat MAbs to the mouse transferrin receptor (TfR), whereas the OX26 is a mouse MAb to the rat TfR. (B) The BBB permeability–surface area (PS) product, the plasma area under the concentration curve (AUC), and brain uptake for the RI7–217, the 8D3, and the OX26 MAb in mice and for the OX26 MAb in rats are shown. Data are mean ± SE ($n = 3$ rats). From Lee et al. (2000) with permission.

RI7 MAb) (Lesley et al., 1984) are both rat IgG_{2a} antibodies against the mouse TfR, whereas the OX26 antibody is a mouse MAb to the rat TfR (Figure 5.6A). The BBB PS product for either the 8D3 or the RI7 MAb in mice is 1–1.5 μl/min per g and these values were comparable to the BBB PS product for the OX26 MAb in rats (Figure 5.6B). The brain uptake of the 8D3 or RI7 MAb in mice was 1.5–3.0%ID/g, which was nearly a log order greater than the brain uptake of the OX26 MAb in rats (Figure 5.6B). However, as discussed above, the higher brain uptake, expressed as %ID/g, of the anti-TfR antibody in mice is a species-scaling effect. Owing to the 10-fold lower body weight of mice relative to rats, the plasma AUC of the antibody is correspondingly 10-fold higher in mice relative to rats, which means the %ID/g will be 10-fold higher (Figure 5.6B). The 8D3 MAb yields continuous immunostaining of the microvasculature in mouse brain (Kissel et al., 1998), and this pattern is similar to that observed with the OX26 MAb in rat brain (Figure 5.5A).

Transcytosis of peptidomimetic monoclonal antibodies through the BBB in vivo

Transcytosis through the BBB has been demonstrated for the 83–14 MAb in rhesus monkeys, the OX26 MAb in rats, and the RI7 MAb in mice (Pardridge et al., 1991, 1995b; Bickel et al., 1994a; Lee et al., 2000). This has been done with a variety of techniques, including the capillary depletion technique, emulsion autoradiography following carotid artery injection, or immunogold electron microscopy following the carotid arterial infusion of 5 nm gold conjugates of the MAb. These studies are reviewed in Chapter 4. However, the principal finding indicative of transcytosis of the MAb through the BBB is the many pharmacologic applications in the brain that are possible with the use of the chimeric peptide technology. The applications with protein-based therapeutics, antisense-based therapeutics, and gene medicines, are discussed in Chapters 7, 8, and 9, respectively. The extension of the chimeric peptide technology to humans and the manufacture of these pharmaceuticals are enabled with the genetic engineering of brain drug-targeting vectors.

Genetically engineered vectors

Chimeric HIR MAb

Characterization of genetically engineered chimeric HIR MAb with soluble HIR

The genes encoding the variable region of the heavy chain (VH) and the variable region of the light chain (VL) of the 83–14 HIR MAb were amplified with the polymerase chain reaction (PCR) using cDNA derived from polyA + mRNA isolated from the 83–14 hybridoma (Coloma et al., 2000). The PCR-amplified VH and VL genes were spliced into eukaryotic expression plasmids containing the constant portions of human IgG_1 heavy chain or human IgG κ light chain. The separate heavy chain and light chain plasmids were electroporated into mouse myeloma cells for permanent transfection and expression of the chimeric HIR MAb. The relative affinity of the chimeric HIR MAb or the original mouse HIR MAb was tested in an enzyme-linked immunosorbent assay (ELISA) format using soluble extracellular domain of the HIR. The latter was produced in Chinese hamster ovary (CHO) cells permanently transfected with a gene encoding the soluble extracellular domain of the HIR (Sparrow et al., 1997). The soluble HIR includes all of the α subunit, which contains the 83–14 epitope (Figure 5.4A), and a portion of the β subunit of the insulin receptor that is extracellular to the transmembrane region. The serum-free CHO cell conditioned media was partially purified with a wheat germ agglutinin (WGA) affinity column and the glycosylated insulin receptor was eluted with N-acetylglucosamine. The partially purified soluble insulin receptor was coated on ELISA plates and the ELISA analysis shows an equal affinity of the chimeric and murine HIR MAbs (Figure 5.7A). Nonlinear regression analysis of the

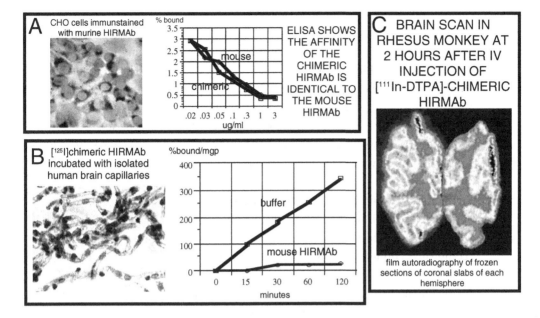

Figure 5.7   (A) Enzyme-linked immunosorbent assay (ELISA) shows equal affinity of the mouse human insulin receptor monoclonal antibody (HIR MAb) and chimeric HIR MAb. The antigen in these studies was affinity purified soluble extracellular domain of the HIR that was produced from Chinese hamster ovary (CHO) cells. Immunocytochemistry was performed with the CHO cells using the 83–14 HIR MAb and the micrograph is shown in the inset. This demonstrates that the CHO cell line secretes functional and soluble HIR that reacts with the HIR MAb. (B) Isolated human brain capillaries were used as an in vitro model system of the human BBB and the binding of the [^{125}I]-chimeric HIR MAb to these capillaries was measured over 120 min in the presence of either buffer alone or buffer plus 10 μg/ml mouse HIR MAb. (C) Film autoradiogram of rhesus monkey brain at 2 h after intravenous injection of chimeric HIR MAb radiolabeled with indium-111 bound to a diethylenetriaminepentaacetic acid (DTPA) chelator moiety conjugated to the chimeric HIR MAb. From Coloma et al. (2000) with permission.

ELISA data demonstrated the K_D of the chimeric HIR MAb binding to the soluble HIR was 0.13 ± 0.06 nmol/l. There was no significant difference in the K_D of binding of either the murine or chimeric HIR MAb to the soluble insulin receptor (Coloma et al., 2000). Western blot analysis was also used to demonstrate comparable binding of the murine 83–14 HIR MAb and the chimeric HIR MAb to the soluble insulin receptor. However, in these Western blot analyses, it was necessary to use a goat antihuman secondary antibody in order to detect the chimeric HIR MAb. Following the genetic engineering, the chimeric MAb was recognized only by secondary antibodies that bind human IgGs and not mouse IgGs (Coloma et al., 2000).

Binding of chimeric HIR MAb to human brain capillaries

The chimeric HIR MAb was radiolabeled with [^{125}I] and added to isolated human brain capillaries, used as an in vitro model system of the human BBB. These studies showed very avid binding of the chimeric HIR MAb to human brain capillaries and the binding exceeded 300% per mg protein at 120 min of incubation. Moreover, the binding was completely suppressed by the addition of 10 μg/ml unlabeled mouse 83–14 HIR MAb (Figure 5.7B). These studies predict the chimeric HIR MAb will be a highly active brain drug-targeting vector in humans, similar to what is observed in vivo with primates (Coloma et al., 2000).

Uptake of the chimeric HIR MAb by the primate brain in vivo

The chimeric HIR MAb was conjugated with diethylenetriaminepentaacetic acid (DTPA) for subsequent radiolabeling with indium-111. The affinity of the DTPA-conjugated chimeric HIR MAb for the insulin receptor was tested in the ELISA analysis and this showed there was no change in the affinity of the chimeric HIR MAb for the insulin receptor following conjugation with DTPA (Coloma et al., 2000). The DTPA-conjugated chimeric HIR MAb that was radiolabeled with indium-111 was injected intravenously in the anesthetized rhesus monkey and brain uptake was measured 2 h later. A pharmacokinetic analysis of the plasma concentration of the chimeric HIR MAb was performed over a 2-h period. The parameters for the plasma clearance of the [^{111}In]-chimeric HIR MAb are listed in Table 5.1 in comparison with the parameters for the [^{125}I]-murine HIR MAb in primates.

The brain scan in the rhesus monkey at 2 h after intravenous injection is shown in Figure 5.7C and this shows avid uptake of the chimeric HIR MAb by the primate brain in vivo (Coloma et al., 2000). There is a greater uptake of the antibody in gray matter relative to white-matter tracks and this is consistent with the greater vascular density in gray matter compared to white matter (Lierse and Horstmann, 1959). Gel filtration fast protein liquid chromatography (FPLC) of the 2-h primate serum demonstrates metabolic stability of the radiolabeled chimeric HIR MAb and the absence of low molecular weight metabolites in the serum (Figure 5.8). The chimeric HIR MAb radiolabeled with indium-111 was somewhat more stable than the murine HIR MAb radiolabeled with iodine-125 (Pardridge et al., 1995b). Although the mouse 83–14 HIR MAb labeled with iodine-125 is relatively metabolically stable, the plasma trichloroacetic acid (TCA) precipitability does decrease from 99% to 94% at 2 h after intravenous injection, which is indicative of formation of low molecular weight metabolites labeled with iodine-125. The brain uptake of radioactivity is generally higher when the peptide is radiolabeled with iodine-125 as opposed to indium-111, as discussed in Chapter 4. The brain uptake of the iodine-125 metabolites explains the slightly higher BBB PS product and brain uptake of the murine HIR MAb labeled with iodine-125, compared to the same

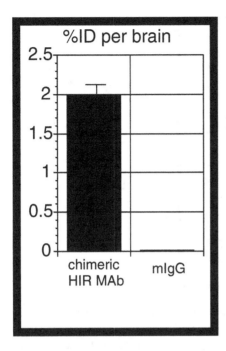 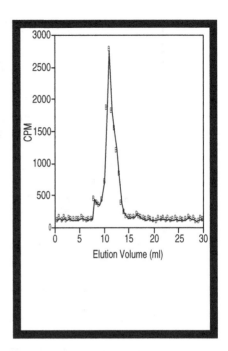

Figure 5.8   Left: Brain uptake in a 32-year-old male at 2 h after intravenous injection of the diethylenetriaminepentaacetic acid (DTPA)-chimeric human insulin receptor monoclonal antibody (HIR MAb) chelated with indium-111 or the comparable brain uptake for a mouse immunoglobulin G (mIgG) isotype control. Right: Gel filtration fast protein liquid chromatography (FPLC) of serum taken from the rhesus monkey 2 h after intravenous injection of the radiolabeled chimeric HIR MAb was performed and shows metabolic stability of the radiolabeled antibody with no formation of low molecular weight metabolites labeled with indium-111. From Coloma et al. (2000) with permission.

values for the chimeric HIR MAb labeled with indium-111 (Table 5.1). Because of the greater metabolic stability of the formulation with the indium-111 radionuclide, the brain-imaging study shown in Figure 5.7C represents a brain scan with literally no "noise" caused by brain uptake of radiolabeled metabolites.

Humanized HIR MAb

The chimeric HIR MAb contains approximately 85% human amino acid sequence and about 15% mouse amino acid sequence, since the entire VH and VL components of the IgG are still of mouse origin. Some chimeric MAbs may be still immunogenic in humans (Bruggemann et al., 1989), owing to the persistence of the murine amino acid sequence in the framework regions (FR) of the VH and VL moieties of the chimeric MAb. The murine framework amino acid regions are

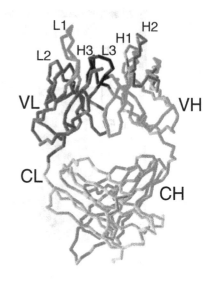

METHODS

Cloning and sequencing of murine
VH and VL

Homology match of murine and
human framework region (FR)

Synthesis of synthetic gene by
PCR overlap extension followed by
subcloning in eurkaryotic
expression vector

Expression, purification, and
characterization of humanized
MAb

Figure 5.9   Left: Method for humanizing a monoclonal antibody (MAb) based on complementarity-determining region (CDR)-grafting. Right: Stick model of a Fab fragment of a human monoclonal antibody. The constant region of the light (CL) and heavy (CH) and the variable regions of the light (VL) and heavy (VH) chains are shown. The three CDRs of the heavy chain (H1, H2, H3) and the light chain (L1, L2, L3) are shown. PCR, polymerase chain receptor. Model from Rodriguez-Romero et al. (1998) with permission.

removed when an MAb is "humanized," a process also called CDR grafting (Jones et al., 1986), where CDR is complementarity-determining region.

The nucleotide sequence of the gene encoding the VH and VL of the antibody is determined, and this allows for prediction of the amino acid sequence of the four FRs and the three CDRs of the VH and VL of the antibody. These framework region sequences are matched to comparable sequences in the human IgG database for selection of a known human IgG with a framework region that is highly homologous to the framework region of either the VH or VL of the MAb to be humanized (Figure 5.9). Synthetic genes encoding either the VH or the VL of the humanized MAb gene are then produced by PCR overlap extension (Horton et al., 1989), followed by subcloning in eukaryotic expression vectors for expression, purification, and characterization of the humanized HIR MAb. The three-dimensional structure of a typical Fab fragment of a human IgG is shown in Figure 5.9. This shows the close association of the CDRs of the light chain (designated L1, L2, L3) with the three CDRs of the heavy chain (designated H1, H2, H3) that form the antigen-binding pocket (Rodriguez-Romero et al., 1998). In a CDR-grafted MAb, only the murine amino acid sequences comprising the six CDRs remain, whereas the murine amino acid sequences comprising the entire VL or VH domains are retained in a chimeric MAb.

It is possible to retain affinity of the MAb following grafting of only the six CDRs of the murine MAb to a homologous human IgG molecule (Roguska et al., 1996). However, invariably there is a loss of affinity of the MAb following CDR grafting (Foote and Winter, 1992). In this case, it is possible to restore affinity by substitution of select amino acid residues from the FR of the VH or VL genes of the original murine MAb into the corresponding area of the FR of the human IgG (Queen et al., 1989). This restores the affinity of the humanized MAb because certain FR amino acids contribute to the conformation of the antigen-binding site in addition to the amino acid residues comprising the CDRs.

Anti-TfR single chain Fv/streptavidin fusion gene and fusion protein

Following the discovery of a suitable transportable peptide for brain drug targeting, it is then necessary to design an appropriate linker strategy, and these are reviewed in Chapter 6. One linker strategy uses avidin-biotin technology (Yoshikawa and Pardridge, 1992). In this approach, the drug is monobiotinylated in parallel with the production of a vector/avidin or vector/streptavidin (SA) fusion protein. Such agents represent universal brain drug-targeting systems since virtually any biotinylated drug could then be delivered through the BBB. Owing to the extremely high affinity of avidin or SA binding of biotin (Chapter 6), there is a nearly instantaneous capture of the biotinylated drug by the vector/avidin or vector/SA conjugate. These proteins could be produced following the initial production of vector/avidin or vector/SA fusion genes with genetic engineering.

Cloning of VH and VL genes of the OX26 MAb

PolyA + mRNA was isolated from the OX26 hybridoma and cDNA was prepared (Li et al., 1999). The VH and VL genes of the OX26 MAb were amplified by PCR using primers specific for murine IgGs (Figure 5.10). The OX26 VH and VL genes were then subcloned into the pSTE bacterial expression vector (Dubel et al., 1995), which contains the sequences for core SA, for the c-myc epitope to the 9E10 MAb, and for a pentahistidine fragment at the carboxyl terminus (Figure 5.10). The pentahistidine carboxyl tail of the recombinant protein expressed in *Escherichia coli* enabled purification of the OX26 single chain Fv antibody from bacterial inclusion bodies using immobilized metal affinity chromatography (IMAC) in the presence of 6 mol/l guanidine followed by renaturation (Kipriyanov et al., 1996).

Characterization with purified rat placental transferrin receptor

The OX26 single chain Fv antibody–SA fusion protein bound the transferrin receptor purified from rat placenta, and this was demonstrated by Western blotting, as

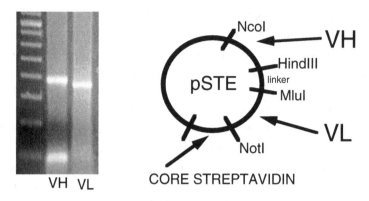

Figure 5.10 Cloning of cDNA and expression of OX26 single chain Fv (ScFv) antibody in *Escherichia coli*. Left: Ethidium bromide-stained agarose gel electrophoresis of variable region of the heavy (VH) and light (VL) genes of the OX26 monoclonal antibody (MAb) amplified by polymerase chain reaction (PCR). Right: The OX26 VH and VL genes were subcloned into the pSTE bacterial expression plasmid that contained a linker separating the VH and VL genes followed by the gene for core streptavidin. From Li et al. (1999) by permission of Oxford University Press.

shown in Figure 5.11A. The purified rat TfR was applied to lanes of sodium dodecylsulfate polyacrylamide gel electrophoresis (SDS-PAGE) gels. Following blotting, the filter was probed with hybridoma-generated OX26 MAb, OX26 single chain Fv/SA fusion protein, or mouse IgG$_{2a}$ isotype control. Both the OX26 MAb and the OX26 single chain Fv/SA fusion protein bind to the 80 kDa rat TfR (Figure 5.11A). Binding of either the OX26 MAb or the OX26 single chain Fv/streptavidin fusion protein to the isolated rat TfR was also demonstrated by ELISA. The OX26 single chain Fv/SA fusion protein expressed in *E. coli* was purified by IMAC to homogeneity, as demonstrated by SDS-PAGE, which is shown in Figure 5.11B. A Coomassie blue stain is shown in lanes 1–3, the 9E10 Western blotting to the c-myc epitope is shown in lanes 5–6, and Western blotting using an antiserum to SA is shown in lanes 8 and 9 of Figure 5.11B. These studies show the single chain Fv/SA fusion protein is purified to homogeneity, which enabled further analysis of the activity of the protein by confocal microscopy and pharmacokinetic studies in rats in vivo (Li et al., 1999).

Amino acid sequence

The amino acid sequence of the OX26 single chain Fv antibody/SA fusion protein is shown in Figure 5.12 (Li et al., 1999). The VH region is comprised of four FRs designated FR1–FR4 and three CDR regions, designated CDR1–CDR3. The VL has a similar structure, with four FRs and three CDR areas. The VH and VL portions of the single chain Fv antibody are separated by a 19 amino acid linker and the

GENETICALLY ENGINEERED BRAIN DRUG DELIVERY VECTORS

Cloning, expression, and confocal microscopy of an antitransferrin receptor single chain antibody-streptavidin fusion gene and protein

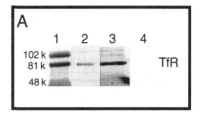

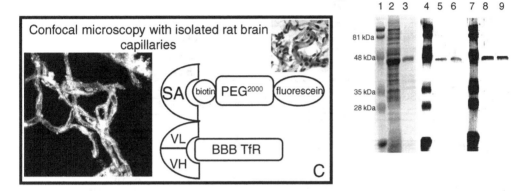

Figure 5.11 (A) Western blotting with rat placental transferrin receptor (TfR) is shown in lanes 2–4, and prestained molecular weight standards are shown in lane 1. The filter was probed with either hybridoma-generated OX26 monoclonal antibody (MAb) (1 μg/ml, lane 2), OX26 single chain Fv/streptavidin fusion protein (1 μg/ml, lane 3), or mouse IgG$_{2a}$ isotype control (1 μg/ml, lane 4). (B) SDS-PAGE of purified OX26 single chain Fv/streptavidin fusion protein expressed in *Escherichia coli*. Coomassie blue stain is shown in lanes 1–3 and 9E-10 Western blotting to the c-myc epitope is shown in lanes 5–6; biotinylated molecular weight standards are shown in lane 4. Western blotting with an antiserum to streptavidin is shown in lanes 8 and 9 along with biotinylated molecular weight standards shown in lane 7. Lane 2 is 10 μg of unfractionated periplasmic inclusion bodies and lane 3 is 1.5 μg of OX26 single chain Fv/streptavidin fusion protein purified by affinity chromatography. Lanes 5 and 8 represent 10 ng of periplasmic inclusion bodies without purification and lanes 6 and 9 represent 2 ng of OX26 single chain Fv antibody/streptavidin fusion protein purified from inclusion bodies. (C) Confocal microscopy of isolated rat brain capillaries (shown in the inset) following incubation of the capillaries with the OX26 single chain Fv/streptavidin (SA) fusion protein that was conjugated with biotin-PEG^{2000}-fluorescein, where PEG^{2000} is polyethylene glycol of 2000 Da molecular weight. The OX26 single chain Fv antibody is comprised of the variable region of the heavy (VH) and light (VL) domain and binds the blood–brain barrier (BBB) TfR. From Li et al. (1999) by permission of Oxford University Press.

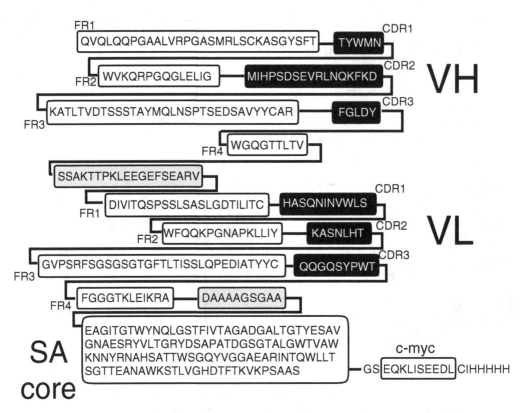

Figure 5.12 Amino acid sequence of the variable portion of the heavy chain (VH) and variable portion of the light chain (VL) of the OX26 single chain Fv antibody fused to core streptavidin (SA). The four framework regions (FR) and three complementary-determining regions (CDR) of the VH and VL domains are shown along with amino acid linkers separating the VH and VL domains and the VL and SA domains. The c-myc epitope that binds the 9E-10 monoclonal antibody is shown at the carboxyl terminus along with a pentahistidine moiety that enables affinity purification by immobilized metal affinity chromatography (IMAC).

single chain Fv antibody is separated from the SA core protein by a 10 amino acid linker (Figure 5.12). The 10 amino acid sequence comprising the c-myc epitope and the pentahistidine sequence at the carboxyl terminus are also shown in the sequence. The amino acids corresponding to residues 14–139 of the SA core protein (Pahler et al., 1987) are shown in italics. The OX26 VH gene corresponds to the murine miscellaneous family subgroup IIB and the VL gene corresponds to the murine κ family XVI, subgroup V, as determined by screening of the IgG database (Kabat et al., 1991). This type of analysis of the amino acid sequence of the CDRs of a peptidomimetic MAb is typical of what is required in the humanization of an MAb, as discussed above.

Binding to the rat brain capillaries: confocal microscopy

The binding of the OX26 single chain Fv antibody/SA fusion protein to the TfR on rat brain capillaries was demonstrated by confocal microscopy, as shown in Figure 5.11C. A light micrograph of the isolated rat brain capillaries is shown in the inset of Figure 5.11C. These microvessels were incubated with the OX26 single chain Fv antibody/SA fusion protein along with biotin-PEG^{2000}-fluorescein, where PEG^{2000} is polyethylene glycol of 2000 Da molecular weight. The use of a biotin/fluorescein conjugate containing a PEG^{2000} linker is preferred over a PEG–fluorescein conjugate with a much shorter linker because binding of the biotin moiety to SA results in fluorescence quenching of the fluorescein (Gruber et al., 1997). This quenching is removed by substitution of the short linker with an extended linker. Other advantages of using extended PEG linkers are discussed in Chapter 6. The confocal microscopy shows continuous immunolabeling of the isolated rat brain capillaries using the conjugate outlined in Figure 5.11C. In contrast, there was no fluorescent signal when the biotin-PEG^{2000}-fluorescein was conjugated to SA and added to the isolated rat brain capillaries (Li et al., 1999). These studies confirm the Western blotting and indicate the cloned single chain Fv antibody derived from the OX26 MAb hybridoma is able to bind the BBB TfR.

Pharmacokinetics and rat brain uptake in vivo

[^{3}H]Biotin was bound to the OX26 single chain Fv antibody/SA fusion protein and injected intravenously in anesthetized rats. This pharmacokinetic study indicated the presence of the SA moiety in the fusion protein delayed the rapid removal of the single chain Fv antibody from the plasma compartment (Li et al., 1999). Previous studies in rats have shown that single Fv chain antibodies are cleared more than 10 times faster than the native IgG (Milenic et al., 1991). However, the clearance of [^{3}H]biotin bound to the OX26 single chain Fv/SA fusion protein was 2.3 ± 0.1 ml/min per kg (Li et al., 1999). This value is comparable to the clearance of [^{3}H]biotin bound to a conjugate of the intact OX26 MAb and neutral light avidin (NLA), and to the systemic clearance of unconjugated OX26 MAb (Li et al., 1999). Therefore, the OX26 single chain Fv antibody/SA fusion protein is cleared from blood at rates equal to that of conjugates of the hybridoma-generated OX26 MAb and recombinant streptavidin, which are formed via a stable thioether linkage between the OX26 MAb and the SA. The fact that the single chain Fv antibody/SA is not cleared rapidly from plasma has distinct advantages for brain drug targeting, where the overall %ID/g of brain is inversely related to the plasma AUC of the vector. In this respect, the formation of a SA fusion protein optimizes the pharmacokinetics of the single chain Fv antibody similar to that observed when an IgG/avidin fusion protein is prepared, as discussed below.

The bifunctionality of the OX26 single chain Fv antibody/SA fusion protein is retained as both biotin and transferrin receptor-binding parameters are intact (Figure 5.11). The BBB PS product in the rat in vivo for the OX26 single chain Fv antibody/SA fusion protein was 0.55 ± 0.04 μl/min per g, which is about half the BBB PS product for the intact OX26 MAb in rats (Figure 5.6B). The reduced affinity of the single chain antibody is expected, since antibody affinity is increased upon bivalent binding of the antibody to the antigen, and the bivalent binding is lost with a single chain Fv antibody.

OX26 MAb/avidin fusion protein

IgG fusion protein

Recombinant fusion proteins have been prepared wherein an IgG molecule is fused to the soluble portion of a membrane-bound receptor (Capon et al., 1989). This was first done for CD4, which was originally believed to be a new therapeutic for the treatment of acquired immune deficiency syndrome (AIDS). A glycoprotein, gp120, on the surface of the human immunodeficiency virus (HIV) binds the CD4 receptor on lymphocytes. The administration of soluble CD4 was believed to saturate the gp120 binding sites on the HIV. However, when CD4 was administered to humans, the protein was rapidly removed from the blood stream (Kahn et al., 1990), probably due to the cationic charge of this protein (Pardridge et al., 1992). The plasma clearance was delayed and the plasma pharmacokinetics were optimized when the CD4 was fused to an IgG molecule to form an "immunoadhesin." A similar phenomenon is observed following the production of IgG/avidin fusion genes and fusion proteins (Shin et al., 1997). A model of an IgG/avidin fusion protein is shown in Figure 5.13A and, in this case, the Fc portion of the IgG is replaced by an avidin monomer. Avidin is a 64 kDa cationic glycoprotein that is a homotetramer of 16 kDa subunits (Green, 1975). Avidin monomers aggregate to form dimers and tetramers, so the aggregation properties of avidin are suited for preparation of IgG/avidin fusion proteins.

Pharmacokinetics and brain uptake of an OX26 MAb/avidin fusion protein

The brain uptake (%ID/g), the BBB PS product, and the plasma AUC are shown in Figure 5.13B for the OX26 MAb, for a chemical conjugate of OX26 and avidin, and for the OX26–avidin fusion protein (Penichet et al., 1999). The plasma AUC of the OX26 MAb is adversely affected by chemical conjugation of this MAb with avidin. As discussed in Chapter 6, avidin is a cationic glycoprotein that is rapidly cleared from plasma within minutes in the rat, principally by liver (Kang et al., 1995b). The presence of the avidin moiety conjugated to the OX26 MAb results in accelerated clearance of the antibody from the blood stream. The reduced plasma AUC causes a marked reduction in the brain uptake of the chemical conjugate of the OX26 MAb

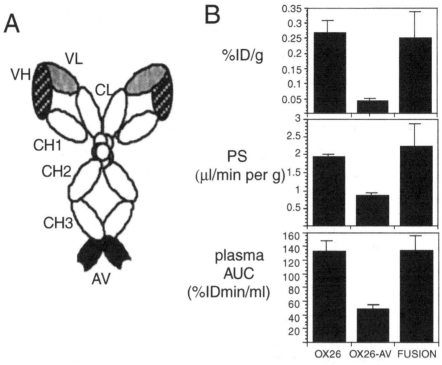

Figure 5.13   Favorable pharmacokinetics of an OX26 monoclonal antibody (MAb)/avidin (AV) fusion protein in rats. (A) Model of immunoglobulin G (IgG)/AV fusion protein showing the domains of the constant region of the heavy chain (CH) and the light chain (CL) and the variable domains of the heavy chain (VH) and light chain (VL). (B) Brain uptake (%ID/g), blood–brain barrier (BBB) permeability–surface area (PS) product, and plasma area under the concentration curve (AUC) for OX26 MAb, for an OX26 MAb/AV conjugate made with a chemical thioether linkage, and the OX26/AV fusion protein. From Penichet et al. (1999) with permission. Copyright (1999) The American Association of Immunologists.

and avidin, as reflected in the reduced %ID/g (Figure 5.13B). These problems of decreased plasma AUC can be obviated by the use of neutral forms of avidin or SA (Kang and Pardridge, 1994b), as discussed in Chapter 6. However, similar to the CD4 immunoadhesins, the plasma clearance of avidin is slowed when the protein is administered in the form of an avidin/IgG fusion protein. The plasma AUC of the fusion protein is identical to the plasma AUC of the intact OX26 MAb. There is also no difference between the BBB PS product between the OX26/avidin fusion protein and the OX26 MAb and the brain uptake of the fusion protein is identical to that of the native OX26 MAb (Figure 5.13B). These studies demonstrate the genetically engineered MAb/avidin fusion genes and fusion proteins may be prepared and these fusion proteins may represent universal brain drug delivery vectors. The MAb/avidin fusion proteins can deliver to brain virtually any biotin-ylated therapeutic. As discussed in Chapter 6, avidin has an extremely high affinity for biotin with a K_D of 10^{-15} mol/l and a dissociation half-time of 89 days (Green, 1975). Therefore, there is instantaneous capture of the biotinylated drug by the avidin fusion protein.

Brain-specific vectors

A brain capillary-enriched protein (BEP) is a protein that is selectively expressed in brain at the microvascular endothelium forming the BBB in vivo (Pardridge, 1991). The BEPs include the *Glut1* glucose transporter or the LAT1 neutral amino acid transporter (Chapter 3). These genes may be expressed in peripheral tissues, but in brain the expression of the BEP gene is generally confined to the brain microvas-culature. In contrast, a BSP is expressed only at the BBB in vivo and not in brain cells and not in peripheral tissues. The discovery of BEP and BSP genes could lead to the identification of novel drug targets and is made possible with the develop-ment of a "BBB genomics" program, as discussed in Chapter 10. An antibody to a BSP would be a potential brain-specific targeting vector, should the BSP be expressed on the plasma membrane of the brain capillary endothelium and should the anti-BSP antibody be an "endocytosing antibody." The latter property enables transcytosis through the BBB in vivo, as discussed above for the peptidomimetic MAbs.

Production of anti-BSP polyclonal antiserum

In order to examine whether BSP antibodies could be generated, capillaries were purified from fresh bovine brain (Figure 5.14A). The plasma membranes of this microvessel preparation were emulsified with complete Freund's adjuvant and injected intradermally in rabbits for production of a polyclonal antiserum (Pardridge et al., 1986, 1990d). This antiserum reacted with many peripheral tissues. However, following absorption of the antiserum with acetone powders of rat liver and rat kidney, the specificity of the antiserum was increased such that it only bound microvessels in brain, as shown in Figure 5.15A. The antiserum strongly bound isolated bovine brain capillaries and the continuous immunostain-ing pattern was indicative of an endothelium origin of the antigen (Figure 5.15C). The endothelial origin of the immunoreactivity was confirmed by immunocyto-chemistry of bovine brain capillary endothelial cells that were released from the capillaries by protease digestion of the basement membrane, and purified by Percoll gradient centrifugation (Pardridge et al., 1986), as shown in Figure 5.15D. There was no immunostaining of either tissue cells or capillaries in heart, liver, or kidney (Pardridge et al., 1986, 1990d). Western blotting of isolated bovine brain

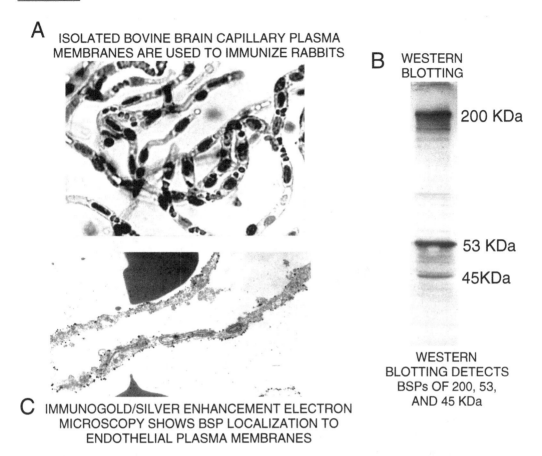

A   ISOLATED BOVINE BRAIN CAPILLARY PLASMA
    MEMBRANES ARE USED TO IMMUNIZE RABBITS

B   WESTERN
    BLOTTING

200 KDa

53 KDa

45KDa

WESTERN
BLOTTING DETECTS
BSPs OF 200, 53,
AND 45 KDa

C   IMMUNOGOLD/SILVER ENHANCEMENT ELECTRON
    MICROSCOPY SHOWS BSP LOCALIZATION TO
    ENDOTHELIAL PLASMA MEMBRANES

Figure 5.14   (A) Light micrograph of isolated bovine brain capillaries. (B) Western blotting with
antibrain capillary-specific protein (anti-BSP) antiserum and the freshly isolated bovine
brain capillaries shown in panel A. (C) Electron micrograph of isolated bovine brain
capillaries in cross-section showing selective staining of the microvessel plasma
membranes using immunogold silver staining technique and a 1:50 dilution of a
secondary antiserum comprised of a 1 nm gold conjugate of a goat antirabbit
immunoglobulin G (IgG) antiserum. The silver enhancement causes the deposition of
electron-dense silver on the binding sites of the secondary antibody which localizes
predominantly to the luminal and abluminal membranes of the microvessel. The bovine
erythrocyte is unstained. The primary antiserum used in these studies was a 1:1000
dilution of the anti-BSP antiserum. From Pardridge et al. (1990d) with permission and
Farrell and Pardridge (1991b) with permission.

capillaries showed that the anti-BSP antiserum reacted with a triplet of 200, 53, and
45 kDa proteins (Figure 5.14B). The anti-BSP antiserum also reacted with the basolateral membrane of choroid plexus epithelium (Figure 5.15B), and Western blotting of choroid plexus showed that the 200 kDa protein was expressed in this cell

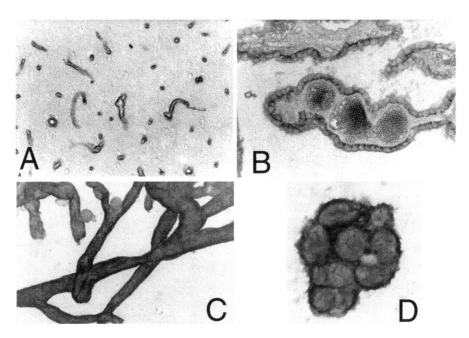

Figure 5.15   Light microscopic immunocytochemistry of bovine brain (A), bovine choroid plexus (B), isolated bovine brain capillaries (C), and freshly isolated bovine brain capillary endothelial cells released from capillaries by protease digestion (D). All specimens were immunostained with an antibrain capillary-specific protein (anti-BSP) antiserum. There is continuous immunostaining of capillary endothelium in either brain sections (A) or isolated brain capillaries (C). In choroid plexus (C) or in isolated brain capillary endothelium (D), there is immunostaining of the basolateral membrane. From Pardridge et al. (1986, 1990d) with permission.

(Pardridge et al., 1990d). However, there was no expression of the 45 or 53 kDa BSPs in the choroid plexus, indicating these proteins were only expressed at the brain microvascular endothelium in vivo. The localization of the 53/45 kDa BSPs at the BBB in vivo was confirmed with immunogold electron microscopy, as shown in Figure 5.14C. Attempts at immunocytochemical localization of the BSP antigens on brain endothelia using preembedding or postembedding microscopic methods and sections of bovine brain were hampered by either poor penetration of the immune reagents or poor ultrastructure in preparations where fixation was light enough to preserve antigenicity (Farrell and Pardridge, 1991b). These problems were eliminated by a method where the primary and secondary antisera were reacted with isolated bovine brain microvessels and the secondary antibody was labeled with conjugates of 1 nm gold particles. Following immunolabeling, the isolated brain capillaries were fixed with glutaraldehyde and osmium, and the size of the gold probe was amplified by silver enhancement. The microvessel pellets were then processed for routine electron microscopy and the BSP antiserum was localized at both the luminal and abluminal plasma membranes of the endothelial cells. There was also immunolabeling of the endothelial tight junction, as shown in Figure 5.14C.

The function of the 53/45 kDa BSP is not known and corresponding cDNAs for these BSPs have not been isolated. However, this study suggests that there are genes that are selectively expressed at the BBB in vivo and that these genes may encode membrane surface proteins. This hypothesis has been confirmed by a BBB genomics program, which identifies BSP genes (Chapter 10). Therefore, endocytosing antibodies directed against the BSPs are potential brain-specific drug-targeting vectors. The advantage of a BSP antibody is that this would provide brain-specific drug targeting. The disadvantage is that a BSP antibody would not enable drug transport across the brain cell membrane, which is needed for intracellular drug targeting of antisense or gene medicines (Chapters 8 and 9). In contrast, ligands to receptors expressed at both the BBB and the BCM enable two-barrier drug targeting, as outlined in Figure 5.2. Both goals of brain-specificity and two-barrier drug targeting could be achieved by the genetic engineering of a bifunctional antibody that recognizes antigens specific for both the BBB and the BCM. Moreover, a "trifunctional" targeting vector could be produced wherein a bifunctional antibody was fused to avidin, as outlined in Figure 5.13A. Such a targeting system would enable transport through both the BBB and the BCM in vivo and enable high-affinity binding of any biotinylated therapeutic. The genetic engineering of multifunctional brain drug-targeting systems can enable both drug targeting and drug conjugation to the targeting system. The diversity of strategies available for linking drugs to BBB transport vectors is discussed in Chapter 6.

Summary

The chimeric peptide technology provides a method for delivering a neuropharmaceutical agent into the brain by transcytosis through the BBB. This involves the formation and administration of a chimeric peptide, which is produced by conjugating or fusing a drug that is not normally transported across the BBB, to a brain drug-targeting vector. The latter can be any one of a group of transportable peptides, which bind endogenous receptors on the BBB. Such receptors normally function in the BBB transcytosis of peptides such as insulin, transferrin, insulin-like growth factors, or leptin. The ligands may also include peptidomimetic MAbs, which undergo transcytosis through the BBB on these same systems, or cationized proteins, such as cationized albumin, which enters brain via absorptive-mediated transcytosis through the BBB.

The discovery of BBB transport vectors is only the first step toward the production of chimeric peptides. The next phase is the identification of suitable linker strategies. The nontransportable drug and the transportable peptide must be joined in such a way that the bifunctionality of the conjugate is maintained. In addition, the plasma pharmacokinetics of the conjugate must be optimized. As discussed in Chapter 3 under the "pharmacokinetic rule," the brain delivery is an equal function of the BBB PS product, which is determined by vector activity, and the plasma AUC, which reflects the underlying pharmacokinetic properties of the chimeric peptide. The various linker strategies that both maintain bifunctionality and optimize plasma pharmacokinetics are discussed in Chapter 6.

6

Linker strategies: the engineering of multifunctional drug formulations

- Introduction
- Avidin-biotin technology
- Pegylation technology
- Liposome technology
- Summary

Introduction

Chimeric peptides are multifunctional drug formulations. Therefore, in linking a drug to a transport vector, it is essential that the bifunctionality of the conjugate be retained. This can be achieved in one of two ways. First, the drug and vector may be conjugated via a noncleavable (amide) linker in such a way that the biological activity of both components is retained. Second, the drug and vector may be conjugated via a cleavable (disulfide) linker, and the biologic activity of the drug may be lost when the drug is in the form of the chimeric peptide. However, the biologic activity of the drug may be restored following cleavage of the drug from the conjugate. Therefore, there are multiple approaches to the creation of multifunctional chimeric peptides and the diversity of the molecular formulations is outlined in Figure 6.1.

The construction of a chimeric peptide starts from three separate platforms that must be given simultaneous consideration. First, a vector discovery program must be initiated for the discovery of species-specific blood–brain barrier (BBB) transport vectors, such as those reviewed in Chapters 4 and 5. Second, the linker strategy must be developed and this might use chemical conjugates, genetically engineered fusion proteins, avidin-biotin technology, pegylation technology, or liposome technology (Figure 6.1). The linker strategy may employ cleavable linkers such as disulfides, or noncleavable linkers such as amides or thioethers. Within the noncleavable amide linker category, the linker may be short, e.g., 14–20 atoms, or extended, e.g., >200 atoms in length. The third area that must be considered is the pharmacokinetics and metabolic stability of the conjugate in vivo. It is not practical to go to considerable lengths to synthesize multifunctional chimeric peptides if

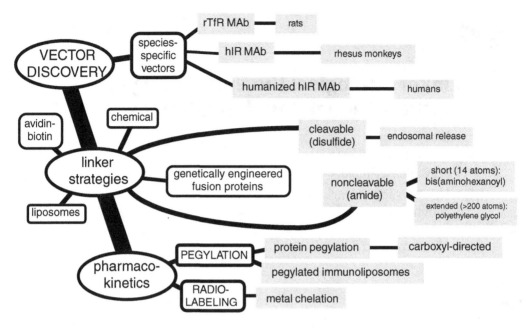

Figure 6.1   The diversity in molecular formulation of chimeric peptides is outlined. This emphasizes three major starting points: vector discovery, linker strategies, and pharmacokinetics. rTFR, rat transferrin receptor; MAb, monoclonal antibody; hIR, human insulin receptor.

the conjugate has an unfavorable pharmacokinetic or metabolic stability profile in vivo. The pharmacokinetics of protein-based therapeutics or liposome formulations may be optimized by pegylation technology. The metabolic stability of a peptide or an antisense radiopharmaceutical may be a function of the radionuclide that is attached, and this could involve radioiodination or the use of indium-111 (Figure 6.1).

The outline in Figure 6.1 shows the diversity in pathways available for synthesizing drug/vector conjugates. The linker strategies that are used to create bifunctional chimeric peptides are crucial to the overall success of the drug-targeting program. Invariably, the areas of vector discovery and drug discovery receive primary emphasis in a drug-targeting program. However, if the proper molecular formulation is not used to link together the drug and vector, then the ultimate pharmacologic activity in the brain in vivo will be suboptimal. The examples illustrated in this chapter will demonstrate that the successful synthesis of biologically active, multifunctional chimeric peptides is strictly a function of the molecular formulation used to build the conjugate. If a neurotrophin, such as brain-derived neurotrophic factor (BDNF), is pegylated on amino residues, then the neurotrophic factor will experience a considerable loss of biologic activity. Conversely, if the protein is pegylated on carboxyl residues, there can be a nearly 100% retention of biologic activity (Sakane and Pardridge, 1997). If the BDNF is conjugated to a BBB drug transport vector without the use of pegylation technology, then the pharmacokinetics of the conjugate will be suboptimal. In this case, the plasma area under the concentration curve (AUC) of the BDNF/vector conjugate will be decreased, and there will be corresponding reduction in the brain uptake (percentage of injected dose per gram brain: %ID/g) of the neurotrophic/vector conjugate. If an epidermal growth factor (EGF) peptide radiopharmaceutical is conjugated to a BBB drug-targeting vector via a short bis-aminohexanoyl (-XX-) 14-atom linker, then the EGF chimeric peptide will not bind to the EGF receptor. Conversely, if the -XX- linker is replaced by a >200 atom linker comprised of polyethylene glycol (PEG), then the EGF chimeric peptide does bind to the EGF receptor with normal affinity (Deguchi et al., 1999). If the EGF peptide radiopharmaceutical is radiolabeled with iodine-125, then the brain scan will have a 10-fold higher "noise" than that achieved when the EGF is radiolabeled with indium-111 (Kurihara et al., 1999). Finally, for industrial scale-up production of chimeric peptides, the ultimate yield of the conjugation reaction is crucial, and this may be optimized by the use of genetically engineered conjugates.

Avidin-biotin technology

Introduction

Chemical conjugates

A conjugate of a drug and BBB transport vector may be prepared with chemical linkers, as outlined in Table 6.1. In this approach, an ε-amino moiety on a surface lysine residue is thiolated with 2-iminothiolane (Traut's reagent). The thiolated drug or vector is then conjugated to the MBS-activated drug or vector to form a stable thioether (-S-) linker that is noncleavable, where MBS is m-maleimidobenzoyl N-hydroxysuccinimide ester (Yoshikawa and Pardridge, 1992). Conversely, an ε-amino group on a lysine residue may be activated with N-succinimidyl-3,2-pyridyldithio(propionate) (SPDP) and conjugated to a thiolated moiety to form a cleavable disulfide (-SS-) linker (Kumagai et al., 1987). However, the use of the chemical conjugation approaches is limited by the inherent low efficiency in chemically conjugating a drug to a transport vector. For this reason, avidin-biotin technology was introduced to BBB drug targeting (Yoshikawa and Pardridge, 1992). In this approach, a conjugate of the transport vector and avidin or neutral forms of avidin, such as neutral light avidin (NLA) or streptavidin (SA), are prepared in parallel with monobiotinylation of the drug. Owing to multivalency of avidin or SA binding of biotin (Green, 1975), a drug that had higher degrees of biotinylation than the

Table 6.1 Strategies for linking drugs to transport vectors

Class	Target AA	Agent	Linkage	Cleavability
Chemical	Lys	MBS	Thio-ether (-S-)	No
	Lys	Traut's		
	Lys	SPDP	Disulphide (-SS-)	Yes
	Lys	Traut's		
Avidin-biotin	Lys	NHS-SS-biotin	Disulfide	Yes
	Lys	NHS-XX-biotin	Amide	No
	Lys	NHS-PEG-biotin	Extended amide	No
	Asp, Glu	Hz-PEG-biotin	Extended hydrazide	No
Genetic		Fusion gene elements:		
engineering		Recombinant protein, recombinant vector		No
		Recombinant vector, recombinant avidin		Flexible

Notes:

AA, amino acid; MBS, *m*-maleimidobenzoyl; *N*-hydroxysuccinimide ester; SPDP, *N*-succinimidyl-3,2-pyridyldithio(propionate); NHS, *N*-hydroxysuccinimide; PEG, polyethylene glycol.

monobiotinylated form would form high molecular weight aggregates upon binding to the vector/avidin or vector/SA conjugate. These aggregates would be rapidly cleared from the blood by cells lining the reticuloendothelial system (RES) and this would result in a degraded plasma pharmacokinetic profile and reduced plasma AUC of the conjugate. Therefore, it is essential that the drug be monobiotinylated for drug targeting.

Avidin or SA have extremely high affinities for biotin with a dissociation constant (K_D) of 10^{-15} mol/l and a dissociation half-time of 89 days (Green, 1975). Therefore, there is essentially instantaneous capture of a biotinylated drug by a vector/avidin or a vector/SA conjugate. This property enables a "two-vial" drug formulation, as outlined in Figure 6.2. In this approach, the vector/avidin or the vector/SA conjugate is produced in one vial. In a second vial, the monobiotinylated drug is produced. The two vials are mixed prior to administration as there is instantaneous capture of the biotinylated drug and formation of the final conjugate, as outlined in Figure 6.2. Since vector/avidin and vector/SA fusion proteins may be mass-produced by genetic engineering (Li et al., 1999; Penichet et al., 1999), the use of avidin-biotin technology reduces the complex synthesis of a chimeric peptide to simple monobiotinylation of the drug.

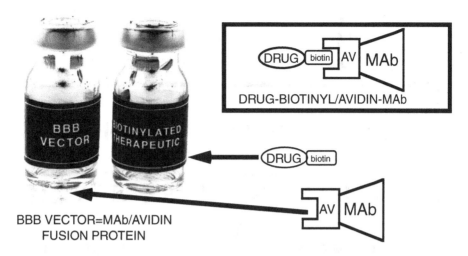

Figure 6.2   "Two vial" format for administration of drug/vector conjugates using avidin-biotin technology. The blood–brain barrier (BBB) transport vector is comprised of a genetically engineered fusion protein of avidin (AV) and a peptidomimetic monoclonal antibody (MAb). Separately, the drug is monobiotinylated. The entire conjugate, which is shown in the inset, is formed instantaneously upon mixture of the two vials. Owing to the very high affinity of avidin binding of biotin, there is instantaneous capture of the biotinylated drug by the MAb/AV fusion protein

Drug monobiotinylation: cleavable vs noncleavable chimeric peptides

Cleavable VIP chimeric peptides

Vasoactive intestinal peptide (VIP) is a principal vasodilator within the central nervous system (CNS) (Bottjer et al., 1984). The topical application of VIP to pial blood vessels of the brain results in vasodilation (McCulloch and Edvinsson, 1980). However, when VIP is infused into the carotid artery, there is no enhancement in cerebral blood flow (CBF) because VIP does not cross the BBB (Wilson et al., 1981). The development of VIP chimeric peptides for enhancement of CBF is discussed further in Chapter 7. VIP is discussed in the present context of linker strategies to exemplify the formulation issues involved in monobiotinylation of a drug using a cleavable, disulfide linker. Mammalian VIP has multiple lysine residues, which are all potential sites of biotinylation. Therefore, biotinylation of mammalian VIP would invariably lead to a multibiotinylated peptide. In order to facilitate mono-biotinylation of VIP, a biologically active VIP analog (VIPa) was synthesized (Bickel et al., 1993a), and the sequence of the VIPa is shown in Figure 6.3. The lysine residues at positions 20 and 21 were converted to arginine residues to prevent biotinylation at these sites. The amino terminus was acetylated to prevent biotinylation

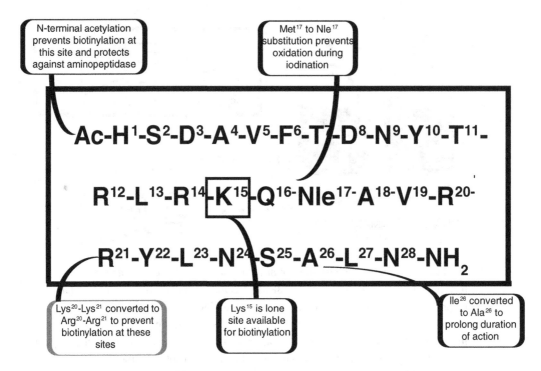

Figure 6.3   Single-letter amino acid sequence of a vasoactive intestinal peptide (VIP) analog designed for monobiotinylation. The single site for biotinylation is the lysine (K) residue at position 15 and modification of this lysine residue is possible with retention of biologic activity of VIP. Ac, acetyl; Nle, norleucine.

at this site and also to protect the peptide against aminopeptidase. These modifications left the lysine residue at position 15 as the single site available for biotinylation, and prior studies had shown that VIP monobiotinylated at Lys[15] was biologically active (Andersson et al., 1991). The methionine residue at position 17 was changed to leucine to prevent oxidation of the peptide since BBB transport of this VIP chimeric peptide was to be investigated using a form of the peptide that was radiolabeled by oxidative iodination. Finally, the isoleucine at position 26 was converted to alanine as prior studies had shown that this modification enhanced the duration of action of VIP (O'Donnell et al., 1991).

The VIPa was then monobiotinylated with NHS-SS-biotin (Bickel et al., 1993a), where NHS is *N*-hydroxysuccinimide, which forms a disulfide linker at the Lys[15] position of the VIPa, and the structure of the biotin-SS-VIPa is shown in Figure 6.4A. Following cleavage of the biotin-SS-VIPa, there is a mecaptopropionate group remaining at the Lys[15] position, as shown in the structure of the cleaved VIPa (Figure 6.4A). The structures of the VIPa, the biotin-SS-VIPa (bioVIPa), and the

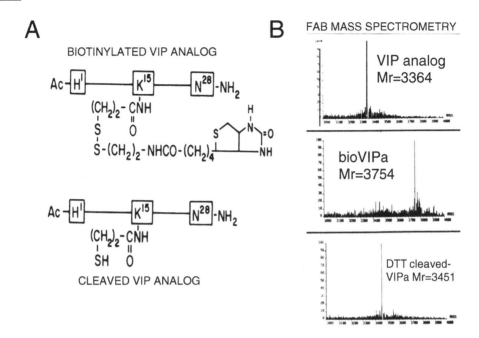

A BIOTINYLATED VIP ANALOG

B FAB MASS SPECTROMETRY

VIP analog Mr=3364

bioVIPa Mr=3754

DTT cleaved-VIPa Mr=3451

CLEAVED VIP ANALOG

Figure 6.4   (A) Structure of biotinylated vasoactive intestinal peptide (VIP) analog (bioVIPa) and the cleaved VIPa following treatment with dithiothreitol (DTT). The biotin moiety is attached to the lysine (K) residue at position 15 following the reaction of the VIPa with N-hydroxysuccinimide (NHS)-SS-biotin. The amino terminal histidine (H) moiety is acetylated (Ac) and the carboxyl terminal asparagine (N) residue is amidated. The molecular mass was determined by fast atom bombardment (FAB) mass spectrometry of high performance liquid chromatography (HPLC) purified VIPa, biotinylated VIPa, and the DTT cleaved VIPa, which is shown in panel B. From Bickel et al. (1993a) with permission.

dithiothreitol (DTT) cleaved VIPa were confirmed by fast atom bombardment (FAB) mass spectrometry, as shown in Figure 6.4B. Radioreceptor assays (RRA) with [^{125}I]mammalian VIP and rat lung membranes demonstrated the cleaved VIPa had a comparable, high affinity for the VIP receptor, as did the original VIPa (Bickel et al., 1993a). As discussed in Chapter 7, the systemic administration of the biotin-SS-VIPa bound to a conjugate of the OX26 monoclonal antibody (MAb) and avidin, designated OX26/AV, and was biologically active in vivo, as the VIP chimeric peptide caused a substantial increase in CBF (Bickel et al., 1993a).

Cleavable opioid chimeric peptides

Opioid peptides represent potential new treatments for heroin addiction because these peptides trigger specific opioid peptide receptor (OR) isoforms in brain whereas morphine, the biologically active product of heroin, binds μ-, δ-, and κ-OR.

However, opioid peptide analogs can be fashioned in such a way that the peptide triggers only one of these specific isoforms (Rapaka and Porreca, 1991). The dermorphins are opioid peptides and a [Lys^7]dermorphin analog, designated K7DA, was synthesized (Bickel et al., 1995a). The K7DA was biotinylated with NHS-SS-biotin to form biotin-SS-K7DA. Following cleavage with DTT, the desbio-K7DA was purified and its biologic activity was assessed in an OR RRA with rat brain synaptosomes using [^{3}H]DAGO as the OR ligand, where DAGO is a specific μ-OR ligand, and DAGO is Tyr-D-Ala-Gly-Phe-(N-methyl)-Gly-ol. Whereas the dissociation constant (K_D) of [^{3}H]DAGO binding to the μ-OR was 0.58 ± 0.08 nmmol/l, and the K_i of K7DA binding was 0.62 ± 0.14 nmol/l, the K_i of the desbio-SS-K7DA was 1.24 ± 0.24 nmol/l (Bickel et al., 1995a). Therefore, these studies showed that the biologic activity of the K7DA opioid peptide was retained following sequential monobiotinylation with NHS-SS-biotin followed by cleavage of the biotin moiety resulting in the formation of K7DA-SH (desbio-K7DA). In parallel, the K7DA was biotinylated with NHS-XX-biotin, where XX is 14 atom bis(aminohexanoyl), noncleavable amide linker. The affinity of the biotin-XX-K7DA analog for the μ-OR was high, with a K_i of 1.6 ± 0.3 nmol/l (Bickel et al., 1995a).

The CNS biologic activity of the K7DA opioid peptides was evaluated in vivo in rats following the intracerebroventricular (ICV) injection of the K7DA opioid peptides with subsequent measurements of pharmacologic activity using the tail-flick analgesia test (Figure 6.5). The unmodified K7DA opioid peptide resulted in a dose-dependent analgesia following the ICV injection of the peptide (Figure 6.5A). As discussed in Chapter 3, the in vivo CNS pharmacologic effect of opioid peptides following ICV injection is due to the fact that the OR mediating the analgesia is situated in the periaqueductal gray (PAG) region of brain that is immediately contiguous with the cerebral aqueduct (Watkins et al., 1992). Therefore, the distance necessary for the opioid peptide to diffuse from the cerebrospinal fluid (CSF) flow tracts in order to reach the end organ is minimal and this accounts for the pharmacologic effects following ICV injection. Similar to the unmodified K7DA, the biotin-XX-K7DA was also biologically active following ICV injection, as shown in Figure 6.5B. However, when the biotin-XX-K7DA was bound to a conjugate of the OX26 MAb and NLA, designated NLA-OX26, there was minimal biologic activity of the opioid chimeric peptide, as shown in Figure 6.5B. The failure to observe an in vivo CNS pharmacologic effect was correlated with the opioid peptide RRA (Bickel et al., 1995a). Although the biotin-XX-K7DA bound to the OR with high affinity, there was insignificant binding of this opioid peptide following conjugation of the biotin-XX-K7DA to NLA-OX26. Similarly, when the biotin-SS-K7DA was bound to NLA-OX26, there was minimal biologic activity in vivo, as shown in Figure 6.5C. Higher doses of the conjugate of biotin-SS-K7DA and the NLA-OX26, designated BioSSK7DA/NLA-OX26, did result in pharmacologic activity with a

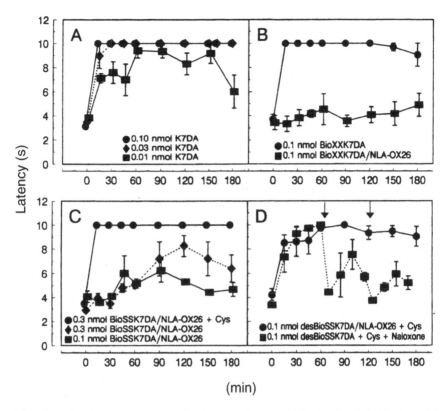

Figure 6.5   Tail-flick analgesia measurements after intracerebroventricular (ICV) administration of the K7DA chimeric opioid peptide. Doses are given in the insets. Panel A shows a dose–response curve following ICV injection of unmodified K7DA. Panel B compares the analgesic effect of biotin (bio)-XX-K7DA with or without conjugation to NLA-OX26. Panel C shows the effect of two different doses of bio-SS-K7DA conjugated to NLA-OX26 and the effect of precleavage of the chimeric peptide with 0.5 mmol/l cysteine (Cys). Panel D shows the naloxone reversibility and time reversibility of the pharmacologic effect of the desbio-SS-K7DA and the effect of the desbio-SS-K7DA in the presence of the vector, NLA-OX26. The arrow in panel D indicates the time of naloxone administration. Data are mean ± SE ($n = 3$ rats). The entire chimeric peptide of biotin-XX-K7DA or biotin-SS-K7DA bound to the conjugate of NLA and the OX26 monoclonal antibody (MAb) is designated BioXXK7DA/NLA-OX26 or BioSSK7DA/NLA-OX26, respectively. From Bickel et al. (1995a) with permission. Copyright (1995) National Academy of Sciences, USA.

delayed reaction time (Figure 6.5C). This suggests there was eventually cleavage of the opioid peptide from the NLA-OX26 resulting in binding of the K7DA-SH to the OR in brain. However, the limiting factor in opioid peptide pharmacologic activity in brain following the ICV injection of this formulation was the cleavage of the disulfide bond. This is demonstrated by showing the profound analgesia observed when the conjugate of the biotin-SS-K7DA and the NLA-OX26 is cleaved with cysteine (Cys) prior to the ICV injection, as shown in Figure 6.5C. The pharmacologic activity achieved with the biotin-SS-K7DA bound to the conjugate of NLA-OX26, following cysteine-mediated cleavage, represented true activation of the μ-OR in brain because this process was reversible with both time and naloxone, as shown in Figure 6.5D.

Disulfide cleavage in brain

The studies with the VIP and opioid chimeric peptides demonstrate that peptide analogs can be produced that enable the facile monobiotinylation using a cleavable disulfide bridge. Moreover, the biotinylated VIP or opioid peptide is biologically active following cleavage of the disulfide linker and release from the MAb/avidin or MAb/NLA conjugate (Bickel et al., 1993a, 1995a). Whereas the VIP-SS-biotin/avidin-OX26 conjugate was biologically active in vivo following systemic administration (Bickel et al., 1993a), there was no central analgesia observed following the intravenous administration of the K7DA-SS-biotin/NLA-OX26 (U. Bickel and W. Pardridge, unpublished observations). These differences in biological activity in vivo occur for two reasons. First, the intact VIPa chimeric peptide binds the VIP receptor even though the disulfide linkage has not been cleaved (Wu and Pardridge, 1996), whereas the opioid chimeric peptide does not bind the OR unless there is cleavage from the conjugate (Bickel et al., 1995a). Second, the cleavage of the disulfide linker is inefficient in brain extracellular space (ECS) in vivo (Bickel et al., 1995a).

The VIPa is still biologically active and still binds the VIP receptor despite conjugation to the NLA-OX26 vector (Chapter 7). This binding of the intact conjugate to the mammalian VIP receptor explains the equal biologic activity of either the VIP-XX-biotin conjugated to SA-OX26 or the VIP-SS-biotin conjugated to AV-OX26. These VIP chimeric peptides were prepared with either the cleavable (disulfide) or the noncleavable (amide) linker, respectively (Bickel et al., 1993a; Wu and Pardridge, 1996). However, in the case of the much smaller opioid peptides, there is no biologic activity of the opioid chimeric peptide when the molecule is presented to the OR in the form of the intact conjugate, K7DA-SS-biotin conjugated to NLA-OX26 (Figure 6.5). In this case, the rate-limiting step in activation of the opioid chimeric peptide is cleavage of the disulfide bond (Figure 6.5).

The cleavage of the disulfide linker in brain may occur in either the intracellular space or the ECS and the steps involved in these two pathways are outlined in Figure 6.6. In the intracellular cleavage pathway, the chimeric peptide must undergo four sequential steps prior to entry of the cleaved peptide into the brain ECS. These steps are: (a) BBB transport of the intact chimeric peptide, (b) transport of the intact chimeric peptide across the brain cell membrane (BCM), (c) intracellular reduction

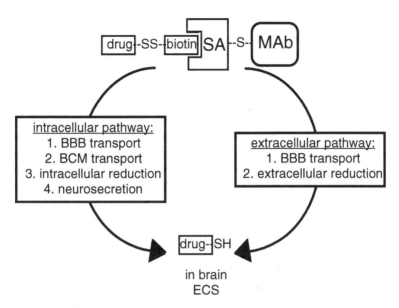

Figure 6.6   Intracellular and extracellular disulfide cleavage of chimeric peptides in brain. SA, streptavidin; MAb, monoclonal antibody; BBB, blood–brain barrier; BCM, brain cell membrane; ECS, extracellular space; S, thioether; SS, disulfide; SH, sulfhydryl. Reprinted with permission from Bickel et al. (1995a). Copyright (1995) American Chemical Society.

and cleavage of the disulfide linker, (d) neurosecretion of the cleaved peptide into the brain ECS. In this case, the VIP-sulfhydryl in the brain ECS may then bind to the VIP receptor on the precapillary arteriolar smooth muscle cells in brain which are situated beyond the BBB. The alternate or extracellular pathway of disulfide cleavage in brain is also outlined in Figure 6.6 and requires the expression of disulfide reductase "ectoenzymes" on the exterior of plasma membranes of brain cells. Although disulfide reductases such as thioredoxin reductase are located strictly in the cytosolic space and not on the plasma membrane, certain disulfide reductases, such as protein disulfide isomerase (PDI), are located on the plasma membrane (Ryser et al., 1994), as depicted in Figure 6.6 for the extracellular cleavage pathway. In order for the extracellular cleavage pathway to cause a successful activation of chimeric peptides in brain, the disulfide reductases would have to be selectively expressed on the plasma membrane of brain cells and not on the plasma membrane of the capillary endothelium comprising the BBB. If the disulfide reductases were expressed on the endothelial plasma membrane, then the chimeric peptide would be cleaved prior to transcytosis through the BBB in vivo.

There is minimal plasma membrane disulfide reductase at the BBB since prior studies have shown that opioid chimeric peptides are stable in the presence of isolated brain capillaries (Bickel et al., 1995a). The stability of the opioid chimeric peptides formed with a cleavable disulfide linker during the process of transcytosis through the BBB in vivo has also been confirmed with in vivo microdialysis experiments (Kang et al., 2000). These findings are consistent with other observations that disulfide reductases are not present in the endosomal compartment of cells (Feener et al., 1990). Instead, the disulfide reductases are in the cytosolic compartments and this accounts for the very high ratio of reduced glutathione to oxidized glutathione in the cytosol (Lodish and Kong, 1993). Because of the selective localization of the cell-reducing power in the cytoplasm, it is rare for cytosolic proteins to have disulfide bridges. Instead, disulfide bonds are formed in the lumen of the endoplasmic reticulum where the concentration of reduced glutathione is low (Lodish and Kong, 1993).

The available evidence to date suggests that the extracellular reduction pathway outlined in Figure 6.6 is not prominent in vivo, at least for the rat. The evidence for this is derived from the studies of the opioid chimeric peptides (Bickel et al., 1995a). First, the cleavage of the disulfide linker following the ICV injection of opioid chimeric peptides is delayed and rate-limiting, as shown in Figure 6.5. Second, the intravenous administration of opioid chimeric peptides did not result in pharmacologic activity in brain. This is explained on the basis of (a) lack of biologic activity of the opioid chimeric peptide when presented to the OR in the form of the intact conjugate, (b) minimal extracellular cleavage pathway, and (c) "short-circuiting" of the intracellular cleavage pathway by metabolism of the opioid chimeric peptide. That is, in order for the intracellular cleavage pathway to be effective, the cleavage and neurosecretion of the cleaved peptide must occur at a rate much faster than intracellular degradation of the opioid peptide.

Given the difficulties inherent in the use of cleavable disulfide linkers, subsequent formulations of chimeric peptides employed noncleavable amide linkers. In this approach, the drug is presented to its cognate receptor in the form of the drug/vector conjugate. With this approach, it is necessary to prepare a chimeric peptide that is biologically active without cleavage of the drug from the transport vector. The use of amide linkers is discussed further in Chapters 7 and 8, which describe the successful pharmacologic applications of chimeric peptides as peptide-based or antisense-based neuropharmaceuticals.

Plasma pharmacokinetics of avidin conjugates

Rapid plasma clearance of avidin

Avidin is a homotetramer comprised of 16 kDa subunits (Green, 1975). The protein is glycosylated and has a highly cationic charge with an isoelectric point (pI) of 10. Both the cationic charge and carbohydrate moiety of avidin appear to play a role in the rapid removal of this protein from the plasma compartment fol-

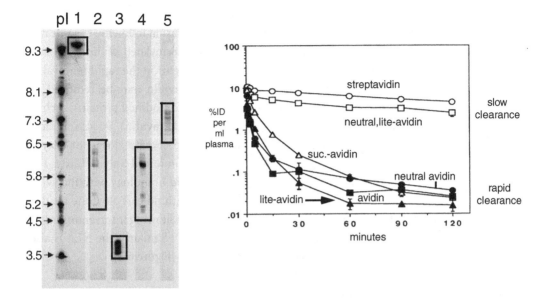

Figure 6.7   Pharmacokinetics of [³H]biotin/avidin clearance from blood is dependent on the charge and glycosylation of avidin. Left: Isoelectric focusing of pI standards and five different avidin analogs. Lanes 1, 2, 3, 4, and 5, respectively, are avidin, neutral avidin, succinylated (suc.) avidin, neutral light (lite) avidin, and streptavidin. The polyacrylamide gel was stained with Coomassie blue prior to photography. The pI of standards is shown on the left. Right: Plasma pharmacokinetics of [³H]biotin bound to one of six different avidin analogs. The percentage of injected dose (ID) per milliliter plasma is plotted versus time after intravenous injection in anesthetized rats. The rate of removal from plasma of the [³H]biotin/avidin complex is strongly influenced by the charge or glycosylation of the avidin protein. Streptavidin and neutral light avidin are both neutral and deglycosylated. From Kang et al. (1995b) with permission.

lowing intravenous injection (Kang et al., 1995b). This is demonstrated by a comparison of the isoelectric focusing (IEF) and plasma pharmacokinetics of avidin and five avidin analogs, including SA, NLA, neutral avidin, succinylated (suc) avidin, and light avidin. NLA is a modified version of avidin in which the carbohydrate content has been removed and the positive charge of the protein has been neutralized (Wilchek and Bayar, 1993). Neutral avidin is an analog of avidin in which the carbohydrate moiety remains intact, but the positive charge has been neutralized. Light avidin is an avidin analog in which the positive charge remains intact, but the carbohydrate moiety is removed. Succinylated avidin is an avidin analog that has an anionic or negative charge following succinylation of the protein.

The pI of avidin and the different avidin analogs is shown in Figure 6.7. The rate of removal from plasma in anesthetized rats of [³H]biotin bound to avidin or one of the avidin analogs is also shown in Figure 6.7. These studies show that the [^{3}H]biotin/avidin complex is rapidly removed from plasma following the intravenous injection of the cationic avidin or the anionic succinylated avidin. This suggests that the positive charge, per se, is not the only factor in the rapid removal of avidin from plasma. Alternatively, the succinylated avidin may be removed by organs such as liver via uptake mechanisms specific for modified proteins, such as succinylated avidin. The deglycosylated avidin (light avidin) is also rapidly removed from plasma, suggesting the carbohydrate moiety does not play a significant role (Kang et al., 1995b). Avidin is a protein found only in birds. The bacterial homolog of avidin, SA, has a 38% amino acid homology with the avian protein (Gitlin et al., 1990). SA is a neutral protein with no carbohydrate residue and is removed slowly from the plasma compartment following intravenous injection in rats (Schechter et al., 1990; Kang et al., 1995b). Similarly, the NLA is also slowly removed from the plasma compartment in rats (Figure 6.7).

Plasma clearance of vector/avidin conjugates

Given the rapid rate of removal of avidin from the plasma compartment (Yoshikawa and Pardridge, 1992), it would be anticipated that a conjugate of a BBB-targeting vector and avidin would also be similarly rapidly removed from plasma. This is demonstrated in Figure 6.8. In these studies, [^{3}H]biotin was bound to a conjugate of avidin (AV) and the OX26 MAb to the transferrin receptor, and this conjugate is alternatively designated AV/OX26 or AV-OX26. The [^{3}H]biotin was also bound to a conjugate of NLA and the OX26 MAb, designated NLA/OX26 or NLA-OX26. The plasma clearance of [^{3}H]biotin bound to AV/OX26 is rapid, with a markedly reduced plasma AUC. In contrast, the rate of plasma clearance of the [^{3}H]biotin bound to the NLA/OX26 is slow, with a higher plasma AUC (Figure 6.8). As discussed in Chapter 3, it is advantageous to optimize the plasma AUC in brain drug targeting because the brain uptake (%ID/g) is directly proportional to both the BBB permeability–surface area (PS) product and to the plasma AUC. The difference in the plasma concentration at prolonged time periods up to 24 h is further magnified in comparing the plasma pharmacokinetics of the NLA and the avidin conjugates (Figure 6.8). In order to optimize the plasma pharmacokinetics, subsequent studies employed conjugates of the peptidomimetic MAb and neutral forms of avidin such as NLA or SA. The attachment of the 50 kDa NLA or SA to the targeting MAb does not reduce the BBB transport of the MAb. Internal carotid artery perfusion experiments demonstrated that the complex of [^{3}H]biotin bound to the conjugate of NLA/OX26 was transcytosed across the BBB in vivo at rates identical to that observed with either transferrin or the unconjugated OX26 MAb (Kang and Pardridge, 1994b), as reviewed in Chapter 4.

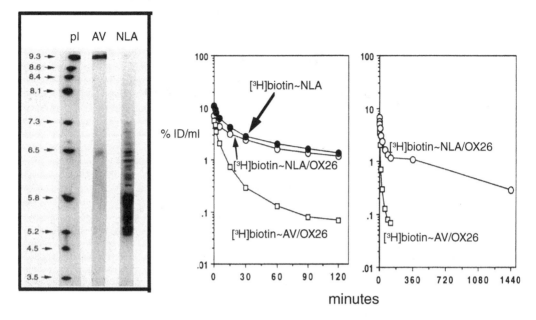

Figure 6.8 Left: Isoelectric focusing of pI standards, avidin (AV) and neutral light avidin (NLA). Right: Pharmacokinetic profile of [³H]biotin bound to (a) NLA, (b) a conjugate of NLA and the OX26 monoclonal antibody (MAb), designated NLA/OX26, or (c) a conjugate of AV and the OX26 MAb, designated AV/OX26. From Kang and Pardridge (1994b) by permission of Gordon and Breach. Copyright (1994) Overseas Publishers Association.

Genetically engineered vector/avidin fusion genes and fusion proteins

The genetic engineering of fusion genes of avidin or SA and BBB drug-targeting vectors is discussed in Chapter 5. In this approach, an avidin monomer is fused to the carboxyl terminus of the heavy chain of the peptidomimetic MAb (Figure 6.9). Owing to the tendency of the avidin or SA monomers to aggregate to form dimers and tetratmers, avidin or SA is an ideal protein for forming immunoglobulin G (IgG) fusion proteins. Moreover, the plasma pharmacokinetic profile of IgG/avidin fusion proteins is quite distinct from that of chemical conjugates of IgGs and avidin. Although IgG/avidin conjugates that are formed chemically with stable thioether linkers are rapidly removed from the plasma compartment (Figure 6.8), the plasma clearance of a genetically engineered IgG/AV fusion protein is delayed, as shown in Figure 5.13. In this respect, IgG/avidin fusion proteins are similar to immunoadhesins formed with other cationic proteins such as CD4, as discussed in Chapter 5. That is, the plasma clearance of the fusion protein of the IgG and the cationic protein is much slower than clearance of the cationic protein, per se.

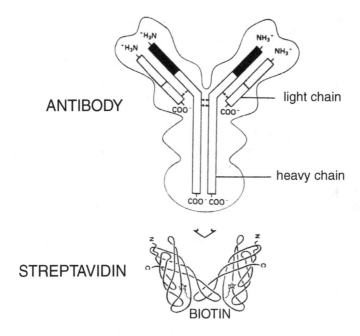

Figure 6.9   Design of an antibody–streptavidin fusion protein. The streptavidin structure is reprinted with permission from Weber, P.C., Ohlendorf, D.H., Wendoloski, J.J. and Salemme, F.R. (1989). Structural origin of high-affinity biotin binding to streptavidin. *Science*, **243**, 85–8. Copyright (1989) American Association for the Advancement of Science.

Immunogenicity of avidin or streptavidin in humans

Avidin is a protein found only in birds and is not produced in humans (Elo, 1980). However, in all western societies humans are fed avidin orally because this protein is abundant in egg whites. Oral antigen feeding is known to induce immune tolerance to proteins (Weiner, 1994), and there is evidence for immune tolerance of avidin in humans. Doses as high as 5–10 mg of avidin have been administered intravenously to humans without toxicity or antibody formation (Samuel et al., 1996). Although SA would be expected to be more immunogenic in humans than avidin, because this protein is not part of the diet, SA has also been administered to humans without immunologic consequences (Rusckowski et al., 1996). Therefore, it is possible that avidin or SA fusion proteins may not be immunogenic in humans.

Drug targeting versus drug sequestration using avidin-biotin technology

In vivo avidin-biotin technology was developed in the 1980s to cause drug sequestration at an end organ (Hnatowich et al., 1987; Klibanov et al., 1988). In this approach, a biotinylated MAb that targets an end organ such as a tumor antigen was administered intravenously. Following a delayed time period that sequestered the

Table 6.2 Drug targeting vs drug sequestration using avidin-biotin technology

	Drug targeting	Drug sequestration
Degrees of biotinylation	Monobiotinylation	Multibiotinylation
Administration of avidin and biotin components	Simultaneous	Sequential
Desired plasma AUC	High	Low

Note:
AUC, area under the concentration curve.

MAb at the end organ, avidin was administered intravenously. This formed a complex between the avidin and the biotinylated MAb and, owing to the rapid removal of avidin from the plasma compartment, there was a corresponding rapid removal of the MAb from the plasma compartment. There was also deposition of avidin at the local tumor site that bound the multibiotinylated MAb. Indeed, the higher degrees of biotinylation of the MAb resulted in enhanced binding of avidin at the site owing to the multivalency of avidin binding of biotin. In a third injection, a biotinylated radionuclide was administered to achieve sequestration of the radionuclide at the tumor site containing the biotinylated MAb and the avidin complex.

Avidin-biotin technology is used differently in drug targeting across biological barriers such as the BBB. In drug targeting, the drug is *monobiotinylated* because the formation of high molecular weight aggregates of avidin or SA with multibiotinylated drugs must be avoided. Otherwise, the aggregated conjugate would be rapidly removed from blood. Whereas rapid removal from blood is desired in drug sequestration, the rapid removal from plasma and reduced plasma AUC is not desired for drug targeting (Table 6.2). Another distinction is that the biotinylated drug/vector–avidin conjugate is administered simultaneously as a single injection for brain drug targeting. In contrast, the biotinylated moiety and the avidin are administered with sequential injections for drug sequestration (Table 6.2).

Pegylation technology

Amino-directed protein pegylation

Protein pegylation involves the conjugation of PEG to surface amino acid residues on proteins. In the 1970s, it was demonstrated that the rapid removal of proteins from the plasma compartment could be delayed by the attachment of PEG polymers to the surface of the protein (Abuchowski et al., 1977a). If the size of the PEG polymer was increased from 2 to 5 kDa, then the plasma clearance was proportionally reduced. Another advantage of protein pegylation is that the immunogenicity of proteins is decreased following protein pegylation (Abuchowski et al., 1977b).

Proteins were uniformly pegylated on the ε-amino groups of lysine residues. In many instances, the biologic activity of the protein was retained following amino-directed protein pegylation. However, in other instances, a considerable amount of biologic activity of the protein was lost following amino-directed protein pegylation (Clark et al., 1996). An alternative to amino-directed pegylation of proteins is carboxyl-directed pegylation. Carboxyl-directed pegylation had been described by Zalipsky (1995). However, nearly all published studies of protein pegylation involved amino-directed pegylation. Indeed, a review article outlined only methods for amino-directed protein pegylation (Chamow et al., 1994). If the biologic activity of a protein is lost following amino-directed protein pegylation, then carboxyl-directed protein pegylation should be considered. This is demonstrated in the case of the nerve growth factor (NGF)-like neurotrophins.

Carboxyl-directed pegylation of BDNF

The NGF-like neurotrophins

Neurotrophins such as NGF, BDNF, neurotrophin (NT)-3, or NT-4/5 are all members of the same family and have similar structures. There is a cationic groove formed by lysine and arginine residues and this cationic groove plays an important role in binding to the respective neurotrophin receptor, abbreviated trk (Ibáñez et al., 1992). For example, NGF binds to trkA and BDNF binds to trkB. The anionic charge on the NGF-like proteins is segregated to the periphery of the cationic groove and there is a preponderance of glutamate and aspartate residues on the periphery of the NGF (Honig and Nicholls, 1995), as revealed by the surface charge model shown in Figure 6.10. Previous studies have shown that modification of lysine residues in NGF results in the loss of biologic activity of the neurotrophin (Rosenberg et al., 1986), and this likely arises from the alteration of crucial lysine residues forming the trkA binding site on the NGF.

Neurotrophins such as NGF or BDNF are rapidly removed from the plasma compartment (Pardridge et al., 1994b), apparently due to the cationic charge of these proteins. Similarly, when a neurotrophin such as BDNF is conjugated to a BBB transport vector, the BDNF/vector conjugate is also rapidly removed from the plasma compartment (Pardridge et al., 1994b), similar to that observed for MAb/avidin conjugates (Figure 6.8). In this setting, the cationic neurotrophin is actually directing the vector to the liver and away from the intended end organ, brain. This results in a reduced plasma AUC and a proportionate reduction in the brain uptake of the neurotrophin/vector conjugate. The rapid uptake of the neurotrophic factor by liver and the rapid removal of the neurotrophin/vector conjugate from plasma can be reversed by protein pegylation. However, the finding that modification of lysine moieties on the NGF-like neurotrophins results in reduced

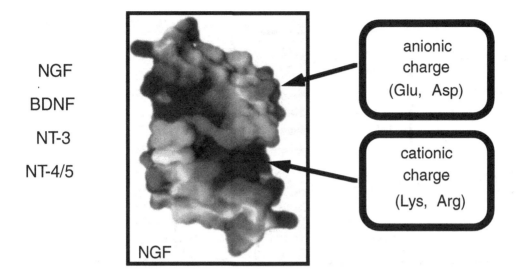

NGF

BDNF

NT-3

NT-4/5

Figure 6.10   Electrostatic charge model of nerve growth factor (NGF) showing the cationic groove as represented by the black coloration in the central part of the molecule. This is comprised of the cationic charges of lysine (Lys) and arginine (Arg) residues. Conversely, the anionic charges shown in gray on the periphery of the molecule are comprised of glutamate (Glu) and aspartate (Asp) residues. The cationic surface charge of the NGF-like neurotrophins causes rapid uptake by liver and kidney, which results in rapid systemic clearance ($t_{1/2} < 5$ min), and poor plasma pharmacokinetics. This can be reversed by protein pegylation. The biologic activity of the neurotrophin can be retained by carboxyl-directed pegylation. BDNF, brain-derived neurotrophic factor; NT, neurotrophin. Reprinted with permission from Honig, B. and Nicholls, A. (1995). Classical electrostatics in biology and chemistry. *Science*, **268**, 1144–9. Copyright (1995) American Association for the Advancement of Science.

biologic activity indicates that amino-directed protein pegylation is not the desired modification.

Carboxyl-directed protein pegylation of BDNF

The scheme for carboxyl-directed pegylation of BDNF is outlined in Figure 6.11. In this approach, the carboxyl moieties of surface glutamate and aspartate residues are pegylated using hydrazide chemistry (Sakane and Pardridge, 1997). Moreover, a biotin moiety may be placed at the tip of the PEG strand using a specially designed bifunctional PEG derivative. This bifunctional PEG contains a hydrazide moiety at one end of the PEG molecule and a biotin moiety at the other end of the PEG molecule (Pardridge et al., 1998b), as shown in Figure 6.11. In these studies, PEG of 2000 Da, designated PEG^{2000}, or PEG of 5000 Da, designated PEG^{5000}, was used. Two different classes of PEG hydrazide compounds were used. The principal class

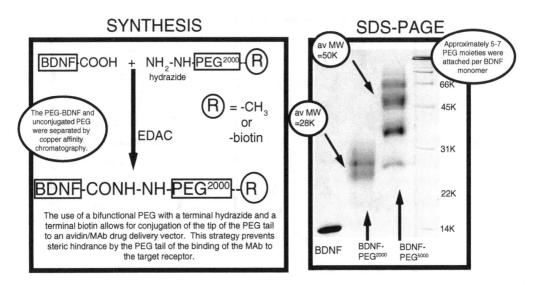

Figure 6.11 Left: Synthesis of pegylated brain-derived neurotrophic factor (BDNF) using carboxyl-directed pegylation and hydrazide conjugate of polyethylene glycol (PEG). Right: Sodium dodecylsulfate polyacrylamide gel electrophoresis (SDS-PAGE) of BDNF, BDNF-PEG2000, and BDNF-PEG5000. MAb, monoclonal antibody; MW, molecular weight. From Sakane and Pardridge (1997) with permission.

contained a methyl moiety at the end opposite the hydrazide linker on the PEG compound. The minor class contained a biotin moiety at the other end of the hydrazide (Hz) linker. The surface carboxyl groups of BDNF were pegylated with PEG-Hz or biotin-PEG-Hz using EDAC as a carboxyl activator, where EDAC is an N-methyl-N'-3-(dimethylaminopropyl)carbodiimide hydrochloride. The attachment of the PEG2000 to the BDNF increased the average molecular weight from 14 to 28 kDa, and attachment of the PEG5000 resulted in an average molecular weight of 50 kDa, as shown by the sodium dodecylsulfate polyacrylamide gel electrophoresis (SDS-PAGE) studies in Figure 6.11. This suggested that approximately five to seven PEG moieties were attached per BDNF monomer (Sakane and Pardridge, 1997). Each BDNF monomer contains a total of 12 glutamates plus aspartate residues (Leibrock et al., 1989); therefore approximately 50–60% of these acidic amino acid residues were pegylated in these studies (Sakane and Pardridge, 1997).

Retention of biologic activity of BDNF

The plasma clearance (Cl) of [125I]BDNF was measured in anesthetized rats in parallel with the plasma clearance of [125I]BDNF-PEG2000 and [125I]BDNF-PEG5000, shown in Figure 6.12. The unconjugated BDNF was rapidly removed from the plasma compartment with a systemic clearance of 4.2 ± 0.1 ml/min per kg (Sakane

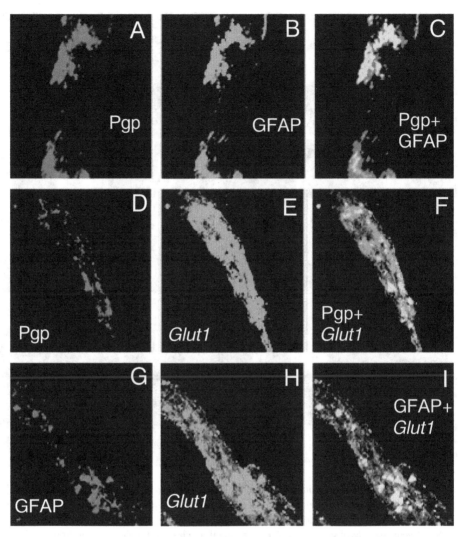

Figure 3.17 Cytocentrifuged human brain capillaries were dual-labeled with antibodies to p-glycoprotein (Pgp) (panels A, D), glial fibrillary acidic protein (GFAP, panels B, G), or the *Glut1* glucose transporter (panels E, H). The overlap of panels A and B is shown in panel C; the overlap of panels D and E is shown in panel F; and the overlap of panels G and H is shown in panel I. Reprinted from *Brain Res.*, **819**, Golden, P.L. and Pardridge, W.M., P-glycoprotein on astrocyte foot processes of unfixed isolated human brain capillaries, 143–6, copyright (1999), with permission from Elsevier Science.

These plates are available for download in colour from www.cambridge.org/9780521154468

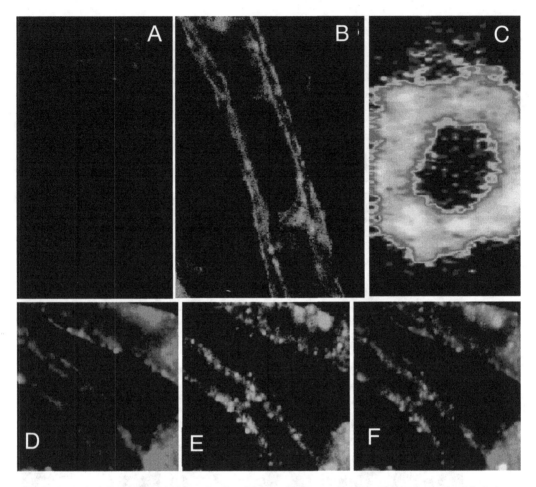

Figure 4.7 (A and B) Freshly isolated, unfixed rat brain capillaries are incubated with rhodamine-labeled pegylated immunoliposomes before confocal analysis. The immunoliposomes contain 20–24 molecules of either the mouse IgG_{2a} isotype control (A) or the OX26 monoclonal antibody (MAb) (B) conjugated at the tip of the polyethylene glycol strands. (C) Cross-section through the rat brain capillary shown in (B) obtained by computer-aided three-dimensional construction of a series of consecutive optical sections. Colors were used to illuminate the capillary lumen (blue/black), luminal and abluminal endothelium plasma membranes (purple), and endothelial cytoplasm (yellow). (D, E, F) Double-labeling of unfixed rat brain capillaries using the OX26 MAb with a fluorescein conjugated secondary polyclonal antibody and a plasma membrane marker, rhodamine-phosphatidyl ethanolamine (PE). The signals for rhodamine-PE alone or OX26 MAb alone are shown in (D) and (E), respectively, and the overlay of these two images is shown in (F). From Huwyler and Pardridge (1998) with permission.

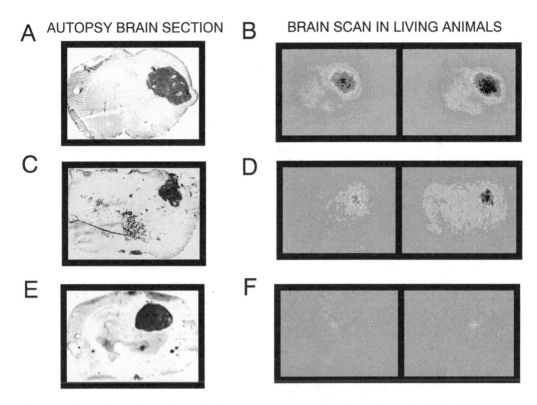

A AUTOPSY BRAIN SECTION
B BRAIN SCAN IN LIVING ANIMALS

C

D

E

F

Figure 7.11 (A, C, E) Experimental U87 brain tumors were grown in nude rats for 16 days. The brain was removed and frozen sections were immunostained with a mouse monoclonal antibody to the human epidermal growth factor (EGF) receptor; these studies used a biotinylated horse antimouse immunoglobulin G (IgG) secondary antibody that had been preabsorbed with rat immunoglobulin. The study shows abundant expression of the immunoreactive EGF receptor in the U87 experimental tumors in brains of nude rats. (B, D, F) Film autoradiography of frozen sections of brain obtained from U87 tumor-bearing nude rats injected intravenously with 100 μCi of either [^{111}In]diethylenetriaminepentaacetic acid (DTPA)-EGF-polyethylene glycol (PEG)^{3400}-biotin conjugated to OX26/streptavidin (B and D) or [^{111}In]DTPA-EGF-PEG^{3400}-biotin without conjugation to the BBB-targeting system (F). The panels on the right (B, D, F) are labeled as brain scan in living animals because the radiolabeled EGF chimeric peptide was administered in vivo and frozen sections were subsequently developed by quantitative autoradiography (QAR), as opposed to in vitro QAR, where the labeled peptide is applied to tissue sections in vitro. From Kurihara and Pardridge (1999) with permission.

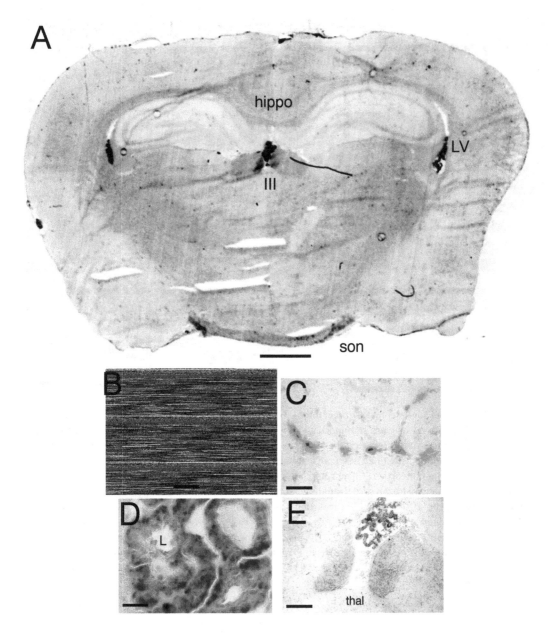

Figure 9.7 (A) β-galactosidase histochemistry in brain at 48 h after intravenous injection of the β-galactosidase gene packaged inside the OX26 pegylated immunoliposomes. hippo, hippocampus; LV, lateral ventricle; III, third ventricle; son, supraoptic nuclei. (B) Control brain from rats receiving no gene administration. (C) Punctate gene expression in intra-parenchymal capillaries is shown and may represent gene expression in either the endothelium or microvascular pericytes. (D) Gene expression in the epithelium of choroid plexus is shown. The lumen (L) of the capillary of the choroid plexus is labeled. The absence of β-galactosidase gene product in the capillary lumen demonstrates the β-galactosidase enzyme activity in the brain does not arise from enzyme in the plasma compartment. (E) The thalamic (thal) nuclei below the choroid plexus of the third ventricle are shown. Magnification bars: (A) 1.5 mm, (B) 2.2 mm, (C) 57 μm, (D) 23 μm, and (E) 230 μm. Panels A and B were not counterstained. From Shi, N. and Pardridge, W.M. (2000). Antisense imaging of gene expression in the brain in vivo. *Proc. Natl Acad. Sci. USA*, **97**, 14709–14. Copyright (2000) National Academy of Sciences, USA.

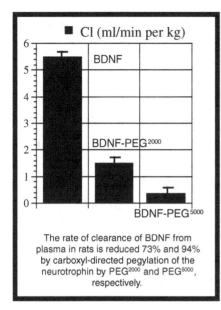

The rate of clearance of BDNF from plasma in rats is reduced 73% and 94% by carboxyl-directed pegylation of the neurotrophin by PEG^{2000} and PEG^{5000}, respectively.

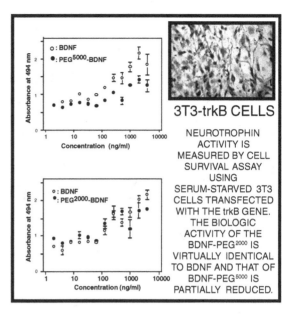

3T3-trkB CELLS

NEUROTROPHIN ACTIVITY IS MEASURED BY CELL SURVIVAL ASSAY USING SERUM-STARVED 3T3 CELLS TRANSFECTED WITH THE trkB GENE. THE BIOLOGIC ACTIVITY OF THE BDNF-PEG^{2000} IS VIRTUALLY IDENTICAL TO BDNF AND THAT OF BDNF-PEG^{5000} IS PARTIALLY REDUCED.

Figure 6.12   Left: Plasma pharmacokinetics showing the rate of clearance (Cl) of [^{125}I] brain-derived neurotrophic factor (BDNF), [^{125}I]BDNF-polyethylene glycol (PEG)^{2000}, and [^{125}I]BDNF-PEG^{5000}. Right: Retention of biologic activity. Cell survival assays of 3T3 cells permanently transfected with the trkB receptor following exposure to BDNF, BDNF-PEG^{2000}, or BDNF-PEG^{5000}. From Sakane and Pardridge (1997) with permission.

and Pardridge, 1997). In contrast, the rates of plasma clearance of the BDNF-PEG^{2000} and the BDNF-PEG^{5000} were reduced to 1.4 ± 0.1 and 0.37 ± 0.01 ml/min per kg (Figure 4.16). Therefore, the carboxyl-directed pegylation of BDNF with either PEG^{2000} or PEG^{5000} resulted in either a 67% or a 91% decrease in the plasma clearance of the BDNF. The hepatic clearance of the BDNF, BDNF-PEG^{2000}, and BDNF-PEG^{5000} was 61 ± 2, 22 ± 3, and 5.1 ± 0.7 μl/min per g, respectively. The reduction in plasma clearance was paralleled exactly by the reduction in hepatic clearance of the BDNF following carboxyl-directed protein pegylation (Sakane and Pardridge, 1997).

The biologic activity of the BDNF following carboxyl-directed protein pegylation with either PEG^{2000} or PEG^{5000} was examined in cell survival assays using National Institute of Health (NIH) 3T3 cells permanently transfected with the BDNF receptor, which is trkB. The expression of immunoreactive trkB in this cell was demonstrated with an anti-trkB antiserum, as shown in the immunocytochemistry studies of Figure 6.12. Although there is a partial reduction in biologic activity of the BDNF following pegylation with PEG^{5000}, there is no reduction in biologic activity of the BDNF following carboxyl-directed protein pegylation with PEG^{2000} (Figure 6.12).

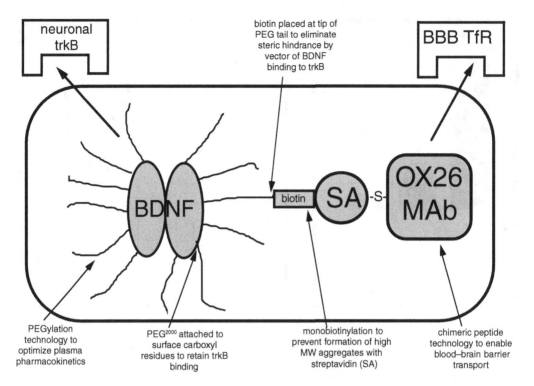

Figure 6.13   Structure of brain-derived neurotrophic factor (BDNF) chimeric peptide that employs
carboxyl-directed protein pegylation technology, avidin-biotin technology, and chimeric
peptide technology. The receptor for BDNF is the neuronal trkB receptor and the receptor
for the OX26 monoclonal antibody (MAb) is the blood–brain barrier (BBB) transferrin
receptor (TfR). The targeting vector is the conjugate of the OX26 monoclonal antibody
(MAb) and streptavidin (SA) joined by a stable thioether (-S-) linker. PEG, polyethylene
glycol; MW, molecular weight.

Formulation of BDNF chimeric peptides

The capture of the BDNF-PEG^{2000}-biotin by a conjugate of the OX26 MAb and SA
results in the formation of the BDNF chimeric peptide shown in Figure 6.13. To
prevent multibiotinylation, it was necessary to place only a single biotin moiety at
the tip of the PEG strand per individual BDNF homodimer. This was achieved by
using a 7% formulation, wherein the amount of Hz-PEG^{2000}-biotin relative to the
total Hz-PEG^{2000}-CH$_3$, was 7% (Pardridge et al., 1998b). There are multiple design
features of the conjugate shown in Figure 6.13. First, protein pegylation technology was used to optimize plasma pharmacokinetics (Figure 6.12). Second, the
PEG^{2000} was attached to surface carboxyl residues, not to amino groups, in order to
retain trkB binding and biologic activity (Figure 6.12). Third, only a single biotin
moiety per BDNF homodimer was present to enable monobiotinylation and

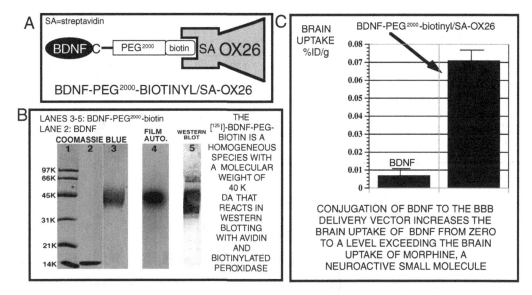

Figure 6.14   (A) Structure of brain-derived neurotrophic factor (BDNF) chimeric peptide. (B) Sodium dodecylsulfate polyacrylamide gel electrophoresis (SDS-PAGE), film autoradiography (auto.), and Western blotting of [^{125}I]BDNF-polyethylene glycol (PEG)^{2000}-biotin. (C) Brain uptake of either the [^{125}I]BDNF or the [^{125}I]BDNF-PEG^{2000}-biotin conjugated to SA-OX26 in anesthetized rats. From Pardridge et al. (1998b) with permission.

prevent the formation of high molecular weight aggregates with SA. Fourth, the chimeric peptide technology was used to enable BBB transport of the complex. Fifth, the biotin moiety was placed at the tip of the PEG tail to eliminate steric hindrance caused by the PEG strands. If the biotin had been conjugated to the surface of the BDNF protein, then the PEG strands would interfere with binding of the OX26/SA to the BDNF-PEG^{2000}-biotin. Similarly, binding of the OX26/SA to the surface of the BDNF protein would cause steric interference with BDNF binding to trkB.

The formulation of the BDNF attached to OX26/SA depicted in Figure 6.14A involves the use of the pegylated BDNF that contains the PEG^{2000} linker between the BDNF carboxyl residue and the biotin moiety. Following attachment of the PEG^{2000} to the BDNF carboxyl residues, the molecular weight of the BDNF monomer was increased from 14 kDa to approximately 40 kDa, as shown by Coomassie blue staining of SDS-PAGE gels (lanes 1–3, Figure 6.14B). Film autoradiography demonstrated the radiolabeled form of BDNF had a molecular weight identical to the BDNF detected by the Coomassie blue staining (lane 4, Figure 6.14B). Western blotting allowed for the detection of the biotin residue on the BDNF-PEG^{2000}-biotin and the molecular weight of the BDNF determined by

ACTIVATION OF AUTOPHOSPHORYLATION OF trkB BY BDNF IS UNAFFECTED BY CARBOXYL-DIRECTED PEGYLATION, BIOTINYLATION, AND CONJUGATION OF BDNF TO OX26/STREPTAVIDIN (SA)

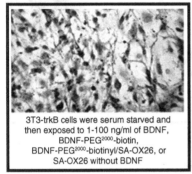

3T3-trkB cells were serum starved and then exposed to 1-100 ng/ml of BDNF, BDNF-PEG^{2000}-biotin, BDNF-PEG^{2000}-biotinyl/SA-OX26, or SA-OX26 without BDNF

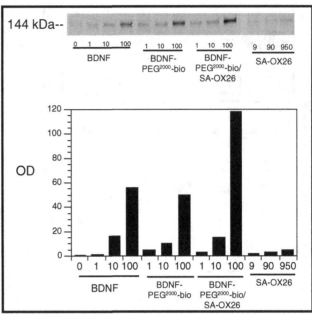

Figure 6.15   Left: 3T3 cells that were permanently transfected with a gene encoding the trkB BDNF receptor are immunostained using an antiserum to trkB, and this shows abundant expression of the trkB in the majority of these cells. Right: The top panel shows the antiphosphotyrosine Western blot. The bottom panel is the densitometric scan of the Western blot and shows retention of the biologic activity of the BDNF following pegylation and conjugation to the SA-OX26 delivery system. From Pardridge et al. (1998b) with permission.

Western blotting (lane 5, Figure 6.14B) was identical to that detected with either Coomassie blue staining or film autoradiography. The [^{125}I]BDNF-PEG^{2000}-biotinyl/SA-OX26 conjugate was injected intravenously into anesthetized rats and the brain uptake was measured 60 min later. These studies show a brain uptake of 0.07%ID/g (Figure 6.14C) which is the level of brain uptake comparable to that of morphine, a neuroactive small molecule (Wu et al., 1997a). Conversely, the brain uptake of the [^{125}I]BDNF was negligible and indicative of a lack of transport of BDNF across the BBB, as discussed in Chapter 4, and shown in Figure 4.16.

The retention of the biologic activity of BDNF following pegylation, biotinylation, and attachment to the SA-OX26 targeting vector was demonstrated with trkB autophosphorylation assays, as outlined in Figure 6.15. In these studies, the 3T3 cells permanently transfected with the trkB receptor were serum-starved and then exposed to 1–100 ng/ml concentrations of BDNF, BDNF-PEG^{2000}-biotin (bio),

BDNF-PEG^{2000}-bio conjugated to SA/OX26, or unconjugated SA/OX26. The molecular weight ratio of the SA/OX26 to BDNF-PEG^{2000}-biotin was 9:1. Therefore, the control experiments with the unconjugated SA/OX26 employed concentrations of the targeting vector at a level of 9–950 ng/ml (Figure 6.15). Following exposure of the cells to the BDNF solutions for 15 min at 37 °C, the media was aspirated, the cells were lysed, and immunoprecipitated with an anti-trkB antiserum followed by protein G affinity chromatography, and SDS-PAGE on 7.5% polyacrylamide gels (Pardridge et al., 1998b). Following SDS-PAGE, the gel was blotted to a filter, which was stained with 2 μg/ml antiphosphotyrosine antibody. The filter was then scanned and the signal quantitated with NIH image software. The molecular size of the trkB immunoprecipitate was estimated with biotinylated molecular weight standards and was 144 kDa, as shown in Figure 6.15. These studies show that the biologic activity of the BDNF was completely retained following carboxyl-directed protein pegylation and conjugation to SA/OX26 (Figure 6.15).

In summary, carboxyl-directed protein pegylation technology and avidin-biotin technology were combined to construct the BDNF chimeric peptide shown in Figure 6.13. All three goals were achieved: (a) optimization of plasma pharmacokinetics with protein pegylation technology, (b) complete retention of biologic activity using carboxyl-directed protein pegylation, (c) bifunctionality of the chimeric peptide with the retention of trkB binding (Figure 6.15) and efficient transport through the BBB via the transferrin receptor (Figure 6.14). The biologic activity of the BDNF chimeric peptide outlined in Figure 6.13 was further proved by the demonstration of in vivo CNS pharmacologic effects in global or regional ischemia, as discussed in Chapter 7.

Use of extended polyethylene glycol linkers

Synthesis of biotinylated EGF with short and extended linkers

A second application of protein pegylation technology in brain drug targeting is the use of PEG strands to form extended linkers between the drug and the targeting vector. When protein pegylation is used to delay the rapid plasma clearance of a protein, and to optimize plasma pharmacokinetics, then it is necessary to attach *multiple* PEG strands per individual drug molecule (Deguchi et al., 1999). However, when protein pegylation technology is used to extend the linker between the drug and the vector, then only a *single* PEG strand is attached to each drug molecule. This is outlined in the case of EGF chimeric peptides, as shown in Figure 6.16A. As discussed in Chapter 7, EGF peptide radiopharmaceuticals are potential new imaging agents for diagnosis of brain tumors, which overexpress the EGF receptor (EGFR). The EGF can be radiolabeled with either iodine-125 or

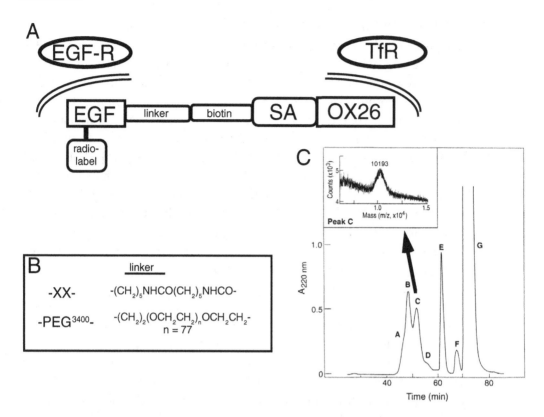

Figure 6.16   (A) Structure of epidermal growth factor (EGF) chimeric peptide with a linker between the
biotin moiety and the EGF. (B) Two types of linkers were used: a 14 atom bis-
aminohexanoyl linker, designated -XX-, and a >200 atom polyethylene glycol (PEG) linker,
designated (PEG)^{3400}. (C) Purification of monobiotinylated diethylenetriaminepentaacetic
acid (DTPA)-EGF-PEG^{3400}-biotin by two gel filtration fast protein liquid chromatography
(FPLC) columns in series. Peak A is EGF-(PEG^{3400}-biotin)$_3$. Peak B is DTPA-EGF-(PEG^{3400}-
biotin)$_2$. Peak C is DTPA-EGF-PEG^{3400}-biotin. Peak D is DTPA-EGF. Peak E is DTPA. Peak F is
N-hydroxysuccinimide (NHS)-PEG^{3400}-biotin. Peak G is a solvent peak. The insert is matrix-
assisted laser desorption ionization (MALDI) mass spectra and shows the molecular mass
(10 193) for peak C. The n designation of the (PEG^{3400}-biotin) $_n$ refers to the number of
PEG^{3400} strands conjugated to the EGF. EGF-R, EGF receptor; SA, streptavidin; TFR,
transferrin receptor. Reprinted with permission from Deguchi et al. (1999). Copyright
(1999) American Chemical Society.

indium-111. The particular advantages of using the indium-111 radionuclide are
discussed in Chapter 4 and shown in Figure 4.17. The EGF is monobiotinylated
with a linker between the ε-amino moiety of a lysine residue on the EGF and the
biotin moiety. The linker is comprised of either the bis-aminohexanoyl or -XX-
linker, which is comprised of 14 atoms, or an extended PEG linker of 3400 Da

molecular weight, designated PEG^{3400}, as shown in Figure 6.16B. The length of the PEG^{3400} linker is >200 atoms. The biotin moiety is then captured by the conjugate of SA and the OX26 MAb, which binds the transferrin receptor (TfR). The EGF-PEG^{3400}-biotin was purified through two Superose 12HR gel filtration fast protein liquid chromatography (FPLC) columns in series and the structure was determined by matrix-assisted laser desorption ionization (MALDI) mass spectrometry, as shown in Figure 6.16C. The EGF-PEG^{3400}-biotin shown in Figure 6.16C also contained a single DTPA moiety for chelation of indium-111, where DTPA is diethylenetriaminepentaacetic acid, and this conjugate is designated DTPA-EGF-PEG^{3400}-biotin. The formulation of the EGF following conjugation with NHS-PEG^{3400}-biotin was analyzed by SDS-PAGE and Western blotting, as shown in Figure 6.17A. The Coomassie blue stain of the SDS-PAGE gel shows the molecular weight of the unconjugated EGF is 6200 Da and a second band is formed on the gel when the NHS-PEG^{3400}-biotin is added. This band is seen in lanes 1–4 of Figure 6.17A, and this migrates at a molecular size of 10 kDa, which approximates the expected molecular weight, 9900 Da, of EGF with a single PEG^{3400}-biotin residue attached (Kurihara et al., 1999). At the higher molar ratio of NHS-PEG^{3400}-biotin:EGF, an additional band is detected which migrates at 16 kDa and approximates the expected molecular weight of EGF with two PEG^{3400}-biotin moieties attached. The incorporation of the biotin residue in the pegylated EGF was confirmed by Western blotting, as shown in Figure 6.17A.

Biologic activity of the EGF chimeric peptides with short and extended linkers

The biologic activity of the EGF chimeric peptide was examined with RRAs C6 rat glioma cells (Deguchi et al., 1999) that had been permanently transfected with a gene encoding the human EGFR (Capala et al., 1997). These cells are designated C6–EGFR cells. In this case, the transgene was under the influence of a dexamethasone-inducible promoter (Capala et al., 1997), and the C6 glioma cells were exposed to 1 μmol/l dexamethasone in tissue culture (Deguchi et al., 1999). When the EGF-XX-biotin was conjugated to OX26/SA, and added to the C6–EGFR cells, there was no significant binding of the EGF chimeric peptide to the EGF receptor. However, when the EGF-XX-biotin, without conjugation to OX26/SA, was added to the C6–EGFR cells, there was full binding of the EGF to its cognate receptor. These studies indicated that biotinylation, per se, did not impair EGF binding to the EGFR, but attachment of the EGF-XX-biotin to the OX26/SA conjugate completely aborted binding of the EGF chimeric peptide to the EGF receptor. This was not particularly surprising because the molecular weight of the EGF is approximately 6 kDa, whereas the molecular weight of the OX26/SA is 200 kDa. Binding of the EGF to the OX26/SA via a short 14-atom -XX-linker resulted in complete steric hindrance of EGF binding to its cognate receptor caused by the OX26/SA (Deguchi et al., 1999). This steric hindrance was eliminated by

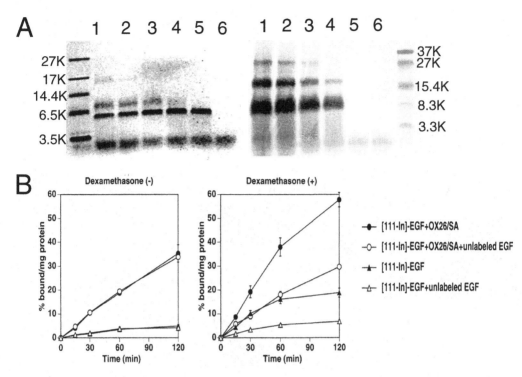

Figure 6.17 (A) Sodium dodecylsulfate polyacrylamide gel electrophoresis (SDS-PAGE) (left) and Western blotting (right) of epidermal growth factor-polyethylene glycol (EGF-PEG)^{3400}-biotin. Reaction mixture of EGF and varying concentrations of N-hydroxysuccinimide (NHS)-PEG^{3400}-biotin was applied to 16.5% SDS-PAGE minigels. The gel slab was either stained with Coomassie blue for protein content (left) or blotted to a nylon membrane followed by staining with avidin and biotinylated peroxidase to visualize attachment of the PEG^{3400}-biotin to the EGF molecule (right). The molar ratio of NHS-PEG^{3400}-biotin:EGF in the reaction mixture was 5:1 (lane 1), 4:1 (lane 2), 2:1 (lane 3), 1:1 (lane 4), 0:1 (lane 5), and 5:0 (lane 6). (B) Radioreceptor assay showing time course of binding of either [^{111}In]diethylenetriaminepentaacetic acid (DTPA)-EGF-PEG^{3400}-biotin conjugated to OX26/SA (circles) or binding of [^{111}In]DTPA-EGF-PEG^{3400}-biotin (triangles) to C6 rat glioma cells transfected with the human EGF receptor gene. Assays were performed in the presence (right panel) or absence (left panel) of prior dexamethasone (1 μmol/l) stimulation and in the presence (open circles) or absence (closed circles) of 1 μmol/l unlabeled EGF. Each point is the mean $\pm$ SE ($n = 3$). Reprinted with permission from Kurihara et al. (1999). Copyright (1999) American Chemical Society.

substitution of the 14-atom -XX-linker with a >200 atom PEG^{3400} linker, as outlined in Figure 6.16B. The biologic activity of the [^{111}In]DTPA-EGF-PEG^{3400}-biotin conjugated to OX26/SA was demonstrated with RRAs using the C6–EGFR cells and these studies are shown in Figure 6.17B. In the absence of dexamethasone pretreatment, there is little induction of the EGF receptor in these cells and there was minimal binding of unconjugated [^{111}In]EGF to the cells. However, there was significant binding of the [^{111}In]EGF-PEG^{3400}-biotin/SA-OX26 to the C6–EGFR cells that were not pretreated with dexamethasone, owing to the expression of the TfR on these cells (Deguchi et al., 1999). The conjugate bound to both the TfR and the EGF receptor on the cells, when the EGF receptor was induced by dexamethasone pretreatment. The saturation analysis demonstrated that the ED$_{50}$ of EGF competition of the binding of [^{111}In]EGF-PEG^{3400}-biotin/SA-OX26 was approximately 1 nmol/l (Deguchi et al., 1999).

In summary, the studies outlined in Figures 6.16 and 6.17 indicate the use of single extended PEG linkers in the construction of chimeric peptides can result in complete restoration of biologic activity despite conjugation to the BBB drug-targeting systems. The utility of EGF chimeric peptides for imaging brain tumors is discussed further in Chapter 7.

Liposome technology

The conjugation of drugs to BBB drug-targeting vectors using chemical linkers, avidin-biotin technology, or genetically engineered fusion proteins, results in the attachment of no more than one to four drug molecules per individual transport vector molecule. However, the use of liposome technology offers the capability of greatly increasing the ratio of drug molecules conjugated to individual vector molecules. More than 10 000 small molecules may be entrapped in a single 100-nm liposome. The lipid/drug ratio of a 100-nm liposome is 3.2 (Mayer et al., 1989). Given approximately 100 000 lipid molecules on the liposome surface, then more than 28 000 small molecules could be packaged within a single 100 nm liposome (Huwyler et al., 1996). Therefore, the use of both liposome technology and chimeric peptide technology could result in a greatly increased ratio of drug molecules conjugated per individual targeting vector (Figure 6.18).

Liposomes, even small unilamellar vesicles, on the order of 50–80 nm are too large to cross the BBB in vivo, as discussed in Chapter 3, in the absence of a BBB drug-targeting system. Moreover, liposomes have very poor plasma pharmacokinetic profiles in vivo. Upon injection of liposomes into the blood stream, the surface of these particles is immediately coated with plasma proteins (Chonn et al., 1992), and this triggers uptake by the RES in vivo. The absorption of plasma proteins to the surface of liposomes can be eliminated with liposome pegylation, as

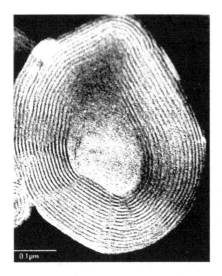

LIPOSOMES, EVEN SMALL UNILAMELLAR VESICLES,
ARE TOO LARGE TO CROSS THE BLOOD–BRAIN
BARRIER (BBB)

LIPOSOMES HAVE POOR PHARMACOKINETICS IN
VIVO OWING TO RAPID REMOVAL FROM THE
BLOOD STREAM BY THE RETICULOENDOTHELIAL
SYSTEM

HYPOTHESIS
BOTH PROBLEMS OF POOR BBB TRANSPORT AND
POOR PLASMA PHARMACOKINETICS (PK) OF
LIPOSOMES MAY BE CIRCUMVENTED WITH THE
USE OF SPECIALLY FORMULATED PEGYLATED
IMMUNOLIPOSOMES.

PEGYLATION TECHNOLOGY OPTIMIZES PK, AND
VECTOR MEDIATION ENABLES BBB TRANSPORT

Figure 6.18 Liposomes as brain drug delivery vehicles. Left: Structure of a multilamellar liposome with a diameter of 400–500 nm. From Gregoriadis (1976) with permission. Right: Hypothesis regarding the use of pegylated immunoliposomes for brain drug targeting.

discussed in Chapter 3. The pegylated liposomes are also referred to as "sterically stabilized" or "stealth" liposomes (Mori et al., 1991; Papahadjopoulos et al., 1991).

The construction of pegylated immunoliposomes designed for drug transport across the BBB was discussed in Chapter 3 and outlined in Figure 3.8. The enhancement of the pharmacokinetic profile with the use of pegylation technology for liposomes is shown in Figure 3.9. The brain uptake of pegylated immunoliposomes using both liposome technology and chimeric peptide technology is demonstrated in Figure 3.9. The binding of OX26 pegylated immunoliposomes to the TfR on isolated rat brain capillaries or the endocytosis of OX26 pegylated immunoliposomes into rat glioma cells bearing the TfR is shown in Figure 3.10.

The use of pegylated immunoliposomes for brain drug targeting was reduced to practice for small molecules such as daunomycin, as discussed in Chapter 3. However, a novel application of pegylated immunoliposomes for brain drug targeting is the use of these formulations for brain drug targeting of gene medicines, which is demonstrated in Chapter 9.

Summary

In the conventional drug discovery and drug development pathway, there is a typical algorithm for the drug discovery process. A similar algorithm exists for drug-targeting technology, as outlined in Figure 6.19. The drug discovery program

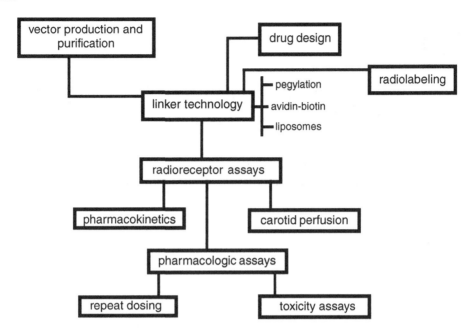

Figure 6.19 Pathway of preclinical evaluation in brain drug-targeting research. From Gregoriadis (1976). Copyright © 1976 Massachusetts Medical Society. All rights reserved.

yields new drug candidates and the vector discovery program yields the targeting vector candidate. However, following initial vector production and purification and initial drug design, the linker technology must then be employed and this could incorporate pegylation technology, avidin-biotin technology, liposome technology, and radionuclide technology, as outlined in Figure 6.19. The bifunctionality of the drug/vector conjugate is verified in radioreceptor assays that analyze the affinity of the conjugate for both the cognate receptor of the drug and the targeting vector. Next, in vivo assays must be performed that examine the pharmacokinetics and metabolic stability of the drug/vector complex in vivo. Additional in vivo studies must be performed to demonstrate BBB transport of the conjugate. Finally, pharmacologic assays are performed in vivo to demonstrate in vivo CNS pharmacologic effects, as well as the pharmacodynamics of the chimeric peptide in the brain in vivo. Toxicity studies and repeat dosing experiments are also performed to complete the preclinical evaluation of the BBB chimeric peptide designated for in vivo CNS applications.

7

Protein neurotherapeutics and peptide radiopharmaceuticals

- Introduction
- Peptide neurotherapeutics
- Peptide radiopharmaceuticals as neurodiagnostics
- Summary

Introduction

The human brain uses less than a dozen monoaminergic or aminoacidergic neurotransmitter systems, but employs hundreds of peptidergic neurotransmission and neuromodulation systems. Therefore, targeting neuropeptide receptor systems in the brain offers numerous opportunities for the development of novel neurotherapeutics and neurodiagnostics for the treatment and diagnosis of brain diseases (Pardridge, 1991). One approach to the development of peptide-based neuropharmaceuticals is the discovery of small molecule peptidomimetics. However, there are two problems with small molecule drug development. First, small molecule peptidomimetic drugs, should they be discovered, tend to be peptide receptor antagonists, not agonists (Hefti, 1997). When the endogenous ligand is more than 10 amino acids in length, there are few, if any, examples of pharmacologically active small molecule peptidomimetics in clinical practice. The second problem is that, even if a small molecule peptidomimetic drug was discovered, the molecule would still need a blood–brain barrier (BBB) drug-targeting system if the molecule did not have the dual molecular characteristics of (a) lipid-solubility, and (b) molecular weight under a threshold of 400–600 Da (Chapter 3).

Given the problems inherent in the drug discovery of functional small molecule peptidomimetics, and given the abundance of known endogenous neuropeptides that are biochemically characterized, one could ask why there is not a single neuropeptide presently in clinical practice as either a neurotherapeutic or neurodiagnostic agent for the central nervous system (CNS)? Neuropeptides have not been developed as neuropharmaceuticals because, with few exceptions, neuropeptides do not cross the BBB in pharmacologically significant amounts. As discussed in Chapter 3, neuropeptides – even an oligopeptide as small as two amino acids – form more than eight to ten hydrogen bonds with solvent water and this greatly restricts BBB transport of the molecule. The addition of each amino acid results in a further log order decrease in BBB transport of a peptide. Therefore, neuropeptides do not cross the BBB unless these molecules have an affinity for particular receptor-mediated transcytosis systems (Chapter 4).

Neuropeptides can be used for the treatment and diagnosis of brain disorders should these molecules be made transportable through the BBB with brain drug-targeting technology. This chapter will review four examples of peptide neuropharmaceuticals – two neurotherapeutics and two neurodiagnostics. The peptides reviewed in this chapter are vasoactive intestinal peptide (VIP), a drug that increases cerebral blood flow (CBF); brain-derived neurotrophic factor (BDNF), a neuroprotection agent; epidermal growth factor (EGF), a peptide radiopharmaceutical for early diagnosis of brain cancer; and $A\beta$ neuropeptide, a potential amyloid imaging agent for the diagnosis of Alzheimer's disease (AD). In each of the four cases, it will be shown that VIP, BDNF, EGF, and $A\beta^{1-40}$ do not cross the BBB and do not cause an in vivo CNS pharmacologic effect without a BBB drug-targeting system. Conversely, in vivo CNS pharmacologic effects can be achieved when these neuropeptides are delivered through the BBB using the chimeric peptide technology for brain drug targeting. These cases also illustrate the inherent amplification when CNS drug development is practiced from a platform of CNS drug targeting. The development of a *single*, multifunctional brain drug-targeting technology enables the creation of *multiple* pathways of CNS drug development. There is virtually an unlimited number of neuropeptide-based drugs that are pharmacologically inactive in the absence of a brain drug-targeting technology, but which have remarkable in vivo CNS pharmacologic effects when delivered through the BBB using brain drug-targeting technology.

Peptide neurotherapeutics

VIP as a cerebral blood flow enhancer

VIP and cerebral blood flow

The principle vasodilator in the human brain is VIP. The expression of both VIP and VIP receptors is abundant throughout the brain and these pathways serve a number of functions in the brain, including the regulation of CBF (Bottjer et al., 1984). When VIP is applied topically to pial vessels, there is vasodilatation (Lindvall and Owan, 1981). However, when VIP is infused into the carotid artery of multiple species, there is no enhancement of CBF (McCulloch and Edvinsson, 1980; Wilson et al., 1981), because VIP does not cross the BBB (Bickel et al., 1993a). VIP is also a principal vasodilator in exocrine and endocrine glands in the periphery, and the intravenous injection of VIP results in an increase in blood flow in salivary gland (Huffman et al., 1988). VIP causes an enhancement of organ blood flow by triggering VIP receptors on precapillary arteriolar smooth muscle cells (Itakura et al., 1984), which results in vasodilatation. These VIP receptors on smooth muscle cells are situated beyond the BBB in brain. Because VIP has a molecular weight of only 5 kDa, the molecule freely traverses the porous endothelial wall in peripheral tissues such as salivary gland and causes an increase in blood flow in that tissue after systemic (intravenous) administration (Huffman et al., 1988). The studies described below will show that VIP can result in substantial increases in CBF following intravenous injection providing the neuropeptide is conjugated to a BBB drug-targeting system. These studies with VIP chimeric peptides will also illustrate the targeting capabilities of the chimeric peptide technology (Wu and Pardridge, 1996). When VIP is conjugated to the BBB drug-targeting system, comprised of a monoclonal antibody (MAb) and streptavidin (SA), the effective molecular weight of the VIP increases from 5 kDa to 205 kDa, because the molecular weight of the MAb/SA conjugate is 200 kDa. This increased size results in a restriction in the free movement of VIP across the capillary wall in peripheral tissue such as salivary gland (Wu and Pardridge, 1996). It will be shown that when VIP is conjugated to the brain drug-targeting system, there is a selective increase in pharmacologic action of the neuropeptide in the targeted end organ (brain). However, conjugation of the VIP to the targeting agent causes an abolition of pharmacologic effects in peripheral tissues (salivary gland), where no pharmacologic effect is desired.

Molecular formulation of VIP chimeric peptide

The amino acid sequence of the VIP analog (VIPa) that was specifically designed for monobiotinylation (Bickel et al., 1993a), was discussed in Chapter 6 and shown in Figure 6.4. The first-generation VIP chimeric peptide employed a cleavable (disulfide) linker between the peptide and the biotin moiety (Figure 6.5). The biotin-SS-VIPa was then bound to a conjugate of the OX26 MAb to the rat transferrin receptor and avidin (AV), designated OX26/AV. The intracarotid infusion of this VIP chimeric peptide in nitrous oxide-ventilated rats resulted in a 65% increase in CBF (Bickel et al., 1993a). This VIP chimeric peptide was administered by intracarotid infusion, because the pharmacokinetic profile of this chimeric peptide would not be optimal owing to the use of the cationic avidin in the conjugate, as described in Chapter 6.

In order to achieve an in vivo CNS pharmacologic effect with VIP chimeric peptides in conscious rats following intravenous administration, it was necessary to make changes in the original formulation. The second-generation VIP chimeric peptide contained a noncleavable (-XX-) linker between the peptide and the biotin, and contained an SA moiety in lieu of the avidin (Wu and Pardridge, 1996). The use of SA instead of avidin results in an optimization of the plasma pharmacoki-

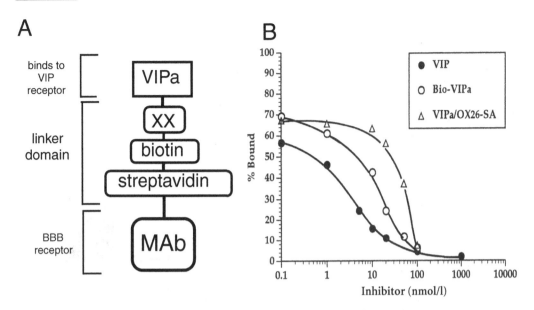

Figure 7.1   Vasoactive intestinal peptide (VIP) radioreceptor assay shows VIP chimeric peptide has high affinity for the mammalian VIP receptor. (A) Structure of the VIP chimeric peptide, which is comprised of three domains. The first domain is the VIP analog (VIPa) that binds the VIP receptor. The second domain is the linker domain, which is comprised of streptavidin, which binds the biotin, which is conjugated to an internal lysine residue on the VIPa via a 14-atom bis-aminohexanoyl (-XX-) linker. The third domain is the targeting domain comprised of a monoclonal antibody (MAb) that targets an endogenous peptide receptor on the BBB such as the transferrin receptor or the insulin receptor. (B) Competition curves of three VIP analogs in a radioreceptor assay using rat lung membranes and [^{125}I]mammalian VIP as the tracer. The ED$_{50}$ values for the VIP, the biotin-XX-VIPa (bioVIPa), and the biotin-XX-VIPa conjugated to OX26/SA (VIPa/OX26–SA) are 3, 12, and 45 nmol/l, respectively. A 100 nmol/l concentration of the OX26/SA conjugate, without VIPa attached, had no effect on the binding of [^{125}I]VIP. Reproduced in part from Wu and Pardridge (1996) with permission and Pardridge (1998c) with permission. © 1998 The Alfred Benzon Foundation, DK-2900 Hellerup, Denmark.

netic profile and an increased plasma area under the concentration curve (AUC), as discussed in Chapter 6. The advantages of using the noncleavable amide linker are also reviewed in Chapter 6. The use of this noncleavable linker requires that the chimeric peptide trigger the VIP receptor when the neuropeptide is presented to the receptor while the bio-XX-VIPa is still bound to OX26/SA.

The structure of the second-generation VIP chimeric peptide is shown in Figure 7.1A. The VIP was monobiotinylated with NHS-XX-biotin, where NHS is N-hydroxysuccinimide, and -XX- is a 14-atom bis-aminohexanoyl linker. A conjugate of the OX26 MAb and SA was formed with a stable thioether linker. Owing to

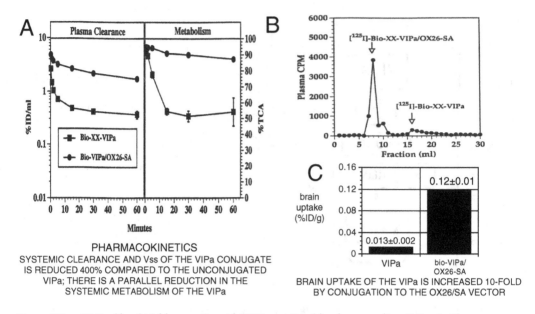

PHARMACOKINETICS
SYSTEMIC CLEARANCE AND Vss OF THE VIPa CONJUGATE
IS REDUCED 400% COMPARED TO THE UNCONJUGATED
VIPa; THERE IS A PARALLEL REDUCTION IN THE
SYSTEMIC METABOLISM OF THE VIPa

BRAIN UPTAKE OF THE VIPa IS INCREASED 10-FOLD
BY CONJUGATION TO THE OX26/SA VECTOR

Figure 7.2   (A) Profile of trichloroacetic acid (TCA)-precipitable plasma radioactivity of either unconjugated [^{125}I]biotin-XX-vasoactive intestinal peptide analog (bio-XX-VIPa) (squares) or [^{125}I]bio-XX-VIPa conjugated to OX26/SA (circles) after intravenous dose of 5 μCi/rat. The plasma radioactivity, expressed as percentage injected dose (%ID)/ml, is shown in the left panel and the percentage of plasma radioactivity that is precipitable by TCA is shown in the right panel. (B) Gel filtration high performance liquid chromatography (HPLC) of pooled plasma samples collected 60 min after intravenous injection of the [^{125}I]bio-XX-VIPa/OX26–SA conjugate in three rats. (C) Brain uptake of either unconjugated VIPa or VIPa chimeric peptide. From Wu and Pardridge (1996) with permission.

the high affinity of SA binding of biotin, there was instantaneous capture of the biotin-XX-VIPa by the OX26/SA to form the conjugate shown in Figure 7.1A. The affinity of the intact conjugate for the mammalian VIP receptor was determined with a VIP radioreceptor assay (RRA) using [^{125}I]VIP as the ligand and rat lung membranes as the source of mammalian VIP receptor (Wu and Pardridge, 1996). The results of the VIP RRA are shown in Figure 7.1B and indicate the biotin-XX-VIPa still binds to the VIP receptor when presented to the receptor in the form of the intact conjugate and bound to OX26/SA.

Pharmacokinetics and metabolic stability

The biotin-XX-[^{125}I]VIPa was injected intravenously into anesthetized rats. A pharmacokinetic analysis was made for both the unconjugated biotin-XX-VIPa and the conjugate of the biotin-XX-VIPa bound to OX26–SA. The pharmacokinetic profiles are shown in Figure 7.2A. The unconjugated biotin-XX-VIPa was rapidly removed from plasma with a plasma clearance of 5.0 ± 1.1 ml/min per kg (Wu and Pardridge, 1996). The unconjugated VIP was taken up by peripheral tissue with a systemic volume of distribution (V_{ss}) of 536 ± 35 ml/kg. The high rate of systemic clearance of the biotin-XX-VIPa is also reflected in the metabolic instability of the peptide as shown by the decrease in total plasma radioactivity that was precipitable by trichloroacetic acid (TCA), and this is shown in the right panel of Figure 7.2A. The plasma clearance and peripheral degradation of the VIPa were decreased following conjugation to OX26/SA as shown in Figure 7.2A. The plasma clearance was reduced nearly fivefold to 1.1 ± 0.1 ml/min per kg and the V_{ss} was also reduced nearly fivefold to 116 ± 14 ml/kg. Similarly, the metabolic stability of the VIP chimeric peptide was enhanced, as indicated by the plasma TCA profile (Figure 7.2A).

The stability of the VIP chimeric peptide following intravenous injection in rats was corroborated by gel filtration high performance liquid chromatography (HPLC) of plasma taken 60 min after intravenous injection of the [^{125}I]-labeled chimeric peptide, and these data are shown in Figure 7.2B. More than 90% of the plasma radioactivity obtained 60 min after intravenous injection migrated at 8 ml through the column, which is an elution volume identical to the biotin-XX-[^{125}I]VIPa/OX26–SA chimeric peptide, whereas residual radioactivity migrated at 16 ml through the column, a volume that approximates the salt volume of the column. Unconjugated biotin-XX-[^{125}I]VIPa that was not conjugated to OX26/SA also migrated at 16 ml in the gel filtration HPLC. These studies indicate the VIP chimeric peptide is metabolically stable throughout the 60-min experimental period and this metabolic stability allows for interpretation of the data on brain uptake of [^{125}I] radioactivity, which is shown in Figure 7.2C. As discussed in Chapter 4, if a neuropeptide is metabolically unstable in vivo, and rapidly converted to radiolabeled metabolites, it is difficult to interpret brain uptake of radioactivity. This is because the brain radioactivity reflects the uptake of labeled metabolites formed in the periphery, and not brain uptake of the intact neuropeptide. The data indicate there is negligible brain uptake of the unconjugated VIP consistent with lack of transport of this neuropeptide through the BBB. Conversely, the brain uptake of the VIP chimeric peptide is 0.12 ± 0.01%ID/g (Figure 7.2C), and this level of brain uptake is more than 50% greater than the brain uptake of morphine, a neuroactive small molecule (Wu et al., 1997a).

In summary, the data in Figure 7.2 indicate that conjugation of the VIP to the BBB drug-targeting system has two beneficial effects. First, the use of the brain drug-targeting system enables transport through the BBB and, second, conjugation to the targeting system slows the uptake of the peptide by peripheral tissues. This retardation of peripheral tissue uptake causes an increase in the metabolic stability of the neuropeptide. Attachment to the vector results in an increased BBB permeability–surface area (PS) product, and the delay in uptake by peripheral tissues results in an increase in the plasma AUC. As discussed in Chapter 3, an increase in the BBB PS product and an increase in the plasma AUC both contribute to an increased brain uptake, expressed as %ID/g.

Biotinidase

The metabolic stability of the VIP chimeric peptide using an avidin-biotin linker (Figure 7.2B) demonstrates that biotinidase activity is not a significant factor, at least in the rat in vivo. Biotinidase converts biocytin, which is a conjugate of biotin and lysine, to free biotin and lysine (Cole et al., 1994). Biocytin is rapidly degraded in plasma in vitro in certain species such as the dog or mouse and must be considered in any in vivo application of biotinylated therapeutics (Rosebrough, 1993; Foulon et al., 1998). However, if biotinidase was a significant factor in vivo in rats, then the metabolic stability of the VIP chimeric peptide formed with an avidin-biotin linker would not be observed. It is conceivable that biotinidase may be a prominent factor in certain species such as mice. In this case, biotin-cysteine analogs (Hashmi and Rosebrough, 1995), which form stable thioether linkers, and have resistance to biotinidase, may be preferred reagents for biotinylation.

VIP and cerebral blood flow in conscious rats

The method for measuring blood flow in conscious rats following intravenous injection of VIP chimeric peptides for both brain and a peripheral tissue, salivary gland, is outlined in Figure 7.3. The external organ technique uses [^{3}H]diazepam as a "fluid microsphere." In order to measure CBF in conscious animals, rats were surgically prepared with a femoral artery and femoral vein catheter by implanting PE50 tubing in the two vessels. These catheters were then exteriorized at the dorsal part of the neck with an adaptor and tubing stoppers under anesthesia (Wu and Pardridge, 1996). After a 24-h period of recovery, the conscious animals were moderately restrained with the use of a plastic holder. Mean arterial blood pressure (MABP) and organ blood flow were measured in a noise-controlled room with a temperature maintained at 26–28 °C, using the external organ technique and [^{3}H]diazepam. Because conscious animals were examined, immediate cardiac arrest was induced with intravenous KCl prior to decapitation. Four treatment groups were studied: control rats, rats given unconjugated biotin-XX-VIPa, rats given biotin-XX-VIPa conjugated to OX26–SA, and rats given OX26–SA without VIP attached. The MABP in the four groups was 107 ± 4, 91 ± 9, 98 ± 13, and 114 ± 7 mmHg, respectively. Both organ vascular conductance, which is a ratio of organ blood flow divided by MABP, and organ blood flow were measured. However, the changes in vascular conductance and organ blood flow were parallel,

METHODS

1. Implant and exteriorize femoral a. and v. cannulae 24 h in advance
2. Mean arterial blood pressure is measured in conscious rats with a tail pulse amplifier (IITC)
3. Inject VIP chimeric peptide intravenous at $t = -20$ min
4. Inject intravenous [^{3}H]diazepam, a "fluid microsphere," at $t = -30$ s, and withdraw femoral artery blood at 2 ml/min via syringe pump
5. Administer intravenous KCl at $t = -5$ s, and decapitate at $t = 0$
6. Measure [^{3}H]diazepam, in brain, salivary gland, and femoral a. "external organ"

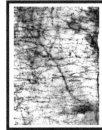

Intraparenchymal arteriolar smooth muscle cells in brain are richly innervated with VIPergic nerve endings that modulate cerebral blood flow

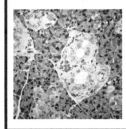

Salivary gland is perfused by porous microvessels that allow for the rapid organ uptake of small oligopeptides such as VIP from the circulation

Figure 7.3   Method for measuring blood flow in brain and salivary gland in conscious rats using the external organ technique. The immunocytochemistry of brain shows abundant vasoactive intestinal peptide (VIP)ergic nerve endings terminating on the smooth muscle cell of precapillary arterioles of brain (upper right), and is from Itakura et al. (1984) with permission. Hematoxylin and eosin stain of rat salivary gland (lower right panel).

because the effect of VIP chimeric peptides on MABP in conscious rats was minimal at the doses used in the study (Wu and Pardridge, 1996).

The effects on organ blood flow in brain and salivary gland following intravenous injection of VIP or VIP chimeric peptide in conscious rats are shown in Figure 7.4. The administration of the unconjugated VIPa, without the delivery system, resulted in a 350% increase in blood flow in salivary gland. Conversely, no effect of VIP on blood flow in brain was observed, because VIP does not cross the BBB (Figure 7.4). However, when the VIP chimeric peptide was administered, there was a 60% increase in CBF, but no change in blood flow in salivary gland (Wu and Pardridge, 1996).

The blood flow studies in Figure 7.4 demonstrate that conjugation of a peptide therapeutic to the BBB drug-targeting system directs the drug to the appropriate target organ (brain) to promote drug action, and restricts drug uptake by a peripheral tissue (salivary gland) and thereby reduces drug toxicity. The overall therapeutic index of a drug is the ratio of drug action/drug toxicity. In the case of VIP, the therapeutic index is proportional to the ratio of CBF/SBF, where SBF is salivary gland blood flow. The CBF/SBF ratio is 0.32 following administration of

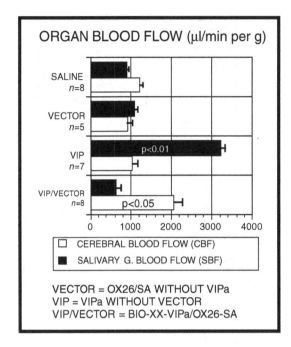
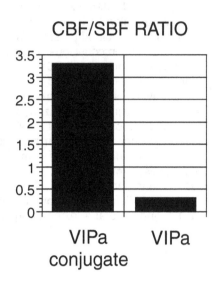

Figure 7.4   Left: Organ blood flow in brain and salivary gland. Right: Ratio of cerebral blood flow (CBF) to salivary gland blood flow (SBF) in rats administered vasoactive intestinal peptide (VIP) alone or VIP chimeric peptide. From Pardridge (1998c) with permission.

unconjugated VIP and is increased 10-fold to 3.3 following the administration of the VIP chimeric peptide (Figure 7.4). Therefore, the BBB drug-targeting system increased the therapeutic index of the VIP by 1000%.

In summary, the data in Figures 7.1–7.4 indicate substantial increases in CBF can be achieved in vivo in conscious rats using VIP chimeric peptides administered intravenously at relatively low doses of 5 µg/rat (Wu and Pardridge, 1996). The results with the VIP chimeric peptide also demonstrate the potential of targeting technology to increase the therapeutic index of a drug by targeting a drug to a specific end organ and restricting the uptake in peripheral tissues (Figure 7.4).

BDNF chimeric peptides and neuroprotection in cerebral ischemia

Neurotrophins and neurologic disease

There are more than 30 different neurotrophic factors discovered to date (Hefti, 1997), and these peptides all have remarkable pharmacologic effects when directly injected into the brain. The neurotrophic factors could be used as neurotherapeutics for the treatment of chronic neurodegenerative disease or for the treatment of acute brain disorders such as stroke or trauma. In the 1990s, a considerable effort was devoted to the development of neurotrophic factors for the treatment of a neurodegenerative condition, amyotrophic lateral sclerosis (ALS), as shown in Figure 1.6. In this instance, the neurotrophins were administered by subcutaneous administration, apparently without consideration as to whether these proteins crossed the BBB (The BDNF Study Group, 1999). Neurotrophic factors such as ciliary neurotrophic factor (CNTF) or insulin-like growth factor (IGF)1 were entered into clinical trials for treatment of ALS based largely on in vitro data obtained in cell culture (Hefti, 1997). The clinical trials went forward with the treatment of ALS patients with BDNF, CNTF, or IGF1 following subcutaneous administration. The phase III clinical trials all failed. None of these neurotrophic factors cross the BBB. BDNF and CNTF do not have BBB transport systems and do not cross the BBB. There is a transport system for IGF1, but owing to the fact that IGF1 is >99.9% bound by serum proteins, there is no transport of the IGF1 across the BBB in vivo in pharmacologically significant amounts (Chapter 4). Since the phase III clinical trials failed for all three neurotrophic factors, one could conclude that BDNF, CNTF, or IGF1 are not effective treatments for neurodegenerative conditions such as ALS. The alternative explanation is that the neurotrophins are not expected to have CNS pharmacologic effects following systemic administration, if a BBB drug-targeting technology is not used. As shown below, the neurotrophic factors have remarkable restorative properties in brain following noninvasive (intravenous) administration, providing the neurotrophic factor is administered as a conjugate of a BBB drug-targeting system.

Blood–brain barrier transport of neurotrophins

The assertion that neurotrophins were not effective in ALS clinical trials because these molecules did not cross the BBB could be countered with the argument that neurotrophins do cross the BBB. There are reports that neurotrophins cross the BBB, based on the finding of brain uptake of radioactivity following the intravenous injection of radiolabeled neurotrophins. In one study, [^{125}I]nerve growth factor (NGF) was administered intravenously to postnatal rats and radioactivity was recorded in brain over the next 1–2 h (Fabian and Hulsebosch, 1993). However, in this study, gel analysis of plasma and brain radioactivity was performed 2 h after intravenous injection and the plasma gel analysis showed extensive degradation of the [^{125}I]NGF. The final degradation products are [^{125}I]iodide and [^{125}I]tyrosine. These molecules, particularly radiolabeled tyrosine, cross the BBB via carrier-mediated transport, as discussed in Chapter 3. However, as discussed in Chapter 4, the brain uptake of radioactivity is only a function of the peripheral degradation of the peptide and subsequent uptake of radiolabeled metabolites. This is shown in the case of BDNF (Figure 4.16). Following intravenous injection of [^{125}I]BDNF, there is a rapid uptake of radioactivity by brain. However, when the peripheral metabolism of the BDNF is inhibited by protein pegylation, the brain radioactivity decreases to a value that is not significantly different from the brain uptake of a plasma volume marker (Figure 4.16). That is, when the peripheral degradation of the neurotrophin is blocked, and there is no formation of low molecular weight metabolites that cross the BBB, there is no apparent "uptake" of the neurotrophic factor. The primary evidence that neurotrophins do not cross the BBB is the series of studies that show these proteins cause pharmacologic effects in brain following intracerebral injection; however, the neurotrophins exert no CNS pharmacologic effects following intravenous administration (Beck et al., 1994; Schabitz et al., 1997; Stroemer and Rothwell, 1997; Hayashi et al., 1998; Miyazawa et al., 1998; Peng et al., 1998; Sakanaka et al., 1998; Justicia and Planas, 1999; Zhang et al., 1999b).

Neurotrophins in cerebral ischemia

Stroke is a leading cause of death and morbidity. Other than antithrombotic therapy, there has been no new treatment in stroke therapy in 30 years despite intensive efforts to develop small molecule neuroprotectives that cross the BBB. However, these small molecule neuroprotectives invariably trigger monoaminergic or aminoacidergic neurotransmission systems in the brain and have significant toxicity. Neurotrophic factors are highly neuroprotective following intracerebral injection and offer the promise of new forms of neuroprotective therapy in stroke with minimal side-effects. The neurotrophic factors that are neuroprotective in either global or regional cerebral ischemia include BDNF (Beck et al., 1994; Schabitz et al., 1997), erythropoietin (EPO) (Sakanaka et al., 1998), neurotrophin (NT)-3 (Zhang et al., 1999b), transforming growth factor (TGF)-α (Justicia and Planas, 1999), vascular endothelial growth factor (VEGF) (Hayashi et al., 1998), hepatocyte growth factor (HGF) (Miyazawa et al., 1998), EGF (Peng et al., 1998), and interleukin-1 receptor antagonist (IL-1ra) (Stroemer and Rothwell, 1997). To date, none of these neurotrophic factors have been shown to cross the BBB. All of the studies reporting the neuroprotective effects of these neurotrophins involve the intracerebral injection of the protein, and in many of these studies, the neurotrophin must be administered *prior* to the ischemic insult. However, in the treatment of stroke patients, the neurotrophin must be administered noninvasively (intravenously) and at a certain window of time *after* the ischemic insult. The studies described below show that neuroprotection in either global or regional cerebral ischemia can be achieved with neurotrophin chimeric peptides that are enabled to cross the BBB in vivo.

Blood–brain barrier disruption in cerebral ischemia

It has been argued that the need for developing neuroprotective drugs that cross the BBB in the treatment of stroke is not necessary because there is BBB disruption in cerebral ischemia. Actually, the BBB is not disrupted in either global or regional cerebral ischemia until the late stages of the ischemic insult wherein the possibilities for achieving reversible neuroprotection are lost. For example, in a regional ischemia model, such as the middle cerebral artery occlusion (MCAO) method, there is no BBB disruption for the first 4–6 h after the ischemic insult (Menzies et al., 1993). It is unlikely that a significant neuroprotection could be achieved following the administration of neuroprotective agents at such a late time point in regional ischemia when the BBB is disrupted. In the case of global cerebral ischemia, such as the transient forebrain ischemia (TFI) model, there is no BBB disruption until 6 h after the transient ischemic insult and this disruption is very minor and only to small molecules such as sucrose (Preston et al., 1998). Nevertheless, the administration of a neuroprotective agent at 6 h following global cerebral ischemia would unlikely result in significant neuroprotection or have any impact on neuronal survival. These considerations indicate that if a neuroprotective agent is to be effective in the treatment of global or regional cerebral ischemia, the neuroprotective agent must be administered within a few hours of the ischemic insult, and this is a period when the BBB is not disrupted. Therefore, the neurotrophin must be enabled to cross the BBB in vivo.

Molecular formulation of BDNF chimeric peptides

The formulation of a BDNF conjugate that is enabled to traverse the BBB via the endogenous BBB transferrin receptor is outlined in Chapter 6 and shown schematically in Figure 6.13. This formulation employs carboxyl-directed protein pegylation to optimize the plasma pharmacokinetics of the neurotrophic factor and also uses the chimeric peptide technology to enable BBB transport (Pardridge et al., 1998b). Protein pegylation will result in an optimal plasma pharmacokinetic profile (Figure 6.12) and this will increase the plasma AUC. The chimeric peptide technology will enable BBB transport of the neurotrophin (Figure 6.14) and will result in an increased BBB PS product. An increase in both the plasma AUC and the BBB PS product will cause an increase in the brain uptake of the neurotrophin chimeric peptide, as discussed in Chapter 6. Carboxyl-directed protein pegylation was used in the case of the NGF-like neurotrophins, such as BDNF, to enable complete retention of biologic activity and trkB receptor binding (Figure 6.11–6.15).

The formulation of the BDNF chimeric peptide outlined in Figure 6.13 aims both to enable BBB transport and to optimize the plasma pharmacokinetics. One of the characteristics of the neurotrophin drug development pathway was that the plasma pharmacokinetics of these drugs was not considered until the very late stage of drug development (Hefti, 1997). At that point, it was found that the neurotrophins were rapidly removed from the plasma compartment following intravenous injection. In humans, plasma NGF was measurable only after the intravenous injection of a dose as high as 1000 μg/kg and then the plasma NGF was only

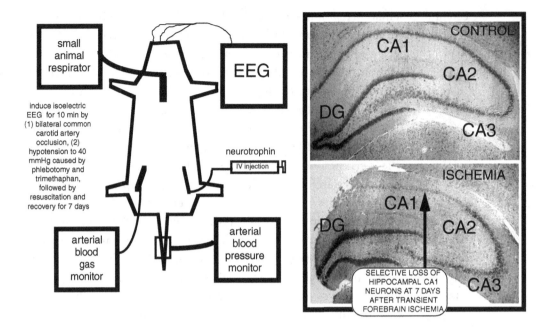

small
animal
respirator

EEG

induce isoelectric
EEG for 10 min by
(1) bilateral common
carotid artery
occlusion, (2)
hypotension to 40
mmHg caused by
phlebotomy and
trimethaphan,
followed by
resuscitation and
recovery for 7 days

neurotrophin
IV injection

arterial
blood
gas
monitor

arterial
blood
pressure
monitor

CONTROL
CA1
CA2
DG
CA3

ISCHEMIA
CA1
DG
CA2
SELECTIVE LOSS OF
HIPPOCAMPAL CA1
NEURONS AT 7 DAYS
AFTER TRANSIENT
FOREBRAIN ISCHEMIA
CA3

Figure 7.5   Transient forebrain ischemia model. EEG, electroencephalogram.

measurable for the first 5 min after intravenous injection (Petty et al., 1994). These observations underscore the very rapid removal from the plasma compartment of the NGF-like neurotrophins. Based on the "pharmacokinetic rule" (Chapter 3), it is not advisable to administer drugs that have degraded plasma pharmacokinetic profiles and reduced plasma AUC, because the brain uptake of the drug (%ID/g) will be reduced in proportion to the decreased plasma AUC.

BDNF chimeric peptides and global cerebral ischemia

The global ischemia method used was the TFI model (Smith et al., 1984), which is outlined in Figure 7.5. The rat is rendered unresponsive with an isoelectric electro-encephalogram (EEG) for a 10-min period owing to a combination of (a) bilateral common carotid artery occlusion, and (b) hypotension caused by phlebotomy and administration of a hypotensive agent, trimethaphan. After a 10-min period of iso-electric EEG, the rat is resuscitated, allowed to recover, and examined 7 days later. At this point, there is nearly complete loss of pyramidal neuron density in the CA1 sector of the hippocampus, as shown by Nissl staining (Figure 7.5).

In order to examine the neuroprotective effects of BDNF chimeric peptides in global ischemia with the TFI model, four treatment groups of rats were evaluated. These groups are: (a) rats administered saline buffer, (b) rats administered uncon-jugated BDNF at a dose of 50 μg/rat intravenously (IV), (c) rats administered

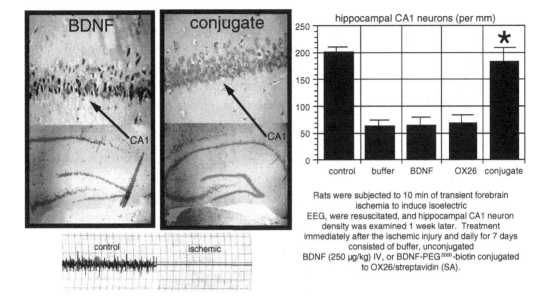

Figure 7.6   Left: Nissl staining at high and low magnification of brain taken from rats subjected to transient forebrain ischemia and treated with either unconjugated brain-derived neurotrophic factor (BDNF) or BDNF conjugate. Right: Density of hippocampal CA1 neurons in control rats and four different groups of treated rats following 10 min of transient forebrain ischemia. EEG, electroencephalogram. From Wu and Pardridge (1999b) with permission. Copyright (1999) National Academy of Sciences, USA.

unconjugated OX26 MAb, and (d) rats administered BDNF chimeric peptide equivalent to 50 μg/rat of BDNF IV (Wu and Pardridge, 1999b). The BDNF chimeric peptide was formed by instantaneous capture of BDNF-PEG^{2000}-biotin by OX26/SA. As shown in Figure 7.6, there was complete neuroprotection of the pyramidal neurons in the CA1 sector of the hippocampus following intravenous administration of the BDNF chimeric peptide. However, there was no neuroprotection following the administration of either unconjugated BDNF or unconjugated OX26 that carried no BDNF. Nissl staining at both low and high magnification showed complete restoration of the CA1 sector and normalization of the pyramidal neuron density in this region of the hippocampus following treatment with the BDNF chimeric peptide (Figure 7.6).

Unconjugated BDNF is neuroprotective in the TFI model following the continuous intracerebroventricular (ICV) infusion of BDNF (Beck et al., 1994). ICV administration of BDNF in the TFI model was neuroprotective because the diffusion distance between the CSF flow tract of the lateral ventricle and the CA1 sector of the hippocampus is minimal. However, in the treatment of patients suffering cardiac arrest and global cerebral ischemia, it is not practical to administer BDNF by ICV administration. Instead, it is necessary to administer the BDNF by noninvasive (intravenous) administration, but this would not be effective if the BDNF does not cross the BBB. Conversely, BDNF chimeric peptides that are enabled to cross the BBB are highly effective neuroprotective agents in global cerebral ischemia following intravenous administration (Figure 7.6).

BDNF chimeric peptides in regional cerebral ischemia

The ICV infusion of BDNF is neuroprotective in a permanent MCAO model, providing the ICV infusion of the neurotrophin is started 24 h *prior* to the ischemic insult (Schabitz et al., 1997). Since it is necessary for the BDNF to diffuse from the CSF flow tracts into the layers of the brain following ICV infusion, the BDNF is not neuroprotective following ICV administration without a significant lead time *before* the ischemic insult. It is not practical to administer BDNF by ICV infusion for the treatment of acute regional stroke, much less 24 h before the ischemic insult. What is needed is the development of BDNF chimeric peptides that are neuroprotective in regional ischemia following the noninvasive (intravenous) administration of the neurotrophin *after* the ischemic insult.

Regional ischemia in rat brain was induced in the area of perfusion of the middle cerebral artery by insertion of an intraluminal suture into this artery in nitrous oxide-anesthetized/ventilated adult rats (Zhang and Pardridge, 2001). The suture was placed for permanent MCAO and the volume of the brain infarction and brain edema was measured 24 h later. Rats were then sacrificed, and 2 mm coronal slabs were prepared, and stained with 2% triphenyltetrazolium chloride (TTC). Physiologic parameters were measured and included arterial blood gases, body temperature, and plasma glucose. Four different treatment groups were examined: (a) rats administered saline, (b) rats administered unconjugated BDNF, (c) rats administered unconjugated OX26 MAb, and (d) rats administered BDNF chimeric peptide using the formulation outlined in Figure 6.13, which is identical to a formulation used in the global cerebral ischemia studies (Figure 7.6). Results of the BDNF neuroprotection in regional cerebral ischemia are shown in Figure 7.7 and show a 65% reduction in the infarct volume. The infarct volume was 350 ± 21 mm^3 in animals treated with the saline, unconjugated MAb, or unconjugated BDNF, but was reduced to 121 ± 23 mm^3 by administration of 50 μg/rat of BDNF chimeric peptide, which was given intravenously *after* the ischemic insult. A significant 45% decrease in infarct volume was observed when the dose of chimeric peptide was reduced 10-fold to 5 μg/rat. No statistically significant effect on infarct volume was observed when the dose of the BDNF chimeric peptide was reduced 50-fold to 1 μg/rat (Zhang and Pardridge, 2001). Neuroprotection in this permanent MCAO model was still observed when the intravenous administration of the BDNF

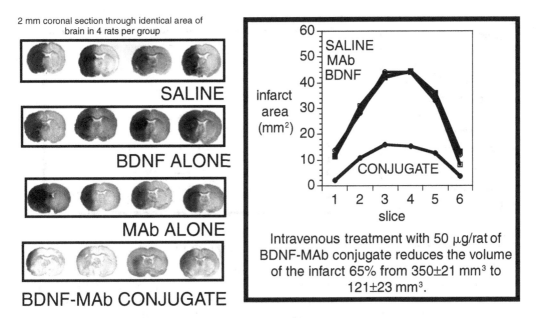

2 mm coronal section through identical area of brain in 4 rats per group

SALINE

BDNF ALONE

MAb ALONE

BDNF-MAb CONJUGATE

Intravenous treatment with 50 μg/rat of BDNF-MAb conjugate reduces the volume of the infarct 65% from 350±21 mm³ to 121±23 mm³.

Figure 7.7   Neuroprotection of brain-derived neurotrophic factor (BDNF) chimeric peptide in regional brain ischemia: permanent middle cerebral artery occlusion (MCAO) (24 h). Left: Triphenyltetrazolium chloride (TTC) stains of coronal sections of rat brain following 24 h permanent MCAO. There were four treatment groups. Right: The infarct area for each of six different coronal slices is shown, and these values were used to compute the volume of the infarct. MAb, monoclonal antibody. From Zhang and Pardridge (2001) with permission.

chimeric peptide was delayed for 1–2 h after occlusion of the middle cerebral artery (Zhang and Pardridge, 2001).

In summary, BDNF chimeric peptides are powerful neuroprotective agents in either global or regional cerebral ischemia and this neuroprotection is achieved with the noninvasive (intravenous) administration of the BDNF chimeric peptide. When the BDNF was administered intravenously without attachment to a BBB drug-targeting system, there is no beneficial pharmacologic effect of the neurotrophin, because BDNF does not cross the BBB (Pardridge et al., 1998b), which is intact in brain ischemia (Menzies et al., 1993; Preston et al., 1998). The neurotrophins are a case study of the development of CNS drugs that do not cross the BBB. If the CNS drug development pathway is allowed to go forward without considerations to BBB transport, then the program will ultimately result in termination (Figure 1.6). Conversely, if CNS drug discovery and CNS drug targeting are merged early in the CNS drug development process, then neuropharmaceuticals that are active in brain following noninvasive (intravenous) administration can be developed.

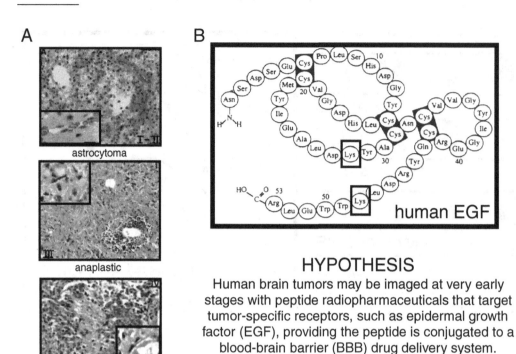

Figure 7.8   (A) Hematoxylin and eosin stain of human gliomas. GBM, glioblastoma multiforme. (B) Amino acid sequence of human epidermal growth factor (EGF). Reprinted from *Peptides*, **16**, Shin, S.Y., Shimizu, M., Ohtaki, T. and Munekata, E., Synthesis and biological activity of N-terminal-truncated derivatives of human epidermal growth factor (h-EGF), 205–10, copyright (1995), with permission from Elsevier Science.

Peptide radiopharmaceuticals as neurodiagnostics

EGF peptide radiopharmaceuticals for diagnosis of brain tumors

Imaging brain tumors with peptide radiopharmaceuticals

The histology of the three types of primary brain gliomas is shown in Figure 7.8A. The least malignant glioma is an astrocytoma, the glioma with moderate malignancy is an anaplastic glioma, and the highest grade malignant glioma is a glioblastoma multiforme (GBM). Some astrocytomas that remain in the brain following neurosurgical extirpation of the tumor can degenerate into anaplastic or GBM tumors with time (Watanabe et al., 1996). These are called secondary GBMs. Brain tumors can be distinguished biochemically because these tumors have specific patterns of gene expression (Wong et al., 1987; Nishikawa et al., 1994). For example, 63% of primary GBMs overexpress immunoreactive epidermal growth factor receptor (EGFR), whereas only 10% of secondary GBMs overexpress the immuno-reactive EGFR. In contrast, 97% of secondary GBMs overexpress the immunoreactive p53 protein (Watanabe et al., 1996).

The selective expression in primary brain tumors of proteins or receptors that are not expressed in normal brain provides the setting for using peptide radiopharmaceuticals for diagnosing brain tumors. For example, an EGF peptide radiopharmaceutical could be used for diagnosing gliomas if the EGF peptide radiopharmaceutical was (a) radiolabeled with an appropriate radionuclide and (b) enabled to cross the BBB in the brain tumor, which is also called the blood–tumor barrier (BTB). Although the BTB may be leaky to small molecules, relative to the normal BBB, in late-stage brain tumors, the BTB is intact early in the course of either primary brain tumors or metastatic brain tumors (Zhang et al., 1992). Moreover, BBB disruption may be observed in a brain tumor when the radionuclide is a small molecule, but the BTB is sufficiently intact to prevent the uptake of a large molecule such as EGF, which has a molecular weight of 6200 Da.

Molecular formulation of EGF chimeric peptides

The primary amino acid sequence of human EGF is shown in Figure 7.8B. Unlike mouse EGF, which has no lysine (Lys) residues, human EGF has two lysine residues (Hommel et al., 1992). Since both mouse and human EGF bind to the rodent or human EGF receptor (Kim et al., 1989), the two lysine residues in human EGF are not crucial for receptor binding. These lysine residues were both conjugated to prepare the formulation of the EGF chimeric peptide described in Chapter 6 and outlined in Figure 6.16. One lysine residue was conjugated with diethylenetriaminepentaacetic acid (DTPA) for chelation with indium-111 and the other lysine residue was conjugated with NHS-PEG^{3400}-biotin (Kurihara et al., 1999). As discussed in Chapter 6, the polyethylene glycol (PEG) linker in this setting is not used to alter the plasma pharmacokinetics of the EGF, but is used as an extended linker between the EGF and the biotin moiety (Deguchi et al., 1999). In this formulation, there is only a *single* PEG strand per EGF molecule.

Imaging C6 experimental gliomas with EGF chimeric peptides

Experimental gliomas in Fischer rats were generated with C6 rat glioma cells (Kurihara et al., 1999). These C6 cells had been permanently transfected with a gene encoding the human EGF receptor (Fenstermaker et al., 1995), and these cells are designated C6–EGFR. These cells were implanted in the caudate putamen nucleus at a dose of 10^5 cells/rat and approximately 4 weeks later, the tumor-bearing rats were anesthetized for intravenous injection of either [^{111}In]DTPA-EGF-PEG^{3400}-biotin conjugated to OX26/SA or [^{111}In]DTPA-EGF-PEG^{3400}-biotin without conjugation to OX26/SA. In these investigations, each group of rats also received an intravenous injection of 16 nmol of unlabeled EGF to saturate hepatic

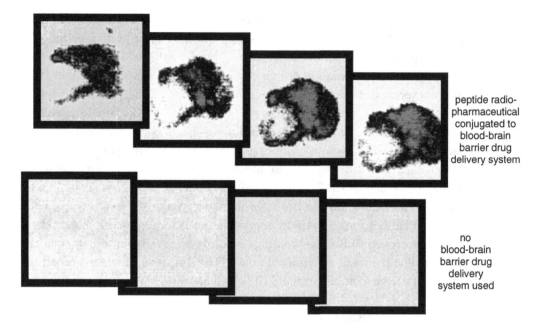

peptide radio-
pharmaceutical
conjugated to
blood-brain
barrier drug
delivery system

no
blood-brain
barrier drug
delivery
system used

Figure 7.9   Film autoradiography of brain sections obtained from C6 epidermal growth factor
receptor (EGFR) tumor-bearing rats injected intravenously with 100 μCi of
[^{111}In]diethylenetriaminepentaacetic acid (DTPA)-EGF-polyethylene glycol (PEG)^{3400}-biotin
with (top panels) or without (bottom panels) conjugation to OX26/streptavidin. Reprinted
with permission from Kurihara et al. (1999). Copyright (1999) American Chemical Society.

uptake of the EGF chimeric peptide (Kurihara et al., 1999). Since the unconjugated
EGF did not cross the BBB or BTB, the EGF loading had no effect on the binding
of the EGF chimeric peptide to the brain tumor EGF receptor. Sixty minutes after
isotope injection, rats were decapitated and the brain was removed and sectioned
into 3-mm slabs. These slabs were frozen and 15 μm sections were prepared and
thaw-mounted on glass coverslips for exposure to Kodak Biomax MS X-ray film for
4 days at −70 °C with intensifying screen. The film was scanned and the image was
cropped in Adobe Photoshop (Figure 7.9). The brain image using the EGF peptide
radiopharmaceutical that was administered without conjugation to the BBB drug-
targeting system is shown in the bottom panel of Figure 7.9. The brain images
obtained following intravenous injection of the [^{111}In]DTPA-EGF-PEG^{3400}-biotin
conjugated to the OX26/SA drug-targeting system are shown in the upper panel of
Figure 7.9. These results indicate there is no measurable transport of the EGF
peptide radiopharmaceutical into either normal brain or the brain tumor when the
EGF is not conjugated to a BBB drug-targeting system.

Conversely, when the EGF peptide radiopharmaceutical is conjugated to

OX26/SA, and injected intravenously into the tumor-bearing rats, there is uptake in normal brain of the peptide radiopharmaceutical owing to transport through the BBB (Kurihara et al., 1999). The regions of the tumor are clearly demarcated because there is reduced uptake of the radiolabeled chimeric peptide in the tumor. The *reduced* uptake of chimeric peptide in the tumor was the opposite of the results anticipated and this observation suggested that the C6–EGFR cells did not express the EGFR transgene in vivo in these brain tumors. This absence of expression of the EGFR transgene in vivo was confirmed by EGFR immunocytochemistry on parallel sections of the tumor (Kurihara et al., 1999). The EGFR transgene was under the influence of a dexamethasone-inducible promoter. To induce expression of the EGFR transgene in cell culture, it was necessary to expose the cells to 1 μmol/l dexamethasone (Fenstermaker et al., 1995). However, this was not possible in the in vivo studies. There was no significant expression within the tumor of the EGFR transgene in the brain tumor in vivo, because this environment lacked the high doses of dexamethasone, which are easily achieved in cell culture.

The signal in the brain tumor region is actually decreased compared to normal brain, and this is due to decreased vascular density in the tumor, relative to normal brain (Kurihara et al., 1999). In parallel, there is decreased density in BTB transferrin receptor in the tumor compared to normal brain. The vascular density in C6 glioma cells is probably comparable to the vascular density in white matter, since the CBF in the C6 glioma is 56% reduced compared to the CBF in gray matter of normal brain (Hiesiger et al., 1986). As shown below, for the Aβ peptide radiopharmaceutical, there are marked differences in brain imaging of gray matter versus white matter and this arises from the differences in vascular density of gray matter and white matter. Therefore, the density of the transferrin receptor or insulin receptor at the BBB in white matter is reduced compared to gray matter.

Imaging U87 experimental gliomas with EGF chimeric peptides

The studies in Figure 7.9 with the C6–EGFR tumor indicate the EGFR transgene is not expressed in vivo. Therefore, an alternate experimental model was established wherein human U87 glioma cells, which do express abundant immunoreactive EGFR (Huang et al., 1997), were implanted in the caudate putamen nucleus of the brain of nude rats (Kurihara and Pardridge, 1999). Prior to the in vivo imaging with the U87 glioma model, the U87 glioma cells were grown in cell culture and the reactivity of the EGF chimeric peptide with the EGFR in this model system was examined with RRAs. The structure of the EGF chimeric peptide is shown in Figure 7.10A, which emphasizes the bifunctionality of the EGF chimeric peptide. The conjugate binds both the EGFR in tumor cells in brain for imaging the tumor, and binds the transferrin receptor on the BTB to enable transport into the tumor region from blood.

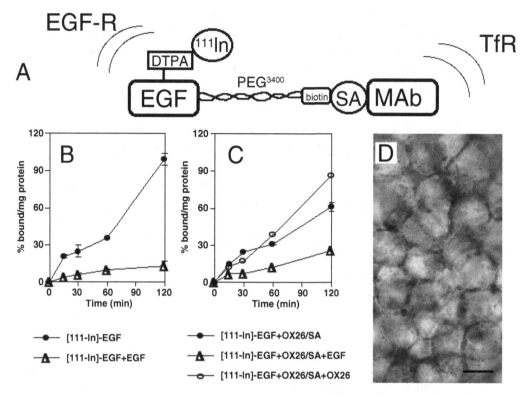

Figure 7.10   (A) The structure of the epidermal growth factor (EGF) chimeric peptide is shown. EGF-R, EGF receptor; DTPA, diethylenetriaminepentaacetic acid; SA, streptavidin; MAb, monoclonal antibody. (B, C) Radioreceptor assays using labeled EGF analogs and U87 human glioma cells in cell culture. (D) Immunocytochemistry of U87 human glioma cells immunostained with a mouse monoclonal antibody to the human EGF receptor. From Kurihara and Pardridge (1999) with permission.

The conjugate retains high-affinity binding to the human EGF receptor on the U87 cells as shown by the RRA in panels B and C of Figure 7.10. There is time-dependent binding of the $[^{111}In]DTPA-EGF-PEG^{3400}$-biotin to the U87 cells in culture and this binding was nearly completely suppressed by unlabeled EGF (Figure 7.10B). When the radiolabeled EGF was conjugated to OX26/SA, there was also a time-dependent increase in binding of the conjugate to U87 cells and this was inhibited by unlabeled EGF, but was not inhibited by unlabeled and unconjugated OX26 MAb (Figure 7.10C). These studies indicate the OX26 MAb to the rat transferrin receptor does not bind to the human transferrin receptor on the human U87 glioma cells. Conversely, the OX26 MAb binds to the rat transferrin receptor expressed on the capillaries that perfuse the experimental human glioma in brains of nude rats. The abundant expression of the immunoreactive human EGFR on the

U87 cells in cell culture is also shown in the immunocytochemistry studies using a mouse monoclonal antibody to the human EGFR (Figure 7.10D). The basolateral pattern of the immunostaining in this study indicates the EGFR is expressed on the plasma membrane of the U87 cells (Kurihara and Pardridge, 1999).

The immunoreactive human EGFR in the U87 cells grown in vivo in the form of experimental brain tumors, was detected by immunocytochemistry of autopsy brain sections of the experimental tumors, as shown in panels A, C, and E of Figure 7.11 (colour plate). The [^{111}In]DTPA-EGF-PEG^{3400}-biotin, without conjugation to OX26/SA, was injected intravenously into the nude rats bearing the U87 gliomas, and there was no imaging of large brain tumors, as shown in Figure 7.11F. The EGF peptide radiopharmaceutical does not image even a large brain tumor because the EGF radiopharmaceutical does not cross the BTB in the absence of a brain drug-targeting system (Kurihara and Pardridge, 1999). Conversely, either small brain tumors (panel D) or large brain tumors (panel B) were imaged with EGF peptide radiopharmaceuticals that were conjugated to the BBB drug-targeting system, as shown in Figure 7.11. Quantitation of these scans showed that the radioactivity in the tumor brain was 20-fold greater than the radioactivity in normal brain following administration of the EGF chimeric peptide (Figure 7.11B). Conversely, the radioactivity in either the tumor or normal brain was not significantly different from the background level when the EGF peptide radiopharmaceutical was administered without conjugation to the BBB drug-targeting system (Figure 7.11F).

The studies in Figure 7.11 show that it is not possible to image experimental brain tumors that express the EGFR with EGF peptide radiopharmaceuticals unless the latter are conjugated to BBB drug-targeting systems. Although the BTB is disrupted in brain tumors such as U87 experimental brain tumors (Yuan et al., 1994), the disruption of the BBB is not sufficient to enable imaging of the tumor with unconjugated peptide radiopharmaceuticals such as EGF that have molecular weights of 6200 Da. Instead, successful tumor imaging requires conjugation of the peptide radiopharmaceutical to a BBB drug-targeting system. Once the EGF peptide radiopharmaceutical is delivered through the BBB via the rat endothelial transferrin receptor, the EGF is then bound to the EGFR on the human tumor cells.

The sustained binding of the EGF chimeric peptide to the tumor may be attributed, in part, to the biological characteristics of EGF binding to its receptor. The human EGFR binds both EGF and TGFα (French et al., 1995). However, there are differences in the pathway of receptor-bound EGF and TGFα. Once internalized, TGFα is rapidly dissociated from the EGFR, but EGF remains bound to the EGFR after internalization (French et al., 1995). Therefore, the prolonged residence time of EGF on its receptor may contribute to the high signal/noise ratio of the EGF chimeric peptide radiopharmaceutical over the U87 tumor. This high tumor signal is due to the EGF part of the chimeric peptide and not to the OX26 MAb part of the chimeric peptide. The tumor binding of the conjugate does not arise from nonspecific binding of the MAb moiety of the conjugate to tumor IgG Fc receptors. If this was the case, then the tumor would still be "hot" in the C6 glioma model despite lack of expression of EGFR, but this is not observed (Figure 7.10). Rather, the OX26 MAb plays its role at the BTB to enable transport of the EGF chimeric peptide into the interstitial space of the tumor so that it can then react with the EGFR on the tumor plasma membrane.

Imaging human brain tumors with EGF chimeric peptides

Prior attempts to image brain tumors overexpressing the EGFR have employed anti-EGFR MAbs (Kalofonos et al., 1989; Dadparvar et al., 1994). However, these antibodies do not cross the BTB unless there is advanced stages of the tumor where the BTB is disrupted (Dadparvar et al., 1994). In this case, there is no significant difference between the tumor uptake of a monoclonal antibody specific to the EGFR and an isotype control antibody (Kalofonos et al., 1989). Conversely, it should be possible to image brain tumors early in tumor development using peptide radiopharmaceuticals that target specific receptors produced on the plasma membrane of the tumor cells as a result of tumor cell-specific gene expression. The studies shown in Figure 7.11 could be extended to imaging human brain tumors, because human gliomas coexpress both the insulin receptor at the BTB and the EGFR on the plasma membrane of the tumor cell, as shown by the immunocyto-chemistry in Figure 7.12. As reviewed in Chapter 5, BBB drug targeting in Old World primates such as rhesus monkeys or humans employs MAbs to the human insulin receptor (HIR), and the HIR MAb has a 10-fold greater BBB transport activity as compared to the transferrin receptor MAb. Therefore, the formulation of the EGF peptide radiopharmaceutical shown in Figure 7.10A would employ an MAb to the HIR, not the transferrin receptor, for studies in humans. The BTB of the human GBM expresses abundant quantities of the HIR at the capillary endo-thelium perfusing the tumor (Figure 7.12A, 7.12C). There is also expression of the immunoreactive EGFR on the tumor plasma membrane with no measurable expression of EGFR in normal brain, as shown by the demarcation of the immu-noreactivity in Figure 7.12B. High magnification of the immunoreactive EGFR in the tumor plasma membrane is shown in Figure 7.12D. Nonspecific immunoreac-tivity using an isotype control is shown in Figure 7.12E. The immunocytochemis-try studies in Figure 7.12 indicate that the biological properties that enable tumor imaging in the U87 experimental glioma (Figure 7.11) are also present in human brain gliomas. That is, there is high expression of the HIR at the capillary endothe-lium perfusing the tumor and high expression of the EGFR on the tumor cell.

A model of the coexpression of the HIR and EGFR in the human brain tumor is shown in Figure 7.13. The HIR on the BBB perfusing the brain tumor is targeted

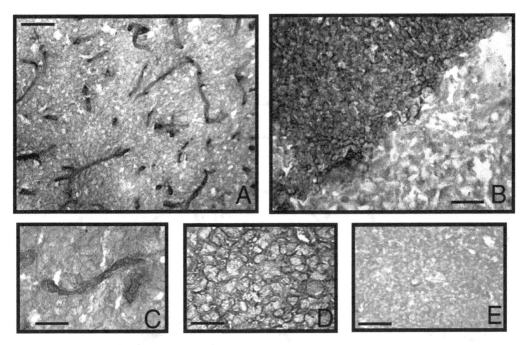

Figure 7.12   Immunocytochemistry of frozen sections of human glioblastoma multiforme immunostained with the 83–14 mouse monoclonal antibody to the human insulin receptor (A and C) or mouse monoclonal antibody to the human epidermal growth factor receptor (B and D) or mouse immunoglobulin G isotype control (E). Magnifications bars are 55 μm (panels A and B) and 14 μm (panels C, D, E).

by the HIR MAb, which enables transport of the EGF chimeric peptide into the tumor interstitium. The EGF chimeric peptide may then bind either the EGFR on the tumor cell membrane (TCM) or the HIR on the brain cell membrane (BCM) of normal cells in brain. However, the EGF chimeric peptide will be rapidly processed in the lysosomal system of normal brain cells followed by lysosomal degradation and export of the radionuclide. Conversely, the EGF chimeric peptide will undergo entry into the lysosomal compartment of the tumor cell at a much slower rate, owing to the tendency of EGF to stay bound to its cognate receptor (French et al., 1995). This differential processing of the EGF chimeric peptide in EGFR-bearing tumor cells and HIR-bearing normal brain cells underlies the high signal/noise ratio in the tumor image relative to normal brain, as shown in Figure 7.11. The hypothesis that the indium-111 radionuclide will be rapidly exported from normal brain following intracellular processing of the chimeric peptides is at odds with studies in cell culture showing that indium-111 radionuclides are sequestered in the intracellular space (Shih et al., 1994; Press et al., 1996). If the indium-111 was sequestered in brain cells despite lysosomal degradation of the EGF

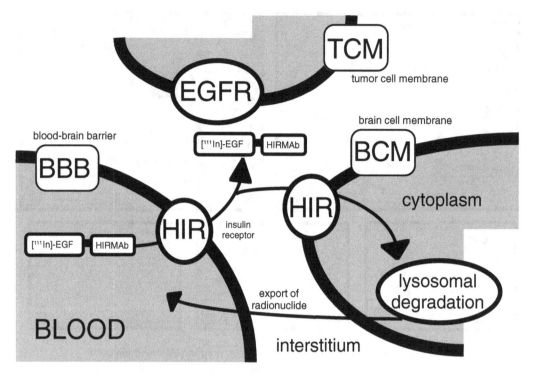

Figure 7.13   Model of pathways involved in imaging human brain tumors using epidermal growth factor (EGF) peptide radiopharmaceuticals and a human insulin receptor (HIR) monoclonal antibody (MAb) as a blood–brain barrier (BBB) drug-targeting system. The HIR is also expressed on the brain cell membrane (BCM) of normal cells in brain, whereas the EGF receptor (EGFR) is selectively expressed on the tumor cell membrane (TCM).

chimeric peptide, then this sequestration would minimize the export of radioactivity from brain and decrease the ratio of radioactivity in the tumor relative to normal brain. However, the studies shown in Figure 7.11 are one of the first in vivo applications of the use of indium-111 peptide radiopharmaceuticals in brain imaging using chimeric peptides. These in vivo experiments demonstrate that the indium-111 radionuclide is exported from normal brain, providing support for the model in Figure 7.13.

Aβ peptide radiopharmaceuticals as neurodiagnostics in Alzheimer's disease

Brain amyloid in Alzheimer's disease

The dementia of AD correlates with the deposition in brain of extracellular amyloid (Cummings and Cotman, 1995). This amyloid is comprised primarily of a 43 amino acid peptide, designated $A\beta^{1-43}$, that has been isolated from AD meningeal

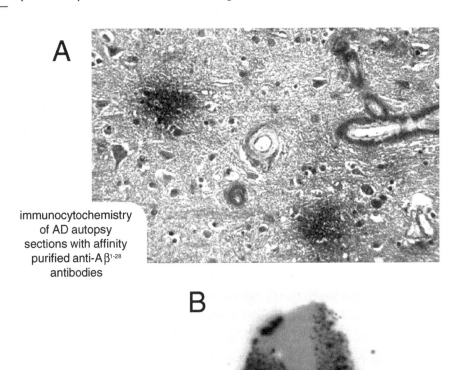

Figure 7.14 (A) Immunocytochemistry of Alzheimer's disease (AD) autopsy sections with affinity-purified anti-Aβ^{1-28} antibodies. The study shows extracellular neuritic (senile) plaque and perivascular amyloid plaque. (B) Film autoradiography of AD autopsy brain sections with [^{125}I]Aβ^{1-40}. There is a preponderance of amyloid plaques in the gray matter tracts with sparing of the central white matter tract.

vessels (Glenner and Wong, 1984), neuritic plaque (Masters et al., 1985), and intracortical microvessels (Pardridge et al., 1987b). Carboxyl terminal truncated forms of Aβ^{1-43}, designated Aβ^{1-40}, are secreted under normal conditions as part of the proteolytic processing of the amyloid peptide precursor (APP), a 695 amino acid protein expressed in brain (Kang et al., 1987). The Aβ^{1-40} is normally secreted into the extracellular fluid, but is not crucial to the formation of the extracellular amyloid in AD (Gravina et al., 1995). In contrast, there is little secretion of soluble Aβ^{1-43}, but this peptide plays a crucial role in initial formation of the extracellular neuritic (senile) plaque or vascular amyloid situated on the brain side of microvessels (Figure 7.14A). For example, antibodies that react to the carboxyl terminus of

$A\beta^{1-43}$ immunolabel amyloid in AD or Down's syndrome brain, whereas antibodies that recognize the carboxyl terminus of $A\beta^{1-40}$ do not recognize the $A\beta$ amyloid (Iwatsubo et al., 1995; Tamaoka et al., 1995). The $A\beta^{1-43}$ has a high degree of β-pleated sheet secondary structure and immediately polymerizes to form fibrils, whereas the formation of fibrils by $A\beta^{1-40}$ is slow (Jarrett and Lansbury, 1993). In contrast, if $A\beta$ amyloid fibrils already exist, then $A\beta^{1-40}$ promptly deposits on the preexisting amyloid fibrils (Jarrett and Lansbury, 1993).

The deposition of $A\beta$ analogs such as $A\beta^{1-42}$ or $A\beta^{1-40}$ on preexisting amyloid plaques forms the basis of methods of detection of amyloid plaques in tissue sections of AD brain. Such methods may use either autoradiography and radiolabeled $A\beta$ isoforms (Maggio et al., 1992), or immunocytochemistry and biotinylated analogs of the $A\beta$ isoforms (Prior et al., 1996). Up to 60% of amyloid plaques in AD brain are recognized with biotinylated forms of $A\beta^{1-42}$, whereas 31% of plaques are labeled with biotinylated forms of $A\beta^{1-40}$ (Prior et al., 1996). The detection of amyloid plaques in frozen sections of AD autopsy brain with either immunocytochemistry or $[^{125}I]A\beta^{1-40}$ and film autoradiography is shown in Figure 7.14. The central white matter tract is relatively spared of amyloid plaque as there is a strong predilection for deposition of amyloid plaques within the gray matter of cortex in AD. Therefore, the detection of $A\beta$ amyloid plaques in AD brain by $A\beta$ peptide radiopharmaceuticals is comparable to the standard detection of $A\beta$ amyloid plaques in autopsy sections of AD brain using immunocytochemistry and antibodies directed against various amino acid sequences of the $A\beta$ peptide (Figure 7.14).

Blood–brain barrier transport of $A\beta^{1-40}$

The deposition of $A\beta^{1-40}$ on preexisting amyloid plaques means that radiolabeled forms of $A\beta^{1-40}$ are potential peptide radiopharmaceuticals for semiquantifying the $A\beta$ amyloid burden in AD brain using brain scan technology in subjects living with AD. Such an AD brain scan could also be a specific tool for diagnosing AD premortem. However, the use of radiolabeled $A\beta^{1-40}$ as a peptide radiopharmaceutical for an amyloid brain scan would require that this neuropeptide is transported through the BBB in vivo. There are reports in the literature that $A\beta^{1-40}$ does cross the BBB, although there is no consensus as to what mechanism could possibly be operating to mediate the BBB transport of $A\beta^{1-40}$. For example, one study reports that $A\beta^{1-40}$ crosses the BBB, but that this transport is nonsaturable (Maness et al., 1994). However, $A\beta^{1-40}$ is too water-soluble to traverse the BBB via free diffusion and nonsaturable lipid mediation (Chapter 3). Another study shows that the brain uptake of $[^{125}I]A\beta^{1-40}$ is directly proportional to the peripheral degradation of the peptide and to the formation of radiolabeled metabolites in plasma that are not precipitable by TCA (Poduslo et al., 1999). The results of this study parallel that of the $[^{125}I]BDNF$ study (Figure 4.16), and both show that when the peripheral metabolism of the labeled neuropeptide is blocked then there is a parallel reduction in the brain uptake of radioactivity. In either case, the $[^{125}I]$peptide is converted in the periphery to $[^{125}I]$tyrosine. The latter can undergo transport across the BBB via LAT1 (Chapter 3) and give rise to radioactivity in brain following intravenous injection of radiolabeled $A\beta^{1-40}$. However, this does not mean that the peptide itself crosses the BBB. Intracarotid arterial perfusion experiments with capillary depletion analysis indicate that radiolabeled $A\beta^{1-40}$ is absorbed to the vascular surface of brain microvessels in vivo, but does not undergo transcytosis through the BBB in vivo (Saito et al., 1995).

If radiolabeled $A\beta^{1-40}$ did cross the BBB, this peptide radiopharmaceutical would presently be in use for quantifying the $A\beta$ amyloid burden in patients with AD with amyloid brain scans. However, when $[^{125}I]A\beta^{1-40}$ was administered via intracarotid arterial infusions of relatively high doses (80–165 μCi/kg) into aged anesthetized squirrel monkeys, there was no radiolabeling of intraparenchymal $A\beta$ amyloid (Walker et al., 1994). The brain amyloid was not labeled because $A\beta^{1-40}$ does not cross the BBB in vivo. In contrast, meningeal vessels were radiolabeled in this study, but these are extracerebral vessels that lack a BBB.

$A\beta^{1-40}$ may not cross the BBB in normal brain, but it may be possible that $A\beta^{1-40}$ crosses the BBB in AD because the BBB is disrupted in this condition. There are some protein abnormalities in the cerebrospinal fluid (CSF) of AD, and these have been interpreted as evidence of BBB disruption in AD. However, CSF protein is not a measure of BBB permeability (Chapter 2). Moreover, the protein changes in CSF of AD are found for only specific proteins (Mattila et al., 1994), and these are not generalized changes. Only generalized increases in CSF protein would be indicative of increased vascular permeability in brain of subjects with AD. Other studies demonstrate that the BBB is not disrupted in AD (Schlageter et al., 1987; Vorbrodt et al., 1997). Therefore, if $A\beta$ peptide radiopharmaceuticals are to be used to image brain amyloid in AD, it will be necessary to conjugate these peptides to brain drug-targeting systems.

Molecular formulation of $A\beta$ chimeric peptides

$A\beta^{1-40}$ was biotinylated with NHS-XX-biotin and bound to a conjugate of the OX26 MAb and SA, designated OX26/SA (Saito et al., 1995). The biotin-XX-$[^{125}I]$-$A\beta^{1-40}$ conjugated to OX26/SA was then applied to frozen sections of autopsy AD brain to examine whether the $A\beta^{1-40}$ peptide radiopharmaceutical still binds to the $A\beta$ amyloid plaques of AD while conjugated to the BBB drug-targeting system. The structure of the $A\beta$ chimeric peptide is shown in Figure 7.15A. The labeling of amyloid plaques in AD tissue sections with the $A\beta$ chimeric peptide was examined by either emulsion autoradiography or film autoradiography, as shown in Figure 7.15C and 7.15D, respectively. The film autoradiography studies show a

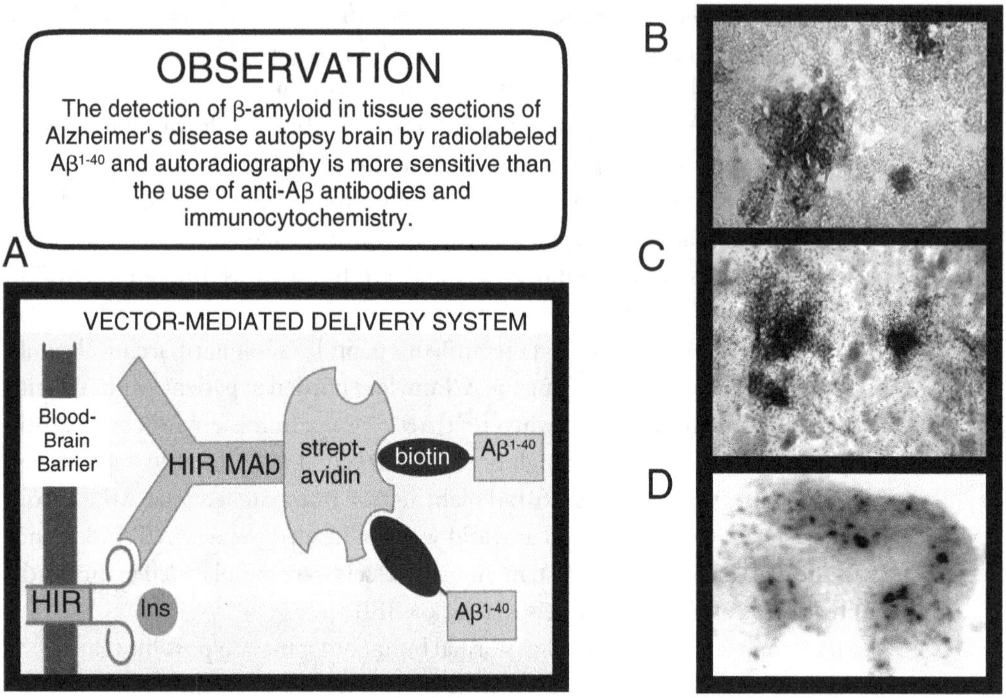

Figure 7.15   Imaging brain amyloid in Alzheimer's disease (AD). (A) Structure of Aβ chimeric peptide comprised of a human insulin receptor monoclonal antibody (HIR MAb) conjugated to streptavidin (SA). The HIR MAb/SA conjugate captures monobiotinylated Aβ$^{1-40}$. Ins, insulin. (B) Immunocytochemistry with an anti-Aβ$^{1-28}$ rabbit polyclonal antiserum and formalin-fixed, formic acid-treated frozen sections of AD brain. Neuritic plaques and vascular amyloid are immunostained with the anti-Aβ$^{1-28}$ antiserum. (C) Emulsion autoradiography shows binding to amyloid plaques of biotinyl [^{125}I]Aβ$^{1-40}$ despite conjugation of the peptide to OX26/SA. (D) Film autoradiography shows binding to amyloid plaques of biotinyl [^{125}I]Aβ$^{1-40}$ despite conjugation of the peptide to OX26/SA. The magnification in panel C is 310-fold greater than the magnification in panel D. From Saito et al. (1995) with permission.

predilection for the amyloid plaques in gray matter with sparing of the central white matter tracts. At the high magnification used with emulsion autoradiography, the size of the amyloid plaques labeled with the Aβ$^{1-40}$ chimeric peptide is comparable to the size of the plaques immunostained with an antibody directed against Aβ$^{1-28}$ (Figure 7.15B). The autoradiography studies in Figure 7.15 are analogous to the radioreceptor assays used for VIP, BDNF, or EGF. These results demonstrate the Aβ$^{1-40}$ peptide radiopharmaceutical still binds to the Aβ amyloid plaque, despite conjugation of the peptide to the BBB drug-targeting system (Figure 7.15A).

Brain imaging in Old World primates

Initial studies in rats demonstrated that unconjugated $A\beta^{1-40}$ did not undergo significant transport through the BBB in vivo. However, $A\beta^{1-40}$ conjugated to OX26/SA was transported through the BBB, and the brain uptake of the $A\beta$ chimeric peptide exceeded the brain uptake of morphine, a neuroactive small molecule (Saito et al., 1995). However, normal rodents do not develop $A\beta$ amyloid in brain. There is a transgenic mouse model of $A\beta$ amyloid (Hsiao et al., 1996), but the OX26 MAb is not active in mice (Lee et al., 2000). Recently, the 8D3 or RI7 MAbs have been developed for brain drug targeting in mice (Lee et al., 2000), and these vectors could be used for imaging the formation of $A\beta$ amyloid plaques in $A\beta$ transgenic mice. Another animal model for imaging brain $A\beta$ amyloid is the aged primate. New World primates such as squirrel monkeys develop amyloid at 16–18 years (Walker et al., 1990; Martin et al., 1991). However, the 83–14 HIR MAb is only effective in Old World primates, such as rhesus monkeys, and not New World primates such as squirrel monkeys (Pardridge et al., 1995b).

Aged (>30 years) rhesus monkeys develop $A\beta$ amyloid plaques in brain (Walker et al., 1990; Gearing et al., 1994). As a first step towards imaging the $A\beta$ amyloid in brain in aged rhesus monkeys, [N-biotinyl] $A\beta^{1-40}$ was radiolabeled with [^{125}I] and the N-biotinyl [^{125}I]$A\beta^{1-40}$ was bound to a conjugate of the 83–14 HIR MAb and SA (Wu et al., 1997b). The radiolabeled $A\beta^{1-40}$ with or without conjugation to the HIR MAb/SA brain drug-targeting system was injected intravenously into young Rhesus monkeys and quantitative autoradiography (QAR) was performed 3 h later. No measurable brain radioactivity was recorded following the intravenous injection of N-biotinyl [^{125}I]$A\beta^{1-40}$, because this neuropeptide does not cross the BBB (Figure 7.16, left panel). Conversely, brain imaging occurred when the N-biotinyl [^{125}I]$A\beta^{1-40}$ was conjugated to the HIR MAb/SA targeting system, as shown in Figure 7.16 (right panel). The gray and white matter tracts are delineated, owing to the threefold greater vascular density in gray matter relative to white matter (Lierse and Horstmann, 1959). The labeling of brain tissue in the 3-h brain scan shown in Figure 7.16 does not reflect imaging of $A\beta$ amyloid because there was no $A\beta$ amyloid in the brains of these young rhesus monkeys. Rather, the image arises from the generalized distribution of the labeled chimeric peptide in brain at this early period after intravenous injection. It is hypothesized that the brain amyloid will be visualized in "late brain scans" taken at 48–72 h after intravenous administration of the radiolabeled chimeric peptide. In analogy with the imaging of brain tumors with chimeric peptides (Figure 7.13), the signal/noise ratio over the amyloid plaque will be enhanced at late imaging times. The rate of decay of brain radioactivity in normal rhesus monkeys following intravenous injection of $A\beta$ chimeric peptides is shown in Figure 7.17. There is a more than 90% reduction in brain radioactivity at 48 h and this radioactivity in brain decays with a $t_{1/2}$ of 16 h in the rhesus monkey in vivo (Figure 7.17).

BRAIN SCANS 3
HOURS AFTER
INTRAVENOUS
INJECTION OF
ISOTOPE

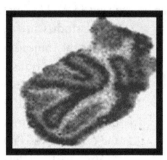

neuropeptide administered
without delivery system

peptide conjugated to
HIR MAb

Figure 7.16　Phosphoimager scans of cerebral hemisphere in rhesus monkeys at 3 h after intravenous injection of 300 μCi of N-biotinyl [^{125}I]Aβ^{1-40} injected either alone (left) or bound to a conjugate of the 83–14 monoclonal antibody to the human insulin receptor (HIR) and streptavidin. Images for occipital lobe are shown. MAb, monoclonal antibody. From Wu et al. (1997b) with permission.

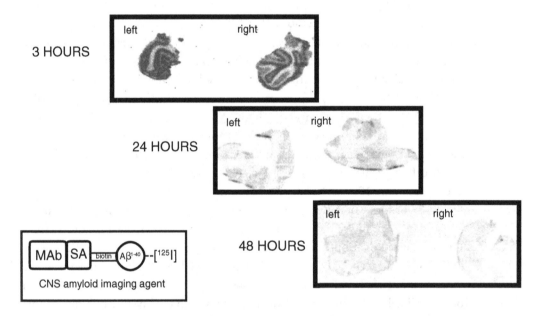

Figure 7.17　Phosphoimager scans of frozen sections of rhesus monkey brain obtained 3, 24, and 48 h after intravenous injection of N-biotinyl [^{125}I]Aβ^{1-40} bound to a conjugate of streptavidin (SA) and a monoclonal antibody (MAb) to the human insulin receptor. The structure of the central nervous system (CNS) amyloid imaging agent is shown in the inset. From Wu et al. (1997b) with permission.

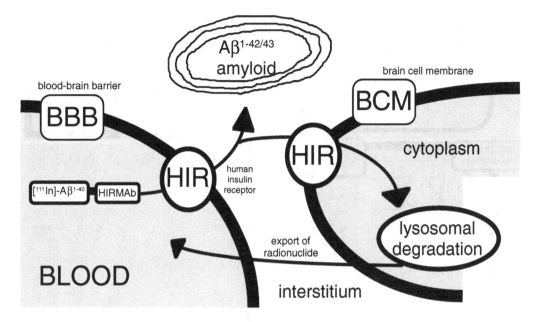

Figure 7.18   Model of imaging of Aβ amyloid in brain. The radiolabeled Aβ peptide radiopharmaceutical is transported through the blood–brain barrier (BBB) via the human insulin receptor (HIR). The HIR is also situated on the brain cell membrane (BCM) of normal cells in brain. Therefore, once inside brain interstitium, the Aβ^{1-40} chimeric peptide may either undergo entry into brain cells via the insulin receptor on the BCM, or bind to Aβ amyloid plaques present in the brain extracellular space. MAb, monoclonal antibody.

The decay in brain radioactivity shown in the time course study in Figure 7.17 indicates there is degradation of the Aβ^{1-40} chimeric peptide and export of the radionuclide from brain back to blood, as depicted in Figure 7.18. Whereas Aβ^{1-40} is normally rapidly degraded in cells, the rate of degradation of the neuropeptide is delayed when Aβ^{1-40} is deposited on to extracellular amyloid (Nordstedt et al., 1994). Therefore, the degradation and export of brain radioactivity in subjects with Aβ brain amyloid will be delayed such that the late brain scans will be "hot" in regions of the brain containing significant quantities of Aβ amyloid, similar to the results obtained with the brain tumor imaging studies (Figure 7.11).

Imaging Aβ amyloid in humans with ^{111}In radiopharmaceuticals

The imaging studies performed in vitro with AD brain sections or in vivo with brain imaging in rhesus monkeys (Figure 7.16) uses Aβ^{1-40} labeled with the iodine-125 radionuclide. However, Aβ amyloid brain scans for use in subjects suspected of having AD might employ external detection methodology such as single photon emission computed tomography (SPECT). Therefore, it would be advantageous to

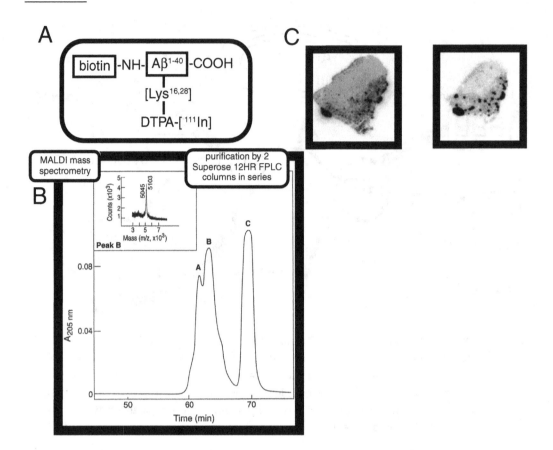

Figure 7.19   (A) Structure of Aβ with dual modifications of biotinylation and conjugation by diethylenetriaminepentaacetic acid (DTPA) on an internal lysine (Lys) residue at position 16 or 28. (B) Purification of Aβ conjugates by gel filtration fast protein liquid chromatography (FPLC) using two Superose 12 HR columns in series. The matrix-assisted laser desorption ionization (MALDI) mass spectrum for peak B is shown in the inset, and corresponds to the [N-biotinyl, Lys-DTPA]Aβ$^{1-40}$. (C) Film autoradiography showing binding of ^{125}I-[N-biotinyl]Aβ$^{1-40}$ (left) or ^{111}In-[N-biotinyl, Lys-DTPA]Aβ$^{1-40}$ (right) to amyloid plaques in frozen sections of Alzheimer's disease brain. The amyloid plaques are small structures with a diameter less than 100 μm (Figure 7.14A, 7.15B). However, when the amyloid plaques are viewed with film autoradiography, there is a coalescence of the plaque signals to yield the large plaque structures that oftentimes have a diameter >1 mm, as shown in Figures 7.15D and 7.19C. Reprinted with permission from Kurihara and Pardridge (2000). Copyright (2000) American Chemical Society.

develop an $A\beta$ peptide radiopharmaceutical amenable to SPECT scanning using radionuclides such as indium-111. The feasibility of developing $A\beta$ analogs that have the dual modifications of (a) biotinylation, for conjugation to BBB drug-targeting systems, and (b) DTPA conjugation, for chelation with indium-111, was examined by preparing a new analog of $A\beta$ (Kurihara and Pardridge, 2000). The $[N\text{-biotinyl, DTPA}]A\beta^{1-40}$ was purified by two Superose 12 HR gel filtration fast protein liquid chromatography (FPLC) columns in series, as shown in Figure 7.19. The structure of the $[N\text{-biotinyl, DTPA}]\text{-}A\beta^{1-40}$ is shown in Figure 7.19 and was confirmed by MALDI mass spectrometry (Figure 7.19, inset). The affinity of this $A\beta$ analog for the $A\beta$ amyloid plaques in tissues sections of autopsy AD brain was examined with film autoradiography. As shown in Figure 7.19 (right panel), the amyloid plaques in gray matter of AD frozen sections were equally visualized with either $^{125}I\text{-}[N\text{-biotinyl}]\text{-}A\beta^{1-40}$ or $^{111}In\text{-}[N\text{-biotinyl, DTPA}]\text{-}A\beta^{1-40}$ (Figure 7.19, right panel).

In summary, it is possible to prepare analogs of $A\beta^{1-40}$ that have the dual modifications of radiolabeling and conjugation to BBB drug-targeting vectors. These $A\beta^{1-40}$ chimeric peptides still bind the amyloid in autopsy sections of AD brain. $A\beta$ chimeric peptides are potential peptide radiopharmaceuticals that may enable the development of a diagnostic AD brain scan. Such a brain scan could also provide a means for semiquantitation of the $A\beta$ amyloid burden in brain of subjects living with AD, which could be useful in evaluation of clinical trials of drugs that alter the formation of $A\beta$ amyloid plaques in AD.

Summary

There currently is an unmet need for the development of new neurotherapeutics for the treatment of neurodegenerative diseases, as reviewed by Shoulson (1998). Despite the advances in the molecular neurosciences during the "decade of the brain," there still is no new treatment for AD, Parkinson's disease, ALS, Huntington's disease (HD), or other neurodegenerative conditions. The patients and family members stricken with HD must be particularly distressed, because the identification of the gene for HD was made nearly 10 years ago, yet no new therapy has been forthcoming. Similarly, there has been no significant new neurotherapeutics for stroke, brain cancer, cerebral acquired immune deficiency syndrome (AIDS), or brain injury. Cytokines have been developed as palliative therapy for multiple sclerosis (MS), but no curative medicines have been developed for MS or any other chronic disease of the brain. Moreover, the cytokines do not cross the BBB, but rather exert pharmacologic actions on the immune system outside of the brain.

It is paradoxical that there should be so much progress in the molecular neurosciences and so little parallel advances in the treatment of cancer and chronic disease of the brain. The explanation to this paradox may be found in the current model of CNS drug development. Twentieth-century CNS drug development relied exclusively on CNS drug discovery and fostered no growth in CNS drug targeting. Since >98% of all drugs do not cross the BBB, this model of brain drug development invariably leads to program termination, and the neurotrophins are a case study of how drugs for the brain were developed. In the 1990s, BDNF, CNTF, and IGF1 were all taken through costly phase III clinical trials for ALS without considering whether these drugs cross the BBB. If the drugs do not cross the BBB, then there is no reason to believe that the drugs will be effective in neurodegenerative disease. The drugs failed as therapeutics for ALS, and it was concluded that these neurotrophins are not effective in this condition. An alternative interpretation is that these drugs should never have entered into clinical trials without some kind of BBB drug-targeting strategy. It is possible that the neurotrophins will prove in the future to be beneficial treatments for ALS, providing the drugs are enabled to cross the BBB.

The idea that drugs, that are normally ineffective following systemic administration, can be converted into highly active neuropharmaceuticals by utilizing brain-targeting technology, is reinforced by the studies reviewed in this chapter. Intravenous BDNF alone is ineffective, but intravenous BDNF chimeric peptide is highly effective as a treatment of either global or regional cerebral ischemia (Figures 7.6 and 7.7). Systemically administered EGF alone is ineffective as a brain tumor-imaging agent, but an EGF chimeric peptide readily images brain cancer (Figure 7.11). Systemically administered VIP alone is ineffective, but a VIP chimeric peptide is effective as a cerebral vasodilator (Figure 7.4). Systemically administered $A\beta^{1-40}$ peptide radiopharmaceutical alone penetrates the brain poorly, but an $A\beta^{1-40}$ chimeric peptide enters the primate brain (Figure 7.16) and can be used as an AD diagnostic agent. These examples demonstrate that CNS drug development need not end in program termination, providing CNS drug discovery and CNS drug targeting are merged early in the overall process of CNS drug development (Chapter 1).

8

Antisense neurotherapeutics and imaging gene expression in vivo

- Introduction
- Phosphodiester oligodeoxynucleotides
- Sulfur-containing oligodeoxynucleotides
- Peptide nucleic acids
- Imaging gene expression in the brain in vivo
- Summary

Introduction

Types of oligodeoxynucleotides

The three most widely utilized classes of oligodeoxynucleotides (ODNs) are phosphodiester (PO)-ODN, phosphorothioate (PS)-ODN, and peptide nucleic acids (PNA), as outlined in Figure 8.1. Antisense ODNs are agents that have the potential to be a new class of neurotherapeutics or neurodiagnostics, should these molecules be made transportable through the blood–brain barrier (BBB). Antisense ODNs hybridize to target mRNA molecules in brain cells via sequence-specific mechanisms based on Watson–Crick base pairing and hydrogen bonding. Therefore, antisense agents could act as neurotherapeutics by binding to a specific target mRNA and eliminating the production of that gene product. Antisense ODN molecules could also be used as radiopharmaceuticals for imaging gene expression in the brain in vivo.

Antisense agents as neurotherapeutics

The neurodegenerative disease that might by most amenable to antisense therapy is Huntington's disease (HD). The HD gene was identified in 1993 and encodes a 343 kDa protein, designated huntingtin, which has polyglutamine repeats owing to a CAG repeat in the huntingtin transcript (Huntington's Disease Collaborative Research Group, 1993). The greater number of CAG repeats in the huntingtin gene and transcript, and the greater number of glutamines added to the huntingtin protein, then the greater the severity of the disease (Gutekunst et al., 1995).

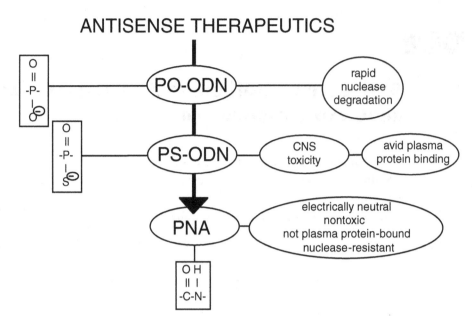

Figure 8.1   Antisense therapeutics. PO-ODN, phosphodiester oligodeoxynucleotide; PS-ODN, phosphorothioate ODN; PNA, peptide nucleic acid; CNS, central nervous system. From Pardridge (1997) with permission.

Polyglutamine repeats are found in a number of transcription factors and serve as binding sites for protein–protein interactions (Stott et al., 1995). For example, glyceraldehyde phosphate dehydrogenase (GAPDH) binds polyglutamine repeats, and GAPDH mRNA increases prior to cellular apoptosis (Burke et al., 1996). Therefore, the polyglutamine repeats in the huntingtin protein could trigger binding of the GAPDH which could lead to an increase in GAPDH mRNA production and induce apoptosis. Either the mRNA for huntingtin or GAPDH are potential targets for antisense neurotherapeutics as novel treatments for HD.

Antisense neurotherapeutics could be used in the treatment of brain cancer or brain viral diseases, such as the cerebral component of acquired immune deficiency syndrome (AIDS). The human immunodeficiency virus (HIV) selectively infects the central nervous system (CNS) in AIDS (Price et al., 1988). As discussed in Chapter 3, none of the drugs comprising the triple therapy of AIDS treatment cross the BBB. Therefore, the HIV harbored within the CNS is presently not eradicated by HIV therapy. An antisense agent specific to one of the HIV mRNA molecules would be a highly specific form of therapy for the treatment of cerebral AIDS. Malignant gliomas produce an aberrant mRNA encoding the epidermal growth factor receptor (EGFR). The EGFR activates glioma cell growth, and this cell growth can be aborted by antisense therapeutics (Moroni et al., 1992; Sugawa et al., 1998).

Antisense agents for imaging gene expression in the brain in vivo

Perhaps the greatest utility of antisense neuropharmaceuticals is the direct imaging of gene expression of the brain in vivo. The sequencing of the human genome will lead to the detection of many genetic abnormalities causing cancer or chronic disease of the brain. However, blood testing of patients will only indicate if the patient carries the mutated gene. Blood testing and genetic counseling will not tell the patient when the gene is actually expressed in the brain. The detection of specific gene expression in the brain using imaging modalities such as single photon emission computed tomography (SPECT) could be achieved with the development of antisense radiopharmaceuticals, should these agents be made transportable through the BBB in vivo. However, all studies of antisense uptake by organs in vivo have uniformly demonstrated that antisense agents do not cross the BBB in vivo (Chem et al., 1990; Vlassov and Yakubov, 1991; Zendegui et al., 1992; Tavitan et al., 1998).

Mechanisms of antisense action

Antisense ODNs bind to target mRNA molecules in a sequence-specific fashion and block translation of the mRNA via one of two mechanisms: (a) translation arrest, or (b) activation of RNAse H and cleavage of the target transcript (Reynolds et al., 1994). The first two classes of antisense agents, the PO-ODNs and the PS-ODNs, both activate RNAse H (Crooke, 1993), although PS-ODNs can inhibit RNAse H at high concentrations (Gao et al., 1992; Stein and Cheng, 1993). In contrast, the PNAs do not activate RNAse H and PNAs exert antisense effects solely through translation arrest (Mollegaard et al., 1994). The lack of activation of RNAse H by PNAs may actually be an advantage in the development of antisense radiopharmaceuticals for imaging gene expression. As discussed below, it is not desirable for an antisense radiopharmaceutical to trigger cleavage of the target transcript during brain imaging. For this and other reasons discussed below, PNAs are the ideal antisense agent for imaging gene expression in the brain in vivo.

Antisense agents do not cross the BBB

Because antisense agents do not cross the BBB, these drugs have been administered to the brain following intracerebroventricular (ICV) infusion. As discussed below, the ICV administration of PS-ODNs results in significant neurotoxicity (Figure 8.1). Another problem with the ICV administration of antisense agents is the very limited penetration of the molecule into brain parenchyma following ICV administration (Grzanna et al., 1998). Antisense agents do not diffuse more than 100 μm from the ependymal surface following 24 h of constant ICV infusion (Haque and Isacson, 1997). The limited distribution of these molecules into brain parenchyma following ICV administration is predicted from the kinetics of diffusion and bulk flow, as described in Chapter 2. ICV infusion is an ideal way of delivering drugs to the ependymal surface of the brain, but is inefficient for delivery of drug into brain parenchyma.

Phosphodiester oligodeoxynucleotides

3'-exonuclease

The primary disadvantage of PO-ODNs is the susceptibility of these molecules to 3'-exonuclease degradation (Mirabelli et al., 1991). The 3'-exonuclease enzyme is abundant in serum which is widely used in tissue culture media. Therefore, early in the development of PO-ODNs, the rapid breakdown of PO-ODNs by serum-derived 3'-exonuclease was observed. However, if the 3'-terminus of a PO-ODN was blocked, then the PO-ODN may be resistant to the 3'-exonuclease in serum and cell culture (Gamper et al., 1992). If the 3'-terminus of PO-ODN was blocked by 3'-biotinylation, then the biotinyl-PO-ODN could be conjugated to an avidin-based BBB drug-targeting system. This hypothesis was tested by preparing a [^{32}P]PO-ODN that was biotinylated at the 3'-terminus and radiolabeled at the 5'-terminus and bound to avidin and added to serum in vitro (Boado and Pardridge, 1992). Similarly, the same PO-ODN, which was a 21-mer antisense to nucleotides 162–182 of the bovine *Glut1* glucose transporter mRNA, was biotinylated at the 5'-terminus and bound to avidin. The protection from serum 3'-exonuclease by avidin binding to the biotinylated PO-ODN was examined. Binding of avidin to the [5'-^{32}P]-5'-biotinylated PO-ODN resulted in no protection of the PO-ODN from serum 3'-exonuclease activity. Conversely, binding of the avidin to the [5'-^{32}P]-3'-biotinylated PO-ODN resulted in complete protection of the PO-ODN from serum 3'-exonuclease (Boado and Pardridge, 1992).

Activation of RNAse H

Biotinylation of a PO-ODN at the 3'-terminus not only provides complete protection against serum 3'-exonuclease, but also enables conjugation to avidin-based BBB drug-targeting systems. However, prior to the in vivo use of "chimeric oligodeoxynucleotides," it was necessary to demonstrate that a 3'-biotinylated PO-ODN conjugated to a BBB drug-targeting system was still biologically active. That is, it was necessary to show that the chimeric oligonucleotide bound to the target mRNA and activated RNAse H. In these initial studies, the targeting system used was a conjugate of avidin (AV) and cationized human serum albumin (cHSA), designated cHSA/AV. The PO-ODN was a 21-mer that was antisense to the nucleotide sequence of the *tat* gene of HIV-1 encompassing nucleotides 5402–5422. This 21-mer PO-ODN was labeled at the 5'-terminus with [^{32}P] and biotinylated at the 3'-terminus (Boado and Pardridge, 1994). Target *tat* mRNA was prepared by in vitro transcription using a *tat* transcription plasmid. The RNAse H assay demonstrated that the [5'-^{32}P]-3'-biotinyl anti-*tat* PO-ODN still activated RNAse H despite conjugation to cHSA/AV (Boado and Pardridge, 1994).

Cellular uptake of chimeric oligonucleotides in cell culture

Having demonstrated that conjugation of 3'-biotinylated PO-ODNs to cellular targeting systems such as cHSA/AV resulted not only in protection against 3'-exonucelase in serum in vitro, but also retention of RNAse H activation, the stability of the chimeric oligonucleotide in cultured cells was then examined. Since cells in tissue culture contain abundant alkaline phosphatase, which would cleave the [^{32}P] label from the 5'-terminus of the PO-ODN, it was necessary to prepare a PO-ODN that was labeled internally. This was synthesized with a template method (Zendegui et al., 1992), by first labeling a PO-ODN that was antisense to the *tat* mRNA with [^{32}P]phosphate at the 5'-terminus using T4 polynucleotide kinase; this PO-ODN was biotinylated at the 3'-terminus (Boado and Pardridge, 1994). This [5'-^{32}P]-3'-biotinylated PO-ODN, and a second antisense PO-ODN, which was a 15-mer complementary to nucleotides 5422–5437 of the *tat* gene, were both hybridized to a third 36-mer PO-ODN, which corresponded to the sense nucleotide sequence encompassing the complementary sequence of both the 15-mer and the 21-mer. Following hybridization of the three PO-ODNs, the 21-mer and the 15-mer were ligated with T4 ligase and the two strands of the duplex were then separated with a 12% sequencing gel (Boado and Pardridge, 1994). This synthesis resulted in the production of a 36-mer biotinylated antisense PO-ODN, designated [^{32}P$_{21}$]-3'-biotinylated PO-ODN, which was internally labeled with [^{32}P] at the 21 position. This PO-ODN was conjugated to cHSA/AV and added to cultured human lymphocytes (Figure 8.2A). At 24 h after adding the chimeric oligonucleotide to the cultured human lymphocytes, the ethanol precipitable cell-associated radioactivity was analyzed on a 12% polyacrylamide sequencing gel, shown in the top panel of Figure 8.2A. The gel shows that there is a retardation in the mobility of the internally labeled 36-mer PO-ODN following biotinylation at the 3'-terminus and this enabled separation from the nonbiotinylated 36-mer (lanes 1–2 of Figure 8.2A). The chimeric oligonucleotide was largely unmetabolized 24 h after incubation with cultured human lymphocytes, as shown in lane 5 of Figure 8.2A. There were some degradation products indicative of minor metabolism. However, when the biotinylated PO-ODN was conjugated to cHSA/AV, the amount of intact PO-ODN in the intracellular compartment of the cultured lymphocyte was 85-fold greater than

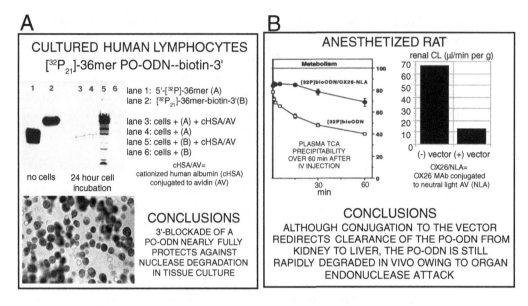

Figure 8.2   3'-Biotinylation and conjugation to blood–brain barrier (BBB) drug-targeting system protects internally labeled phosphodiester oligodeoxynucleotide (PO-ODN) from 3'-exonuclease in tissue culture, but not from endogenous nuclease in vivo in the anesthetized rat. (A) An internally labeled 36-mer PO-ODN, that was biotinylated at the 3'-terminus, was added to cultured human lymphocytes, which are shown in the inset. In these studies, the drug-targeting system was a conjugate of cationized human serum albumin (cHSA) and avidin (AV). From Boado and Pardridge (1994) with permission. (B) The internally labeled biotinylated PO-ODN was injected intravenously into anesthetized rats in either the free form or conjugated to OX26–neutral light avidin (NLA) and the plasma trichloroacetic acid (TCA) precipitability is shown in the left-hand panel. The renal clearance of the unconjugated PO-ODN or the PO-ODN conjugate is shown in the right-hand panel. From Kang et al. (1995a) with permission.

when the biotinylated PO-ODN was added to the cultured lymphocyte without conjugation to the targeting system (lane 6 of Figure 8.2A). Conversely, there was no measurable intracellular PO-ODN if the 3'-terminus was free and not biotinylated (lanes 3 and 4, Figure 8.2A). These studies demonstrate the use of avidin-biotin technology has several advantages in mediating the cellular uptake of PO-ODNs (Boado and Pardridge, 1992, 1994). First, biotinylation at the 3'-terminus results in nearly complete protection against 3'-exonuclease in either serum in vitro or in cells in tissue culture. Second, 3'-biotinylation enables conjugation to targeting systems such as cHSA/AV and this conjugation does not inhibit the biologic activity of the PO-ODN. Despite conjugation to cHSA/AV, the 3'-biotinylated PO-ODN still hybridizes to the target mRNA and activates RNAse H.

Endonuclease activity is rate-limiting in vivo

The experiments in Figure 8.2A demonstrate that the conjugation of 3'-biotiny-lated PO-ODNs to BBB drug-targeting systems results in the desired effects in cell culture, with respect to mediating cellular uptake and resistance to 3'-exonuclease. The stability of the chimeric PO-ODNs was then examined in vivo, wherein the chimeric oligonucleotide was injected intravenously into anesthetized rats and the uptake by brain and other organs was measured (Kang et al., 1995a). In these studies, the PO-ODN was a 36-mer antisense to the *tat* gene of HIV1 and contained a single internally labeled [^{32}P]-labeled nucleotide at the 21 position, and a biotin moiety at the 3'-terminus. This [^{32}P$_{21}$]-3'-biotinylated PO-ODN was bound to a conjugate of the OX26 MAb and neutral light avidin (NLA), and the entire conju-gate is designated [^{32}P]-bio-ODN/OX26–NLA, as shown in Figure 8.2B. In parallel studies, the [^{32}P$_{21}$]-3'-biotinylated PO-ODN was injected into anesthetized rats without conjugation to OX26–NLA. The measurement of plasma radioactivity that was precipitable by trichloroacetic acid (TCA) demonstrated that the internally labeled PO-ODN was rapidly degraded in vivo, despite biotinylation at the 3'-ter-minus (Figure 8.2B). The vast majority of the [^{32}P]-bio-PO-ODN was cleared by liver and kidney during the first 60 min after intravenous injection with 23% cleared by the liver and 41% cleared by the kidney (Kang et al., 1995a). In order to quantify renal clearance accurately, it was necessary to measure both organ and urine radioactivity, as the majority of the [^{32}P] radioactivity was found in the urine during 60 min after intravenous injection. Conjugation of the internally labeled 3'-biotinylated PO-ODN to the OX26–NLA targeting system resulted in a 50% reduc-tion in the systemic clearance of the PO-ODN, from 9.2 ± 0.5 to 4.6 ± 0.3 ml/min per kg. There was also a reduction in the renal clearance of the PO-ODN following conjugation to the OX26–NLA targeting system, as shown in Figure 8.2B. The effective molecular weight of the PO-ODN 36-mer is 10 800 Da and the effective molecular weight of this PO-ODN conjugated to OX26–NLA is 210 800 Da, since the molecular weight of the OX26–NLA conjugate is 200 kDa. This increase in molecular size of the chimeric oligonucleotide causes the decrease in glomerular filtration and renal clearance of the PO-ODN. The chimeric PO-ODN conjugated to OX26–NLA was redirected from kidney to liver, as the hepatic clearance increased threefold following conjugation to OX26–NLA and 65% of the injected dose of the conjugate was cleared by liver (Kang et al., 1995a).

The delayed degradation of the 3'-bio-PO-ODN following conjugation to the OX26–NLA vector is also shown by the amount of plasma [^{32}P] radioactivity that is precipitated by TCA (Figure 8.2B). Nevertheless, the 3'-bio-PO-ODN, in this conjugated form, is still subject to relatively rapid systemic degradation, as one-third of the plasma [^{32}P] radioactivity is TCA-soluble at 60 min after intravenous injection. For example, the systemic clearance of the 3'-bio-PO-ODN/OX26–NLA is 16-fold greater than the systemic clearance of [³H]biotin/OX26–NLA (Kang et al., 1995a). The rapid rate of systemic clearance of the 3′-bio-PO-ODN conjugated to OX26–NLA results in a reduction in the plasma AUC and a proportionate decrease in the brain uptake (percentage of injected dose per gram brain: %ID/g) of the chimeric oligonucleotide. The rapid systemic clearance of the PO-ODN, despite conjugation to OX26–NLA, is due to the high activity of tissue endonuclease activity that is present in vivo (Figure 8.2B). This high endonuclease activity in vivo was unexpected, because there is minimal endonuclease activity in cell culture (Figure 8.2A). The high activity of endonuclease in vivo and low activity of endonuclease in cell culture is an example of the different behavior of drugs in vivo relative to cell culture.

The degradation of internally labeled PO-ODNs by endonuclease in vivo results in the rapid formation of the [³²P]phosphate anion. Although the BBB permeability to the phosphate anion is relatively low, there is a phosphate transporter at the BBB (Dallaire et al., 1992), and the BBB PS product for [³²P]phosphate anion in vivo in the anesthetized rat is 1.0 ± 0.1 μl/min per g (Kang et al., 1995a). The PS product for the phosphate anion in peripheral tissues is many-fold higher than the PS product at the BBB. Therefore, when internally labeled PO-ODNs are injected intravenously into rats, endonuclease activity in the peripheral tissues results in the rapid formation of radiolabeled metabolites and these are taken up by brain and other tissues (Kang et al., 1995a). This uptake of the radiolabeled metabolites confounds interpretation of brain uptake data similar to that of radiolabeled peptides, as discussed in Chapter 4.

The rapid degradation of chimeric PO-ODNs, despite conjugation to BBB drug-targeting systems, indicates that PO-ODNs are not the ideal antisense molecule for in vivo applications. Accordingly, PS-ODNs, which are resistant to exo- and endonuclease activity, were next evaluated as candidates for development of antisense therapeutics for the brain.

Sulfur-containing oligodeoxynucleotides

Phosphorothioate oligodeoxynucleotides

Molecular formulation

The model PS-ODN was an 18-mer complementary to the *rev* gene of HIV-1 and nucleotides 5551–5568 of the HIV-1 genome. The PS-ODN was synthesized with a biotin group at the 3′-terminus and a primary amino group at the 5′-terminus (Figure 8.3A). The [3′-bio-5′-amino]-PS-ODN was tritiated at the 5′-terminus with [³H]-*N*-succinimidyl propionate (NSP). The TCA precipitability of the [³H]-bio-PS-ODN was >99% and the specific activity was 0.68 μCi/μg. This PS-ODN

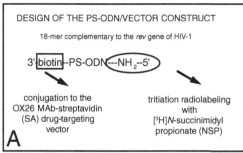

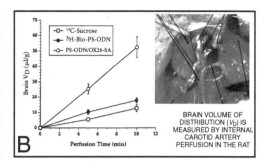

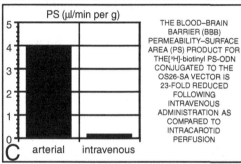

Figure 8.3   (A) Design of a phosphodiester oligodeoxynucleotide (PS-ODN) that contains a biotin at the 3′-terminus and an amino group at the 5′-terminus to enable radiolabeling with [³H]-N-succinimidyl propionate (NSP). (B) Internal carotid artery perfusion of [¹⁴C]sucrose, [³H]-biotinylated-PS-ODN, or the [³H]-biotinylated-PS-ODN conjugated to OX26/streptavidin (SA) was performed for 5 or 10 min, and the brain volume of distribution (V_D) is shown. (C) The BBB permeability–surface area (PS) product for the [³H]biotinyl PS-ODN conjugated to OX26/SA was measured at 10 min following an internal carotid arterial infusion or at 60 min following intravenous injection. From Wu et al. (1996) with permission.

was bound to a conjugate of OX26 and streptavidin, designated OX26–SA (Boado et al., 1995).

BBB transport of chimeric PS-ODNs

The transport of the [³H]-bio-PS-ODN across the BBB in anesthetized rats was measured with the internal carotid artery perfusion (ICAP) technique (Wu et al., 1996), and these results are shown in Figure 8.3B. With the ICAP method, a PE50 catheter is placed into the internal carotid artery, as shown in the inset of Figure 8.3B. The BBB transport was measured after 5- and 10-min ICAP. The ICAP method allows for measurement of brain uptake of the PS-ODN in the absence of mixture of the perfusate with serum proteins. The data show that in the absence of conjugation to a drug-targeting system, the BBB transport of the PS-ODN is not significantly different from the BBB transport of sucrose. However, the brain volume of distribution (V_D) of the [³H]-bio-PS-ODN was increased fivefold above the sucrose volume by conjugation to the OX26–SA vector (Figure 8.3B). The metabolic stability of the [³H]-bio-PS-ODN after a 10-min ICAP was investigated by measuring the TCA precipitability of the brain homogenate [³H] radioactivity. The brain radioactivity that was TCA precipitable after a 10-min carotid artery perfusion was 99 ± 1%. This indicates the increase in BBB transport of the PS-ODN mediated by conjugation to OX26–SA reflected actual BBB transport of the chimeric oligonucleotide conjugate and not the brain uptake of a metabolite (Wu et al., 1996).

The BBB PS product of the [³H]-bio-PS-ODN conjugated to OX26–SA was 4.0 μl/min per g, following ICAP (Figure 8.3B). However, the BBB PS product was much lower when this chimeric oligonucleotide was injected intravenously into anesthetized rats. As shown in Figure 8.3C, the BBB PS product was 23-fold lower after intravenous injection, compared to the PS product recorded with ICAP. The BBB permeability–surface area (PS) product measured with arterial perfusion reflects BBB permeability in the absence of serum proteins. Conversely, the BBB PS product measured after intravenous injection reflects the permeability in the presence of plasma proteins. PS-ODNs are bound to plasma proteins, principally albumin and α_2-macroglobulin (Cossum et al., 1993). Therefore, in order to investigate the effects of serum protein binding on the BBB transport of the bio-PS-ODN bound to OX26–SA, the BBB PS product of the PS-ODN chimeric oligonucleotide was measured following ICAP with rat serum. The brain V_D was reduced to 14 ± 1 μl/g in the presence of 100% rat serum and this V_D value was not significantly different from the brain V_D for [¹⁴C]sucrose, 11 ± 3 μl/g (Figure 8.3B). Therefore, the presence of serum in the internal carotid artery perfusate completely aborted the BBB transport of the PS-ODN that was mediated by conjugation to OX26–SA (Wu et al., 1996). The serum binding of the PS-ODN and the serum inhibition explain the 23-fold reduction in PS product of the chimeric PS-ODN following intravenous administration (Figure 8.3C).

The binding of PS-ODNs to serum proteins, such as albumin or α_2-macroglobulin, completely neutralizes the beneficial effects of conjugation of PS-ODNs to BBB drug-targeting systems (Wu et al., 1996). The binding of PS-ODNs to serum proteins is a mirror image of the avid binding of PS-ODNs to a wide variety of cellular proteins (Brown et al., 1994; Beltinger et al., 1995). Replacement of the oxygen atom with the sulfur atom in the phosphodiester backbone of an ODN results in a greatly increased reactivity of the sulfurated ODN with serum and cellular proteins. Indeed, this high avidity of PS-ODNs for cellular proteins explains many of the pharmacologic effects of PS-ODNs observed in cell culture and these pharmacologic effects are mediated via nonantisense mechanisms (Burgess et al., 1995; Rockwel et al., 1997). Apart from the binding of PS-ODNs to plasma proteins, another consideration in the development of PS-ODNs as neuropharmaceutics is the neurotoxicity of these molecules.

Neurotoxicity of PS-ODNs

The chronic intrathecal infusion of a PS-ODN that is antisense to a sequence of the cytokine responsive gene-2/IP-10 results in spinal cord necrosis and paralysis in rats (Wojcik et al., 1996). In these studies, the PS-ODN was infused intrathecally at a rate of 0.18–1.8 nmol/h. Conversely, no cord necrosis or neurotoxicity was observed following the intrathecal infusion of PO-ODNs (Wojcik et al., 1996). PO-ODNs are not neurotoxic because these molecules are rapidly broken down by exo- and endo-nucleases in vivo (Whitesell et al., 1993). PS-ODNs are neurotoxic because (a) these molecules are more resistant to nucleases, and (b) the sulfur atoms of the PS-ODNs cause a strong reactivity with multiple cellular proteins (Brown et al., 1994; Beltinger et al., 1995). The neurotoxicity of PS-ODNs was also observed when these molecules were administered by infusion into the lateral ventricle of rats (Whitesell et al., 1993). The ICV infusion of PS-ODNs is lethal when the infusion dose exceeds 3 nmol/h. Rates of infusion under 2 nmol/h are better tolerated in rats. The higher infusion rates probably produce a cerebrospinal fluid (CSF) concentration of the PS-ODN that exceeds the normal albumin concentration in CSF. That is, the high binding of PS-ODNs to albumin, and the presence of albumin in CSF, provides a buffer protecting brain cells against the toxic effects of PS-ODNs following ICV infusion. However, the binding of the PS-ODN to CSF albumin greatly increases the effective molecular weight of the PS-ODN, and thereby restricts the diffusion of the PS-ODN into brain parenchyma from the CSF flow tracts (Whitesell et al., 1993). PS-ODNs are also neurotoxic following the peripheral administration of very large doses (Agrawal, 1991).

The buffering of the toxic effects of the PS-ODNs by binding to serum proteins is also seen in cell culture. The concentration of PS-ODN that results in a 50% toxicity in cultured cells is 1.2, 2.8, and 9.5 μmol/l, in the presence of 2.5%, 5%, and 10% of fetal calf serum, respectively (Crooke, 1991). Moreover, early studies noted that physiological concentrations of albumin completely block the pharmacologic effects of PS-ODNs in cell culture (Matsukura et al., 1991).

Nonantisense effects of PS-ODNs

The strong but nonspecific binding of PS-ODNs to a variety of serum and cellular proteins results in many pharmacologic effects that are not mediated via antisense mechanisms. For example, PS-ODNs, but not PO-ODNs, inhibit the binding of basic fibroblast growth factor (bFGF) to its receptor in a manner that is actually sequence-specific (Fennewald and Rando, 1995). However, this is not an antisense mechanism, but is a function of the binding of the polyanionic PS-ODN to the bFGF receptor in a heparin-like manner. In another study, PS-ODNs were shown to bind to the CD4 receptor of lymphocytes, which is the HIV receptor, and thereby block the uptake of HIV by lymphocytes in cell culture (Yakubov et al., 1993). This is a sequence-unrelated nonantisense pharmacologic effect of the PS-ODN. It is probable that many of the reports of pharmacologic effects of PS-ODNs in cultured cells are instances of nonantisense actions of these highly reactive compounds. The high reactivity of a PS-ODN with multiple cellular proteins results in cellular uptake of these nuclease-resistant compounds and rapid and multiple pharmaco-logic effects that are not antisense-mediated. In contrast, electrically neutral mole-cules such as PNAs are not taken up by cells and no pharmacologic effects are seen in tissue culture when PNAs are used as antisense agents. For these reasons, the PS-ODNs are the favored antisense agent for work in cell culture whereas few studies use PNAs. However, the significant problems associated with the use of PS-ODNs, such as nonantisense pharmacologic activity, serum protein binding, and neuro-toxicity, are not characteristic of PNAs as antisense agents. The rapid breakdown of PO-ODNs by exo- and endo-nucleases is also not observed with PNAs, since these polyamide molecules are resistant to nuclease activity.

Phosphorothioate/phosphodiester hybrid oligodeoxynucleotides

Since PS-ODNs bind and cross-link multiple cellular proteins, hybrid ODNs were introduced to minimize the disadvantages involved with the use of fully sulfurated PS-ODN molecules (Agrawal et al., 1997). A PS/PO hybrid ODN is a PO-ODN with several PS moieties at either the 5′- or 3′-terminus, which are inserted to provide resistance to exonuclease (Bishop et al., 1996). However, given the suscep-tibility of PO-ODNs to endonuclease action in vivo, it was hypothesized that PS/PO-ODN hybrids would also be susceptible to endonuclease activity in vivo. This hypothesis was tested by preparing a PS/PO-ODN hybrid that was fully sulfu-rated, with the exception of a single internal PO linkage (Boado et al., 1995).

Molecular formulation

The synthesis of a $[^{32}PO_{21}]$-PS-ODN hybrid is outlined in Figure 8.4A. A 21-mer PS-ODN was synthesized with a biotin moiety at the 3′-terminus and the 5′-ter-minus was phosphorylated with $[^{32}P]$ and T4 polynucleotide kinase. In parallel, a 15-mer PS-ODN was synthesized, and both the 15-mer PS-ODN and the 21-mer PS-ODN were hybridized to a complementary 36-mer PO-ODN template (Boado et al., 1995). Following annealing and ligation with T4 ligase, the 36-mer PS-ODN with a single internal PO linkage was eluted from a urea/polyacrylamide sequenc-ing gel (Figure 8.4A). The conversion of the $[^{32}P]$-labeled 21-mer to the internally labeled 36-mer was demonstrated by sequencing gel electrophoresis and auto-radiography, as shown in Figure 8.4B. In parallel, a 21-mer-PS-ODN that was bio-

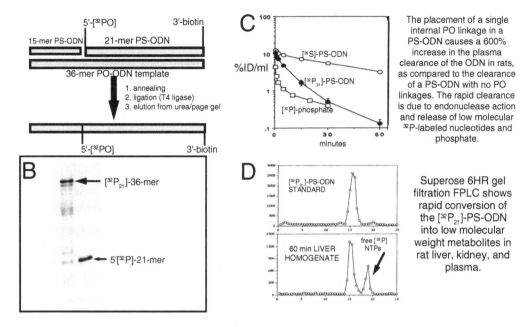

Figure 8.4   (A) Method for production of a 36-mer PS-ODN containing a single internally labeled phosphodiester (PO) linkage. (B) Film autoradiography of a urea gel shows conversion of the 5'-[^{32}P]-21-mer to the [^{32}P] internally labeled 36-mer PS-ODN with a single PO bond at position 21 and a biotin residue at the 3'-terminus. Other gels demonstrated the separation of the PS-ODN antisense and the PO-ODN sense strands. (C) Plasma concentration, expressed as percentage injected dose (ID) per milliliter, is plotted versus time following intravenous injection in anesthetized rats. The [^{35}S]-PS-ODN is fully sulfurated whereas the [^{32}P$_{21}$]-PS-ODN is a 36-mer PS-ODN that contains a single PO linkage at position 21. (D) Gel filtration fast protein liquid chromatography (FPLC) demonstrates conversion in liver of the PS-ODN containing a single PO linkage to [^{32}P]-labeled nucleotide triphosphates (NTP) or [^{32}P]phosphate. From Boado et al. (1995) with permission.

tinylated at the 3'-terminus (Figure 8.4A) was labeled with [^{35}S] by sulfuration, and this fully sulfurated PS-ODN contained no internal PO linkages (Boado et al., 1995).

Plasma clearance and metabolism

The plasma concentrations of the [^{32}PO$_{21}$]-PS-ODN hybrid and the fully sulfurated [^{35}S]-PS-ODN are shown in Figure 8.4C. The fully sulfurated PS-ODN was removed from plasma slowly with a systemic clearance of 0.94 ± 0.07 ml/min per kg (Boado et al., 1995). The major organs responsible for clearance of the PS-ODN from blood were liver and kidney. In contrast, the rate of plasma clearance of the internally labeled PS-ODN that contained a single internal PO linkage was increased fivefold to 4.5 ± 0.4 ml/min per kg. The increased plasma clearance of the PS-ODN that contained a single internal PO linkage was paralleled by a decrease in the metabolic stability of the ODN. The plasma radioactivity at 60 min after intravenous injection that was precipitable by TCA is >95% following intravenous injection of the fully sulfurated PS-ODN, but is <70% following intravenous injection of the PS-ODN containing a single internal PO linkage. These studies indicate that the PS-ODN containing a single internal PO linkage is rapidly degraded by phosphodiester endonucleases and the [^{32}P] radioactivity is then removed by either alkaline phosphatase or 3'-exonuclease (Boado et al., 1995). This results in the formation of [^{32}P]phosphate anion, which is rapidly removed from the blood stream, as shown in Figure 8.4C. The conversion of the PS-ODN to free [^{32}P]phosphate anion and the rapid clearance of the phosphate anion explain the rapid clearance of plasma radioactivity following the injection of the PS/PO hybrid ODN. The conversion of the internally labeled PS-ODN into low molecular weight metabolite was demonstrated by gel filtration fast protein liquid chromatography (FPLC) of liver homogenate obtained 60 min after intravenous injection of the hybrid ODN (Figure 8.4D).

The development of antisense therapeutics is a case study of the importance of rapid entry of pharmaceutical candidates into in vivo testing of pharmacokinetics and metabolism, and the importance of not relying strictly on experiments performed in cell culture. Although PO-ODNs are rapidly degraded in cell culture by 3'-exonuclease, this can be completely eliminated by biotinylation of the 3'-terminus. Other modifications of the 3'-terminus will similarly eliminate the susceptibility of PO-ODNs to 3'-exonuclease in cell culture (Gamper et al., 1992). However, when 3'-protected PO-ODNs are administered in vivo, these molecules are rapidly degraded by endonucleases (Kang et al., 1995a). Similarly, PS-PO hybrid ODNs are also rapidly degraded by endonucleases in vivo. In contrast, fully sulfurated PS-ODNs are much less susceptible to endonuclease activity in either cell culture or in vivo. The PS-ODNs are highly reactive with multiple cellular proteins and this high reactivity probably explains many of the pharmacologic effects recorded with these molecules in either cell culture or following intracerebral injection of PS-ODNs. In the majority of cases, these pharmacologic actions may be mediated via nonantisense mechanisms. In the absence of buffering by serum proteins, PS-ODNs are toxic to cells in culture and are neurotoxic following in vivo administration in brain or spinal cord. Finally, the avid binding of PS-ODNs to serum proteins completely eliminates the ability of brain drug-targeting systems to mediate the transport of these molecules across the BBB in vivo (Figure 8.3C). For these reasons, subsequent development of antisense agents as neuropharmaceuticals focused on peptide nucleic acids.

Peptide nucleic acids

PNAs have a polyamide backbone (Nielsen et al., 1991), in contrast to the phosphodiester or phosphorothioate backbone of PO-ODN or PS-ODNs, respectively (Figure 8.1). The electrically neutral PNAs lack the susceptibility of PO-ODNs to exo- or endo-nucleases and are metabolically stable in serum or in cell culture (Demidov et al., 1994). Similarly, the PNAs are not strongly bound by plasma or cellular proteins, as is the case with PS-ODNs. Indeed, PNAs are so inert that these molecules are not taken up by cells in culture. In order to observe antisense effects with PNAs in cultured cells, it is necessary physically to inject the PNA into the cytoplasm of the cell (Hanvey et al., 1992). Another advantage of PNAs is the very strong hybridization of these antisense molecules to target DNA or mRNA sequences. The melting point (T_m) of a PNA/DNA duplex is approximately 1°C per base pair higher than the T_m of the duplex formed with PO-ODN/DNA hybrids and the T_m of PNA/RNA hybrids is even higher (Nielsen et al., 1994). Another advantage of PNAs, which is important for the development of antisense radiopharmaceuticals, is that amino acid groups can be added to the amino or carboxyl terminus of the PNA. Therefore, a carboxyl terminal tyrosine residue can be added to the sequence to enable radiolabeling with [^{125}I]. A carboxyl terminal lysine residue can be added to enable conjugation with diethylenetriaminepentaacetic acid (DTPA) for radiolabeling with indium-111. The placement of a lysine residue at the carboxyl terminus also reduces the tendency of PNAs to aggregate (Nielsen et al., 1993), and the lysine residue does not interfere with PNA hybridization to target nucleic acid sequences (Egholm et al., 1993).

Molecular formulation

The model PNA used in initial studies was an 18-mer that is antisense to nucleotides 5980–5997 of the genome of HIV-1, which encodes the region of the *rev* mRNA around the methionine initiation codon (Pardridge et al., 1995a). The PNA was synthesized with a biotin moiety at the amino terminus and a tyrosine/lysine sequence at the carboxyl terminus. The carboxyl terminus was amidated to make the PNA resistant to carboxypeptidases. The biotin moiety at the amino terminus makes the PNA resistant to aminopeptidases. The PNA was iodinated on the tyrosine residue with chloramine T. The radiolabeled, biotinylated PNA was bound to a conjugate of the OX26 monoclonal antibody (MAb) to the rat transferrin receptor

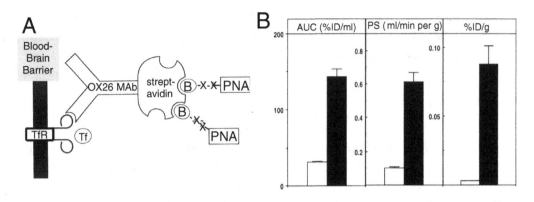

Figure 8.5   Vector-mediated delivery of a peptide nucleic acid through the blood–brain barrier (BBB). (A) A peptide nucleic acid (PNA) that contains a sequence antisense to the *rev* mRNA of human immunodeficiency virus-1 (HIV-1) is attached to a conjugate of OX26 and streptavidin (SA) via a biotin moiety placed at the amino terminus of the PNA. The OX26 monoclonal antibody (MAb) targets the BBB transferrin receptor (TfR). (B) The plasma area under the concentration curve (AUC), the BBB permeability–surface area (PS) product, and the brain uptake, expressed as percentage injected dose (ID) per gram brain, is shown for the unconjugated PNA (open columns) and for the PNA bound to the OX26/SA conjugate (closed columns). From Pardridge et al. (1995a) with permission. Copyright (1995) National Academy of Sciences, USA.

and streptavidin (SA). The structure of the PNA chimeric peptide is shown in Figure 8.5A. The binding of the radiolabeled biotinylated PNA to OX26/SA was confirmed by gel filtration FPLC.

Blood–brain barrier transport

The radiolabeled biotinylated PNA was injected intravenously into anesthetized rats in either the unconjugated form or as a conjugate with OX26/SA (Pardridge et al., 1995a). The plasma area under the concentration curve (AUC), the BBB PS product, and the brain uptake (%ID/g) of the unconjugated PNA or of the PNA conjugate was measured at 60 min after administration and these results are shown in Figure 8.5B. Conjugation of the PNA to OX26/SA resulted in a sevenfold reduction in plasma clearance and this was reflected in the increase in the plasma AUC of the PNA chimeric peptide relative to the unconjugated PNA (Figure 8.5B). The systemic clearance, 8.6 ± 0.3 ml/min per kg, of the unconjugated PNA approximated the systemic clearance of sucrose, 10.8 ± 0.4 ml/min per kg. This indicated the mechanism of systemic clearance of the unconjugated PNA was primarily glomerular filtration and renal clearance. The effective molecular weight of the PNA was increased from 5500 Da to 205 kDa following conjugation to OX26/SA, since the molecular weight of OX26/SA is 200 kDa. This increase in effective molecular size of the PNA chimeric peptide explains the reduction in renal clearance, the reduction in systemic clearance, and the increase in plasma AUC.

The BBB PS product of the unconjugated PNA was 0.10 ± 0.10 µl/min per g and the brain uptake of the unconjugated PNA was 0.0031 ± 0.0002%ID/g and these values are indicative of background brain uptake and absence of BBB transport of the unconjugated PNA. Conversely, the BBB PS product and the brain uptake of the PNA chimeric peptide were increased following conjugation to the BBB drug-targeting system (Figure 8.5B). Brain uptake was increased 28-fold when the biotinylated PNA was conjugated to OX26/SA (Pardridge et al., 1995a), and the level of brain uptake of the PNA chimeric peptide exceeded the brain uptake of morphine, a neuroactive small molecule (Wu et al., 1997a). Capillary depletion analysis demonstrated that the PNA chimeric peptide was transcytosed through the BBB in vivo and was not sequestered in the capillary compartment (Pardridge et al., 1995a).

The metabolic stability of the PNA chimeric peptide was measured both with assays of TCA precipitability of plasma radioactivity and with gel filtration FPLC of serum taken at 60 min after intravenous injection in anesthetized rats. The plasma TCA precipitability of the 60-min plasma radioactivity was >95% and the gel filtration FPLC analysis showed that no low molecular weight metabolites were present in the 60-min plasma. The only radiochemical species detected in plasma at 60 min migrated at the same elution volume as the uninjected PNA chimeric peptide conjugated to OX26/SA (Pardridge et al., 1995a).

The findings in Figure 8.5 show that PNAs do not cross the BBB. These results are in accord with prior work in cell culture, which showed that PNAs do not cross cell membranes, and exert biological activity in cultured cells only when the molecules are physically injected into the intracellular compartment (Hanvey et al., 1992). PNAs, like the PO-ODNs or the PS-ODNs, are highly water-soluble molecules with molecular weights of 5–10 kDa, and are too large to traverse the BBB via lipid-mediated transport (Chapter 3). Tyler et al. (1999) report that unconjugated PNAs do cross the BBB in vivo. In this study the uptake of the PNA by rat brain was measured with a gel shift analysis of extracts of saline-perfused brain. However, this report shows the brain uptake of the PNA is <0.0001%ID/g (Tyler et al., 1999), which is a level of brain uptake comparable to that of sucrose, a molecule that traverses the BBB at the lower limit of detection (Chapter 3). This level of brain uptake is so low, a small contamination of the brain blood pool that was incompletely removed by the saline perfusion could account for the PNA content in brain. The brain uptake of the PNA chimeric peptide (Figure 8.5) is approximately 3 log orders of magnitude greater than the brain uptake of the unconjugated PNA reported by Tyler et al. (1999).

RNAse protection assay

The PNA was conjugated to OX26/SA via a noncleavable (amide) linker between the PNA amino terminus and the biotin moiety (Figure 8.5A). The ability of the intact PNA conjugate to hybridize with its target mRNA was investigated with an RNAse protection assay (RPA). A *rev* transcription plasmid was prepared and this enabled the production of sense and antisense *rev* mRNA using T7 and T3 RNA polymerases, respectively, following linearization of the transcription plasmid with either Pst I or Xba I restriction endonucleases, respectively (Figure 8.6A). The sense or antisense RNA was radiolabeled with [^{32}P] by incorporation of [α-^{32}P]adenosine triphosphate (ATP) during the in vitro transcription (Pardridge et al., 1995a). For the RPA, 0.5 pmol of either biotinylated or nonbiotinylated PNA (Figure 8.6B) was incubated with or without 10 pmol of OX26–SA for 5 min and this was followed by addition of 10^5 cpm of [^{32}P]-labeled sense or antisense *rev* RNA. Following annealing at 42 °C, RNAse T1 and RNAse A were added followed by incubation for 30 min at 37 °C. RNA fragments were analyzed by 7 mol/l urea/20% polyacrylamide gel electrophoresis and autoradiography. The results of the gel analysis are shown in Figure 8.6C. Both the free PNA and the PNA conjugated to OX26/SA hybridized to the target *rev* mRNA, as shown by the generation of an RNAse A/T1 protected fragment. No RNAse protected fragment was observed when the *rev* antisense mRNA was used (Figure 8.6C). The RPA shows that conjugation of the PNA to OX26/SA does not interfere with hybridization of the PNA to the target mRNA sequence (Pardridge et al., 1995a).

Translation arrest

The RPA studies shown in Figure 8.6 indicate the PNA chimeric peptide still hybridizes to the target mRNA despite conjugation to the BBB drug-targeting system. Another indicator of pharmaceutical activity of the chimeric PNA is a translation arrest assay and these results are shown in Figure 8.7. The *rev* mRNA was prepared by in vitro transcription using the *rev* transcription plasmid and T7 RNA polymerase, as shown in Figure 8.6A. PNAs were synthesized with either a biotin moiety at the amino terminus, or with no biotin moiety at the amino terminus, and were complementary to nucleotides 5980–5997 of the HIV-1 genome (Figure 8.6B), which corresponds to the region around the methionine initiation codon of the *rev* mRNA. The outline of the translation arrest assay is shown in the left-hand panel of Figure 8.7. The PNAs, with or without the biotin attached and with or without conjugation to the OX26/SA delivery system, were hybridized to 2 μg of *rev* mRNA (Boado et al., 1998b). Translation was performed in a rabbit reticulocyte lysate with [^{3}H]leucine and production of the translated *rev* protein was analyzed by immunoprecipitation using an anti-*rev* antibody followed by sodium dodecylsulfate polyacrylamide gel electrophoresis (SDS-PAGE) and film autoradiography. The

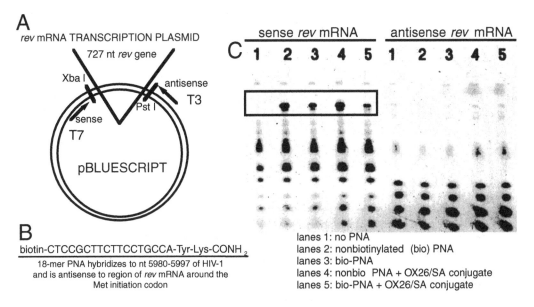

A

rev mRNA TRANSCRIPTION PLASMID

727 nt rev gene

Xba I

antisense

Pst I

T3

sense

T7

pBLUESCRIPT

C

sense rev mRNA | antisense rev mRNA

1 2 3 4 5 1 2 3 4 5

B

biotin-CTCCGCTTCTTCCTGCCA-Tyr-Lys-CONH$_2$

18-mer PNA hybridizes to nt 5980-5997 of HIV-1
and is antisense to region of rev mRNA around the
Met initiation codon

lanes 1: no PNA
lanes 2: nonbiotinylated (bio) PNA
lanes 3: bio-PNA
lanes 4: nonbio PNA + OX26/SA conjugate
lanes 5: bio-PNA + OX26/SA conjugate

Figure 8.6   Retention of biologic activity of anti-rev peptide nucleic acid (PNA) following conjugation to the OX26/streptavidin (SA) vector: RNAse protection assay. (A) rev mRNA transcription plasmid. (B) Sequence of a rev PNA that is antisense to the rev gene of human immunodeficiency virus-1 (HIV-1). (C) RNAse protection assay (RPA) with rev [^{32}P]-labeled mRNA and the PNA antisense to the rev mRNA. Both sense and antisense radiolabeled rev RNA were prepared and used in the RNAse protection assay. The effect of binding of the OX26/SA conjugate to the rev PNA was examined with the RPA. For either sense or antisense rev RNA: lane 1, [^{32}P]-labeled RNA alone; lane 2, [^{32}P]-labeled RNA plus nonbiotinylated PNA; lane 3, [^{32}P]-labeled RNA plus biotinylated PNA; lane 4, [^{32}P]-labeled RNA plus nonbiotinylated PNA and OX26–SA; lane 5, [^{32}P]-labeled RNA plus biotinylated PNA conjugated to OX26–SA. Incubation of the biotinylated PNA or the nonbiotinylated PNA with a sense RNA produced a similar RNAse-resistant fragment and the formation of this fragment was not modified by the addition of OX26/SA (see lanes 3 and 4 for sense RNA). No RNAse-resistant fragment was seen with antisense RNA incubated with or without the PNA or with sense RNA incubated without the PNA, indicating that the RNAse protection was exerted through a sequence-specific mechanism. The autoradiogram was exposed for 3 days at −70 °C. From Pardridge et al. (1995a) with permission. Copyright (1995) National Academy of Sciences, USA.

synthesis of a single band of 19 kDa corresponding to the mature rev protein is shown in lane 2 of Figure 8.7. Translation of the 19 kDa rev protein is completely arrested by the addition of the anti-rev PNA in either its biotinylated form (lane 4) or nonbiotinylated form (lane 3), as shown in Figure 8.7. The addition of OX26/SA alone did not alter translation of the rev protein, as demonstrated in lane 5 of Figure 8.7. Conjugation of the PNA to OX26/SA did not modify the biologic activity of the

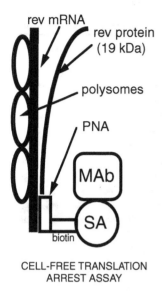

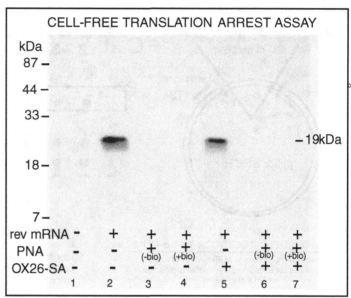

Figure 8.7   Biotinylated peptide nucleic acid (PNA) conjugated to OX26 monoclonal antibody (MAb)/streptavidin (SA) binds to target *rev* mRNA and arrests translation of *rev* protein. Left: The *rev* mRNA was translated on polysomes present in rabbit reticulocyte lysate to generate the 19 kDa *rev* protein. Translation arrest occurred when the PNA hybridized to the *rev* mRNA around the methionine initiation codon, and prevented translation of the *rev* mRNA. The PNA was conjugated to OX26/SA via a biotin linker. Right: Cell-free translation arrest assay: *rev* mRNA was prepared with an in vitro transcription using the *rev* transcription plasmid described in Figure 8.6A. Both biotinylated and nonbiotinylated anti-*rev* PNA (37.5 pmol) were incubated with 2 μg of *rev* mRNA in the presence or absence of the OX26/SA targeting system (75 pmol). From Drug delivery of antisense molecules to the brain for treatment of Alzheimer's disease and cerebral AIDS, Boado, R.J., Tsukamoto, H. and Pardridge, W.M., *J. Pharm. Sci.*, copyright © (1998). Reprinted by permission of Wiley-Liss, a subsidiary of John Wiley & Sons, Inc.

PNA. There was still translation arrest of the *rev* protein, as shown in lanes 6 and 7 of Figure 8.7.

The RPA and translation arrest assays (Figures 8.6 and 8.7) demonstrate that the biologic activity and ability of the PNA to hybridize to the target mRNA is unimpaired following conjugation of the biotinylated PNA to the OX26/SA drug-targeting system using a noncleavable amide linker. These assays are analogous to the radioreceptor assays discussed in Chapter 7, which demonstrate retention of biologic activity of peptides despite conjugation to BBB drug-targeting systems. The initial in vivo application of PNA antisense agents was the in vivo imaging of gene expression in the brain with PNA chimeric peptides used as antisense radiopharmaceuticals.

Imaging gene expression in the brain in vivo

Indirect and direct imaging of organ gene expression

Direct imaging of gene expression

The only direct way to image gene expression in vivo is with the use of antisense radiopharmaceuticals that hybridize to a target mRNA. This hybridization seques-ters the antisense imaging agent in the cytosol and delays the degradation of the agent. This results in a local enhancement of radioactivity that can be imaged with standard external detection modalities such as single photon emission computed tomography (SPECT) or positron emission tomography (PET) in humans or quantitative autoradiography (QAR) in experimental animals. Imaging gene expression has been done in vitro in the laboratory for decades using Northern blotting analysis or in situ hybridization and these methods are based on the com-plementary hybridization of sense and antisense nucleic acids that form a duplex on the basis of Watson–Crick base pairing. The problem with imaging gene expres-sion in vivo is that the target mRNA molecules are buried within the cytoplasm of the cells. These mRNA molecules cannot be accessed by antisense radiopharmaceu-ticals because these agents do not cross the BBB in vivo. Because the mRNA mole-cules are inside the cell, the targeting of antisense agents to brain cells is a "two-barrier" targeting problem because the antisense agent must be targeted not only through the BBB, but also through the brain cell membrane (BCM).

Indirect imaging of gene expression

Given the inability of antisense agents to cross biological membranes, prior attempts to image gene expression have used indirect approaches that are based on diffusible small molecules, and are essentially derivatives of existing imaging tech-nology. For example, the activity of hexokinase in brain is imaged with PET using radiolabeled 2-fluoro-2-deoxyglucose (FDG). The phosphorylation and entrap-ment of the FDG within brain cells is proportional to the activity of hexokinase. One could say this is an image of hexokinase gene expression in brain. However, the final enzyme activity is a function of multiple factors other than gene expres-sion, such as FDG transport at the BBB (Chapter 3), hexokinase compartmental-ization within the cyoplasm and the mitochondria, hexokinase degradation, and other factors.

In the indirect approach, a reporter gene encoding an enzyme is delivered to an organ by a viral vector, and a radiolabeled small molecule substrate that is metab-olized by the reporter enzyme is then administered. In one study, RG2 rat glioma cells were implanted in nude animals as flank tumors (Tjuvajev et al., 1998). Following formation of these flank tumors, a retrovirus containing the herpes simplex virus thymidine kinase (HSV-tk) gene was injected. [^{124}I]-2′-Fluoro-1-β-

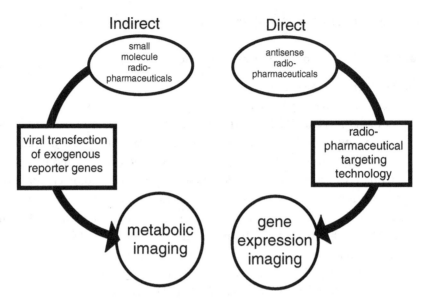

Figure 8.8   Indirect and direct methods for imaging gene expression in vivo.

D-arabinofuranosyl-uracil (FIAU) was administered followed by PET scanning. The [^{124}I]FIAU was trapped in the tumor cells expressing the thymidine kinase and this resulted in imaging of the cells containing the exogenously administered transgene. In a parallel approach to indirect imaging of gene expression, mouse liver was transfected in vivo with adenovirus carrying the HSV-tK reporter gene (Gambhir et al., 1999a). Gene expression was imaged with PET using a different small molecule substrate of HSV-tk, [^{18}F]ganciclovir (FGCV). In another study, the liver of nude mice was transfected with adenovirus and a reporter gene for the dopamine-2 receptor (D2R), and imaging was performed with positron-labeled D2R ligands (Gambhir et al., 1999b).

The indirect approach to imaging gene expression uses a small molecule radionuclide that crosses biological membranes by free diffusion (Figure 8.8). The entrapment of the radioactivity within the tissue is a function of the activity of the enzyme translated from the exogenous transgene. The enzymatic activity of the gene product is directly proportional to the amount of protein produced in the cell and this is a function not only of the transcription of the transgene, but also of the translation efficiency of the transgene mRNA, of the metabolic turnover of the enzyme, and of the transport properties of the small molecule tracer. However, the main problem with the indirect approach for imaging gene expression is that this method can only be applied to subjects that have been administered an exogenous transgene. The indirect approach cannot be used to "image any gene in any person," which is the goal of imaging technology devoted to the analysis of gene expression in vivo.

Direct imaging of gene expression using a lipidized PS-ODN

The gene expression for glial fibrillary acidic protein (GFAP) was imaged in experimental brain tumors with a 25-mer PS-ODN that contained a 5′-amino group (Kobori et al., 1999), similar to that shown in Figure 8.3A. This amino group was then labeled with [^{11}C] for PET imaging of experimental brain tumors in rats. The PS-ODN also contained a cholesterol moiety at the 3′-terminus to enable transport of the PS-ODN across the cellular barriers separating the PS-ODN in blood from the GFAP mRNA within the tumor cells in brain. Prior work had shown that the addition of a cholesterol group to the terminus of an ODN increases cellular uptake of the ODN in cell culture (de Smidt et al., 1991; Krieg et al., 1993).

The addition of a cholesterol moiety to the 3′-terminus of a PS-ODN is a lipidization strategy designed to mediate the transport of the antisense radiopharmaceutical across the BBB and the tumor cell membrane in vivo. As reviewed in Chapter 3, there are some limitations with such a lipidization strategy. First, the cholesterol conjugate is rapidly removed from plasma, which reduces the plasma AUC and causes a proportional reduction in the brain %ID/g, as predicted by the "pharmacokinetic rule" (Chapter 3). This necessitates the administration of very large doses of radioactivity (Kobori et al., 1999). Second, the addition of a cholesterol moiety to a 7500 Da PS-ODN would not be expected to cause a substantial increase in the BBB permeability of the PS-ODN, because the size of this compound exceeds the 400–600 Da threshold of lipid-mediated transport through the BBB in vivo (Chapter 3). Therefore, considering PS-ODNs do not cross the BBB (Wu et al., 1996), it is somewhat surprising that brain uptake of the PS-ODN was reported (Kobori et al., 1999). Third, the addition of the cholesterol conjugate to the PS-ODN eliminates the solubility of the compound in aqueous solution. It was necessary to solubilize the PS-ODN in dichloromethane, and the dose of dichloromethane administered intravenously in the antisense imaging studies is not reported (Kobori et al., 1999).

The solubilization of the cholesterol adduct of a PS-ODN in a harsh solvent such as dichloromethane is analogous to the solubilization of a cholesterol adduct of an oligopeptide in high concentrations of ethanol and dimethylsulfoxide (DMSO), as reviewed in Chapter 3. The administration of the drug/solvent mixture results in the coinjection of sufficient doses (1 g/kg) of the ethanol or DMSO solvents to cause solvent-mediated BBB disruption (Brink and Stein, 1967; Hanig et al., 1972). This phenomenon of solvent disruption of the BBB was also demonstrated for nanoparticles. In this case, the nanoparticles were formulated in Tween 80 and the dose of Tween 80 that was administered was sufficient to cause BBB disruption such that BBB transport of drug was mediated by the detergent solvent, not the nano-particles (Olivier et al., 1999). In an another example of solvent-mediated BBB transport, initial studies showed that interleukin-2 (IL-2) enables BBB transport, and it was subsequently demonstrated that the BBB transport was actually caused by the coadministration of SDS, used to solubilize the IL-2 (Ellison et al., 1990). Doses of solvents such as SDS as low as 30 ng per mouse are sufficient to cause a transient opening of the BBB (Kobiler et al., 1989). These studies show that solvents such as ethanol, DMSO, Tween 80, SDS, and possibly dichloromethane cause BBB disruption, and the potential effect of such solvents on brain uptake in vivo needs to be considered.

Direct imaging of gene expression using the chimeric peptide technology

The direct imaging of gene expression in the brain in vivo with antisense radio-pharmaceuticals will require the application of a drug-targeting technology, because antisense agents do not cross the BBB (Chem et al., 1990; Vlassov and Yakubov, 1991; Tavitan et al., 1998). Therefore, the problem of targeting antisense therapeutics to brain is similar to targeting peptides to brain, except antisense drugs must be targeted through both the BBB and the BCM in vivo, because the target mRNA resides in the cytoplasm of brain cells. The limitations of targeting drugs to the brain with either craniotomy or lipidization strategies are reviewed in Chapters 2 and 3. The alternative approach is to target antisense drugs to the brain by access-ing endogenous transport systems that are expressed at both the BBB and the BCM, using the chimeric peptide technology. Given the limitations in using PO-ODNs or PS-ODNs as antisense agents in vivo (Figures 8.2–8.4), and given the advantages of PNAs as antisense agents (Figures 8.5–8.7), the first application of the chimeric peptide technology to in vivo imaging of gene expression in the brain utilized a chi-meric PNA. This chimeric PNA enabled the imaging of gene expression in an experimental C6 brain glioma (Shi et al., 2000). The antisense radiopharmaceuti-cal was a [^{125}I]-labeled PNA, which was conjugated to a peptidomimetic MAb to the transferrin receptor (TfR). The TfR is expressed not only at the BBB (Chapter 4), but is also widely expressed on brain cells (Mash et al., 1990), an on the plasma membrane of C6 glioma cells (Kurihara et al., 1999).

Brain tumor model

C6 glioma cells were permanently tranfected with a gene encoding the luciferase enzyme (Boado and Pardridge, 1998), and the transfection plasmid is shown in Figure 8.9B. The expression of the luciferase gene was driven by an SV40 promoter at the 5'-end and SV40 3'-untranslated region (UTR) elements at the 3'-end of the gene. In order to optimize gene expression, a 200 nucleotide fragment from the bovine *Glut1* glucose transporter mRNA 3'-UTR was inserted within the SV40 3'-

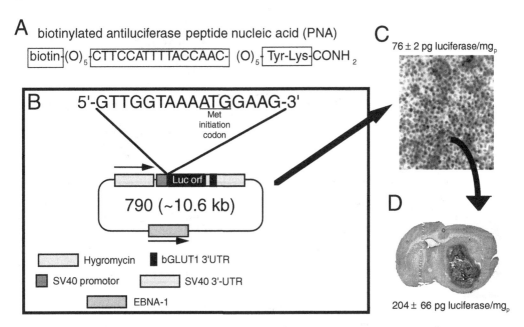

Figure 8.9 (A) Sequence of a peptide nucleic acid (PNA) that is antisense to the region of the luciferase mRNA around the methionine (Met) initiation codon. There is a biotin moiety at the amino terminus and a tyrosine-lysine residue at the carboxyl terminus, which is also amidated. (B) Structure of plasmid, designated clone 790, used to transfect permanently C6 rat glioma cells with the gene encoding the luciferase (Luc) open reading frame (orf). UTR, untranslated region; EBNA-1, Epstein–Barr virus nuclear antigen, which enables episomal replication of the transgene. (C) Luciferase activity in permanently transfected C6 rat glioma cells grown in cell culture. (D) Luciferase activity in the C6 experimental tumors in the brain of Fischer rats. mg_p, milligram cell protein. From Shi et al. (2000) with permission.

UTR. Prior studies demonstrated that this insert optimizes expression of the luciferase transgene in C6 cells (Boado and Pardridge, 1998). The expression of the luciferase transgene in the cultured C6 glioma cells was demonstrated by measuring luciferase enzyme activity in the cells, which was 76 ± 2 pg luciferase/mg cell protein, as shown in Figure 8.9C. These C6 rat glioma cells were then implanted in the caudate putamen nucleus of Fischer rats and experimental brain tumors developed approximately 14 days later. The expression of the luciferase transgene persisted following growth of the C6 brain tumors and the level of luciferase enzyme activity in the experimental tumor was threefold greater than the luciferase enzyme activity in the cultured C6 cells (Figure 8.9D). The antisense imaging agent was then administered to the tumor-bearing animals.

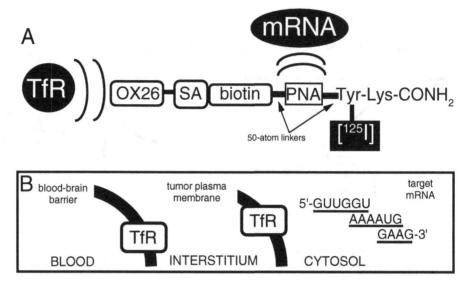

Figure 8.10   (A) Antisense imaging agent is comprised of a blood–brain barrier receptor-specific monoclonal antibody (MAb), streptavidin (SA), and a peptide nucleic acid (PNA) which contains a tyrosine (Tyr) and lysine (Lys) residue at the amidated carboxyl terminus. In this case, the OX26 MAb to the rat transferrin receptor (TfR) was used. (B) Transport of the antisense imaging agent through the blood–brain barrier and the tumor plasma membrane by targeting the TfR on both membranes. Targeting through the two barriers enables delivery of the PNA imaging agent to the target mRNA buried within the cytosol of the tumor cell.

Antisense imaging agent

A PNA with a sequence that was antisense around the methionine initiation codon of the luciferase mRNA was synthesized (Shi et al., 2000). At the carboxyl terminus of the PNA, there are tyrosine and lysine residues to enable radiolabeling with either [^{125}I] or [^{111}In], respectively. The PNA is a 16-mer that contains a 55-atom linker situated between the biotin residue at the amino terminus and the nucleic acid sequence and a 55-atom linker at the near carboxyl terminus between the antisense sequence and the carboxyl terminal amino acid residues. The PNA was radio-iodinated with [^{125}I] to a specific activity of 75–90 μCi/μg and a TCA precipitability of 95–98%. In parallel, a conjugate of the OX26 MAb and recombinant SA was prepared using a stable thioether linkage. There was immediate capture of the [^{125}I]biotinyl-PNA by the OX26/SA, as determined by gel filtration FPLC.

The structure of the intact PNA conjugate is shown in Figure 8.10A. The imaging agent is comprised of four domains. The first domain is the peptidomimetic mono-clonal antibody that targets the TfR, which is expressed on both the BBB and the tumor plasma membrane (Figure 8.10B). Transport through both of these membranes is required because the target of the antisense imaging agent, the luciferase mRNA, is localized in the cytoplasm of the tumor cells. The second domain of the imaging agent is the linker moiety which is comprised of the SA, which is attached to the MAb through a stable thioether linkage, and the biotin moiety, which is incorporated at the amino terminus of the PNA (Figure 8.10A). The third domain of the imaging agent is the tyrosine–lysine sequence at the carboxyl terminus of the PNA, which enables incorporation of a radionuclide. In the present case, the tyrosine was radiolabeled with [^{125}I]. The fourth domain of the mRNA imaging agent is the antisense sequence of the PNA (Figure 8.9A) which hybridizes with the target mRNA.

Characterization of the PNA antisense imaging agent

The [^{125}I]antiluciferase PNA, with or without conjugation to the OX26/SA drug-targeting system, was injected intravenously into adult anesthetized rats that did not have brain tumors (Shi et al., 2000). Organ uptake of the radiolabeled PNA or PNA–conjugate was measured 60 min after intravenous injection. There was no measurable transport of the unconjugated PNA into brain, confirming earlier studies, which are shown in Figure 8.5B. However, there was an increase in the brain uptake of the PNA following conjugation to the OX26/SA drug-targeting system and this level of brain uptake, 0.08%ID/g brain, is in excess of the brain uptake of a neuroactive small molecule such as morphine (Wu et al., 1997a). There was no specific targeting of the PNA–conjugate to heart, although there was increased uptake of the PNA–conjugate in liver, owing to expression of the TfR on hepatocytes in vivo (Wu and Pardridge, 1998). There was a decrease in the renal uptake of the PNA–conjugate, because conjugation of the PNA to the OX26/SA vector eliminates glomerular filtration of the smaller-sized PNA. The pharmacokinetic parameters of the antiluciferase PNA conjugated to OX26/SA were virtually identical to that reported previously for a *rev* PNA conjugated to the same delivery system (Pardridge et al., 1995a; Shi et al., 2000).

The ability of the antiluciferase PNA to hybridize to the target mRNA following biotinylation and binding to the OX26/SA drug-targeting system was demonstrated by a RNAse A/T1 protection assay that was similar to that described in Figure 8.6. The luciferase mRNA was prepared with a luciferase transcription plasmid, designated clone 760, which was derived from the pGL2 promoter luciferase reporter plasmid (Tsukamoto et al., 1997). The sense RNA was synthesized with T7 RNA polymerase following linearization of the plasmid with EcoR I. The size of the plasmid following linearization was 5.7 kb. The transcribed RNA was radiolabeled with [^{32}P] and the correct size of the radiolabeled transcribed RNA was determined by electrophoresis and autoradiography. Both the unconjugated

PNA and the PNA–conjugate hybridized to the luciferase sense RNA and resulted in protection of the same 16-mer RNA fragments, similar to that described for the *rev* system (Figure 8.6). These studies indicate that conjugation of the antiluciferase PNA to the OX26/SA drug-targeting system did not impair the hybridization of the PNA to the target mRNA (Shi et al., 2000).

Imaging gene expression in brain in vivo

The brain scans and autopsy stains for three different groups of adult Fischer rats bearing the C6 gliomas expressing the luciferase transgene are shown in Figure 8.11. There are three rats in each group and group A rats received the radiolabeled antiluciferase PNA conjugated to the OX26/SA drug-targeting system, which is designated SA-MAb in Figure 8.11. Group B rats received the anti-luciferase PNA without conjugation to the drug-targeting system. Group C rats received the anti-*rev* PNA that was conjugated to the OX26/SA drug-targeting system. The autopsy stains show that all rats formed medium to large tumors, with the exception of rat 2 in group B (Figure 8.11). There was no imaging of either normal brain or brain tumor in the group B rats following intravenous injection of the luciferase PNA without conjugation to the drug-targeting system, because the PNA does not cross the BBB in either normal brain or in the tumor. Conversely, there was imaging of luciferase gene expression in the brain tumor in all group A rats following intravenous injection of the luciferase PNA conjugated to the drug-targeting system. The size of the tumor imaged with the antisense radiopharmaceutical is comparable to the size of the tumor shown on the autopsy stain (Figure 8.11). There was no specific imaging of brain tumor following conjugation of the *rev* antisense PNA to the drug-targeting system, as shown in the Group C rats (Figure 8.11).

These studies show that successful imaging of gene expression in the brain in vivo requires at least two conditions. First, a correct sequence in the antisense domain of the imaging agent must be utilized and, second, the antisense imaging agent must be conjugated to a targeting system that enables transport through both the BBB and the BCM. As outlined in Figure 8.10B, the target mRNA is situated behind two barriers, the BBB and the brain cell or tumor cell plasma membrane. Owing to expression of the TfR on both the BBB and the tumor cell plasma membrane, the OX26 MAb is able to target the PNA to the intracellular compartment of the tumor cells where the target mRNA molecules reside (Shi et al., 2000).

Imaging gene expression in the human brain in vivo

The imaging of gene expression in vivo in the brain that is demonstrated in Figure 8.11 for rats could also be performed in humans by replacement of the anti-TfR MAb with an MAb to the human insulin receptor (HIR). As discussed in Chapters 4 and 5, the HIR MAb is specific for humans and is nearly 10 times more active as

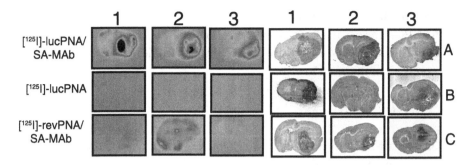

Figure 8.11   Brain scans (left) and autopsy stains (right) are shown for three groups of rats designated A, B, and C. Group A rats received an intravenous injection of the [^{125}I]anti-luciferase peptide nucleic acid (PNA) bound to a conjugate of the OX26 monoclonal antibody (MAb) and streptavidin (SA), which is designated SA-OX26. Group B rats received [^{125}I]antiluciferase PNA without conjugation to SA-OX26. Group C rats received an intravenous injection of [^{125}I]anti-*rev* PNA conjugated to SA-OX26. From Shi et al. (2000) with permission.

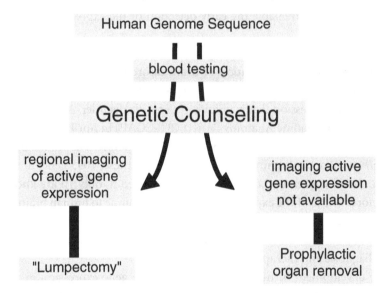

Figure 8.12   Two pathways of genetic counseling based on the availability of technology to enable gene expression in vivo.

a BBB drug-targeting system than anti-TfR MAbs. Moreover, the HIR is also expressed on tumor cells and the expression of the HIR on the tumor cell plasma membrane is demonstrated by the basolateral staining pattern using a murine HIR MAb, as shown in Figure 7.12C. Murine HIR MAbs cannot be administered to humans and the humanization of HIR MAbs is described in Chapter 5. A chimeric

HIR MAb has been prepared (Coloma et al., 2000), and has an identical affinity for the HIR as the original murine antibody (Figure 5.7). Therefore, either a chimeric or humanized HIR MAb could be used for human studies to enable imaging of gene expression in the brain in vivo.

Summary

The availability of the human genome sequence will accelerate the pace of the discovery of pathologic genes that cause cancer or chronic disease in the brain or other organs. However, this sequence information will only enable genetic counselors to advise an individual as to the *presence* of a pathologic gene in their chromosomes, but will not permit counseling as to the *expression* of the pathologic gene at a given point in time. If genetic counseling is based solely on blood testing of the presence of a mutated gene, then the genetic counseling invariably leads to recommendations of prophylactic organ removal (Figure 8.12). In practice, however, pathologic genes are not expressed until later in life, and it would be advantageous to have an imaging modality to enable the early detection of the expression of a pathologic gene.

In addition to genetic counseling, the availability of gene-imaging technology will facilitate the characterization of brain disorders at the molecular level. The expressed sequence tag (EST) databases continue to expand and uncover the existence of gene expression that is unique to a specific disorder. A review of the Brain Tumor Cancer Genome Anatomy Project (BT-CGAP) in April 2000, indicates that, to date, a total of 13 985 expressed genes have been detected in human brain cancer (http://www2.ncbi.nlm.nih.gov/CGAP/hTGI). Of these, 1095 genes are unique to human brain cancer, and of these 1095 unique genes, only 10 are known genes. Therefore, 99.5% of the expressed genes that are unique to human brain cancer are unknown genes! If the expression of these unique genes could be imaged in vivo, then brain cancers could be classified at the molecular level, and this could guide both diagnosis and therapy.

The development of new technology to enable gene expression in vivo in the brain or other organs will take on urgency in the future with the availability of the human genome sequence. The goal of "imaging any gene in any person" will require the development of antisense radiopharmaceuticals, and the only way that such agents can be used to image gene expression in vivo is the adaptation of the antisense radiopharmaceuticals to drug-targeting technology.

9

Gene therapy of the brain

Introduction

Gene therapy is a paradigm shift in the development of pharmaceuticals, and much more so than any changes brought about by the introduction of biotechnology to classical pharmaceutics. As discussed in the Preface, present-day pharmaceutics is a chemistry-driven science that originated early in the twentieth century (Drews, 2000), and is based almost singularly on drug discovery of small molecules. The introduction of recombinant DNA technology and biotechnology represent only changes in the methodology of drug discovery. The large pharmaceutical industry uses biotechnology to clone receptors and establish high-throughput screening (HTS) programs to identify classical organic small molecules. The singular focus on organic small molecules, and the belief that these molecules are able to diffuse freely across biological membranes, underlies the persistent inattention to drug-targeting science on the part of the pharmaceutical industry. The reason that gene therapy is such a paradigm shift is that gene therapy requires a primary emphasis in drug development on biology, not chemistry. The development of genes as drugs also brings into focus the need for new technologies that enable the targeting of genes, or drugs, through the biological membrane barriers of the body.

Four barriers in gene targeting

Gene therapy, should it be implemented successfully, could obviate the need for classical organic small molecules for many types of chronic disease or cancer. However, gene therapy will not be widely used unless the gene formulations are incorporated into a targeting technology that enables the gene medicine to traverse the various biological barriers that exist between blood and brain. The goal of gene

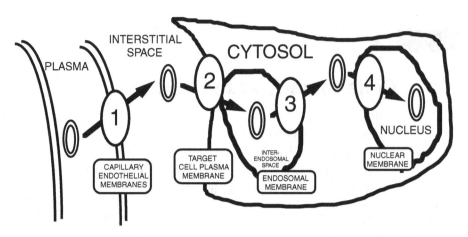

Figure 9.1   Four barriers separating the gene formulation in the blood from the nuclear compartment in brain cells.

therapy is the tissue- and cell-specific expression of a gene following noninvasive administration of the gene medicine. For this to take place, the gene medicine must move from the blood stream to the nuclear compartment of the target cell in the brain. The barriers that must be navigated in gene targeting are outlined in Figure 9.1 and include: (a) the capillary endothelial membrane, which is the blood–brain barrier (BBB) in brain, (b) the target cell plasma membrane, (c) the endosomal membrane, and (d) the nuclear membrane. Until genes are formulated in such a way that these four biological barriers can be circumvented, it will be difficult to achieve cell-specific gene expression in the brain following the intravenous administration of a gene pharmaceutical. As discussed later in this chapter, the tissue-specificity of gene expression can be largely influenced by gene fragments inserted in either the 5′- or 3′-end of the therapeutic gene. However, unless the gene formulation is actually delivered to the interior of the target cell, these 5′- and 3′-promoter and enhancer elements cannot be put to work to bring about the desired tissue- and cell-specific gene expression.

Gene therapy of the central nervous system

As outlined by Martin (1995), many clinical disorders of the brain can now be classified on the basis of the genetic mutations underlying these diseases of the central nervous system (CNS). Intractable brain disorders include Huntington's disease, familial Alzheimer's disease, amyotrophic lateral sclerosis (ALS), myotonic dystrophy, Friedreich's ataxia, Wilson's disease, Tay–Sachs disease and other lysosomal storage disorders, muscular dystrophy, fragile X syndrome, and brain tumors. It is difficult for the patients and family members afflicted with these disorders to know that the gene underlying the cause of their disease has been known

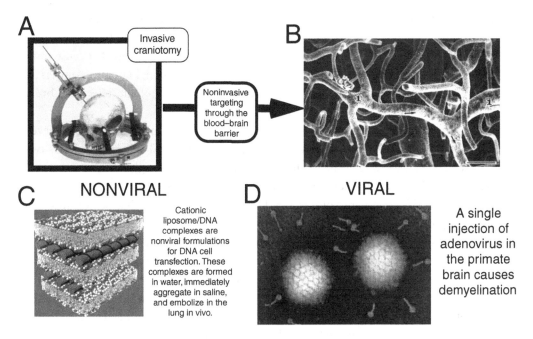

Figure 9.2   Gene therapy of the brain. (A) Craniotomy-based gene delivery to the brain. (B) Scanning electron micrograph of a vascular cast of the human cerebellar cortex. From Duvernoy et al. (1983) with permission. (C) Cationic liposome/DNA complexes. Reprinted with permission from Radler et al. (1997). Structure of DNA-cationic liposome complexes: DNA intercalation in multilamellar membranes in distant interhelical packing regimes. *Science*, **275**, 810–14. Copyright (1997) American Association for the Advancement of Science. (D) Adenovirus.

for years, but there has been no significant progress in the treatment of their disease. This imbalance between the neuroscience knowledge and the clinical benefits will only further expand in the future with the elucidation of the complete sequence for the human genome. The transfer from the laboratory to the clinic of present-day methods for brain gene therapy has not been rapid, and has been delayed by the lack of noninvasive methods for targeting therapeutic genes widely throughout the CNS following intravenous administration.

Present-day approaches to gene therapy of the brain

The evolution of methods for delivering genes to the brain has followed a pattern identical to the methods for delivering drugs to the brain, as outlined in Figure 1.7. The most widely applied method of brain gene delivery is craniotomy, and the intracerebral introduction of therapeutic genes formulated in either viruses or cationic liposomes. Alternatively, cells may be transfected in tissue culture with retroviruses in an ex vivo approach. These permanently transfected cells may then be implanted in brain following craniotomy (Figure 9.2).

In parallel with the craniotomy-based methods of drug or gene delivery to the brain, there is a line of investigation aimed at disrupting the BBB by the intraarterial infusion of either hyperosmolar substances or noxious agents that cause transitory BBB disruption (Nilaver et al., 1995). BBB disruption, like craniotomy, is an invasive procedure and may induce chronic neuropathologic effects in brain (Chapter 2).

The noninvasive administration of gene medicines to the brain can be achieved with targeting of BBB endogenous transport systems, and this approach has two advantages. First, the gene medicine can be delivered throughout the entire brain proper. In contrast, when gene medicines are delivered by craniotomy approaches, the effective treatment volume is <1 mm^3 owing to the limitations of diffusion within the brain (Chapter 2). The second advantage of targeting drugs through the BBB is that the gene formulation can be given by an intravenous or subcutaneous route of administration that is no more invasive than that used by millions of individuals with diabetes mellitus taking insulin injections every day.

The formulations of gene medicines that are used in present practice are based on viruses, cationic liposomes, or naked DNA/polylysine conjugates. The DNA is packaged in the interior of the viral formulations, whereas the DNA is exposed and adsorbed to the exterior of cationic liposome complexes and the DNA is also exposed in the formation of polylysine conjugates. As discussed later in this chapter, a fourth approach used for targeting gene medicines to the brain involves receptor-mediated targeting of pegylated immunoliposomes carrying DNA in the *interior* of the liposome. Each of these approaches has distinct advantages and disadvantages that must be considered in the development of practical methods for gene therapy of the brain in humans.

Gene therapy with viral vectors

Retrovirus

The earliest approaches of gene therapy for the brain involved the treatment of brain tumors using an ex vivo retroviral approach (Culver et al., 1992; Chen et al., 1994). Since retroviruses only infect replicating cells, it is necessary permanently to alter the host genome of a replicating cell such as the fibroblast in tissue culture. The type 1 herpes simplex virus (HSV) thymidine kinase (tk) gene was incorporated into a retroviral vector and fibroblasts were transfected in cell culture. These altered cells were then implanted into the cranial cavity around a brain tumor and a small molecule such as ganciclovir was administered (Culver et al., 1992; Chen et al., 1994). This form of gene therapy is called "suicide gene therapy" because the ganciclovir is taken up by transfected cells and is selectively phosphorylated in the presence of the HSV-tk enzyme to form ganciclovir phosphate. This phosphorylated drug terminates DNA transcription, leading to cessation of cell division. The drug terminates DNA synthesis in the neighboring tumor cell owing to a "bystander effect." Although the ganciclovir phosphate was formed within the fibroblast, and not within the brain tumor cell, there apparently was some diffusion of the ganciclovir phosphate into the neighboring tumor cell. Subsequent studies suggest that the molecular basis of the bystander effect involved the gene expression of connexins and the formation of gap junctions between the fibroblast and the tumor cell (Mesnil et al., 1996).

While suicide gene therapy had some success in small tumors in rodent brain, where diffusion distances are small, subsequent clinical trials were less effective (Ram et al., 1997). Only tumor cells immediately contiguous with the transfected HSV-tk-bearing cell are susceptible to the ganciclovir phosphate, and then only if there is significant diffusion of this polar drug between gap junctions between the transfected cell and the tumor cell. Apparently, the extent of gap junction formation is minimal in human brain tumors (Ram et al., 1997). Even if gap junctions were formed to a significant degree, it is unlikely this approach would cause a significant tumor kill. The transfected cells would have to be in physical contact with virtually all tumor cells, and this is not possible by delivery of cells to the tumor via craniotomy. As reviewed in Chapter 2, the effective treatment volume with craniotomy-based delivery of drugs or genes is <1 mm^3, owing to the limitations of diffusion, which decreases with the square of the distance. On the other hand, it is possible to achieve widespread distribution of a therapeutic gene throughout the brain using BBB drug-targeting technology, as discussed later in this chapter. Therapeutic genes are distributed widely throughout the brain when a BBB drug-targeting strategy is used because the gene medicine is transported through the brain microvascular barrier. Since capillaries are about 40 μm apart in the human brain (Figure 9.2B), the diffusion distance is insignificant once the gene medicine traverses the BBB. Once inside brain cells, gene expression can then be regulated with 5'- or 3'-gene elements that control cell-specific expression of the therapeutic gene.

A concern related to the use of retroviruses is the permanent alteration of the host genome involved with the use of this type of virus. This provided the basis for the development of other types of viruses as vectors for gene therapy of the brain including adenovirus, herpes simplex virus, and adeno-associated virus (AAV).

Adenovirus

The adenovirus can infect cells without replication, and does not integrate into the host genome. The adenovirus genome is sufficiently large to accommodate host genes up to 7.5 kb (La Salle et al., 1993). Replication-defective adenovirus can be produced in high titers in cell culture and the intracerebral injection of adenovirus into the brain has demonstrated gene expression at the local site of injection (Choi-Lundberg et al., 1997; Bemelmans et al., 1999). However, the principal problem with adenovirus is the preexisting immunity to this virus (Kajiwara et al., 2000). Therefore, the injection of even relatively small amounts of adenovirus into the brain results in inflammation, gliosis, perivascular cuffing of small lymphocytes analogous to early lesions seen in multiple sclerosis, and demyelination (Wood et al., 1996; Smith et al., 1997; Driesse et al., 1998; Dewey et al., 1999; Lawrence et al., 1999). Demyelination occurs in the primate brain following a single intracerebral injection of adenovirus (Driesse et al., 1998). Human brains subjected to adenovirus gene therapy show inflammation and demyelination in the region of injection of the adenovirus (Dewey et al., 1999). In rhesus monkeys, the intracerebral injection of adenovirus is lethal at high doses (Smith et al., 1997). The toxicity appears to be dose-related as the intracerebral injection of low-dose adenovirus in rats results in inflammation, whereas necrosis is observed with the intracerebral injection of high doses of adenovirus (Smith et al., 1997). Given these disadvantages of adenoviruses as a vector for gene therapy to the brain, the use of HSV as a viral vector has been investigated.

Herpes simplex virus

The HSV-1 is a large double-stranded DNA virus of about 150 kb in size that is comprised of approximately 75 viral genes (Freese et al., 1990). The HSV-1 protein fuses with the plasma membrane of a target cell and dispenses the viral genome into the cytoplasm. Therefore, HSV-1 infects a wide variety of cells, including neurons (During et al., 1994). When HSV-1 replicates within the brain, a herpes viral encephalitis ensues (McMenamin et al., 1998). Replication-deficient forms of HSV-1 can be generated in the laboratory which do not cause encephalitis. However, the replication-deficient HSV-1 is still toxic to the brain (Kramm et al., 1996; Herrlinger et al., 1998; McMenamin et al., 1998). Similar to adenovirus, the intracerebral injection of HSV-1 results in inflammation, increased expression of antigen-presenting cells, lymphocyte cuffing around microvessels similar to the early lesions of multiple sclerosis, and demyelination (McMenamin et al., 1998). Brain inflammation also occurs following the intrathecal administration of HSV-1 (Kramm et al., 1996). The toxicity of HSV-1 may be related to a preexisting immunity, as the toxic effect of HSV-1 administration can be reduced by elimination of the preexisting immunity to the virus (Herrlinger et al., 1998).

Adeno-associated virus

AAV is a human parvovirus with a small genome that is nonpathologic in humans. The AAV infects neurons at the site of intracerebral injection (Skorupa et al., 1999). Craniotomy-based routes of AAV delivery to the brain are necessary because the

AAV does not cross the BBB (Elliger et al., 1999; Leff et al., 1999). One report involving the intravenous administration of AAV in 2-day-old mice suggests the AAV can cross the BBB (Daly et al., 1999). In this study, the AAV carried the gene encoding β-glucuronidase (GUSB), which is deficient in the type VII mucopolysaccharidosis. The evidence for AAV transport across the BBB was the finding of GUSB enzyme activity in a perivascular pattern in the brain (Daly et al., 1999). However, the GUSB is a glycoprotein substrate of the mannose-6-phosphate (M6P) receptor, also known as the type 2 insulin-like growth factor (IGF)-2 receptor. As reviewed in Chapter 4, the M6P/IGF2 receptor is present on the BBB of rodents, but is not expressed at the human BBB. The BBB M6P/IGF2 receptor may be upregulated in newborn mice, similar to the upregulation of the BBB insulin receptor in development (Chapter 4). Therefore, the GUSB in brain may have originated from blood via receptor-mediated transcytosis of the enzyme across the BBB of the developing mouse, and not from AAV transport through the BBB. The extent to which humans have a preexisting immunity to AAV, similar to adenovirus or HSV-1, has not yet been investigated.

Gene therapy with cationic liposomes

The significant neurotoxicity associated with the use of either adenovirus or HSV-1 has prompted the development of nonviral approaches to gene therapy, which is based on the use of cationic liposomes. These form complexes with anionic DNA (Figure 9.2). Transgenes have been expressed in brain following the intracerebral injection of cationic liposome/DNA complexes (Zhu et al., 1996; Imaoka et al., 1998; Zou et al., 1999). These formulations must be administered by craniotomy because cationic liposomes do not cross the BBB (Osaka et al., 1996).

Aggregation properties of cationic liposome/DNA complexes

Cationic lipids form complexes with DNA and the transfection of cells in culture with these cationic lipid/DNA complexes is widely used in the laboratory (Felgner and Ringold, 1989). Cationic lipids and the anionic DNA form highly ordered structures with diameters less than 200 nm when there is a preponderance of either positive or negative charge in the overall structure (Radler et al., 1997). For example, if the weight ratio of lipid to DNA is >5, then the complex has a net positive charge, owing to the excess of the cationic lipid, and the diameter of the structure is <200 nm. If the weight ratio of lipid to DNA is <5, then the complex has a net negative charge, owing to the excess of the DNA and the complex has a diameter <200 nm. If the weight ratio of lipid to DNA is 5, then the complex has a neutral charge because of equal molar ratio of anionic and cationic charges, and the complex aggregates into large globules of 2–5 μm in size (Radler et al., 1997).

The cationic liposome/DNA complexes are uniformly formulated in water. When physiological concentrations of saline are added, the complex becomes electrically neutral and immediately aggregates into large micron size globules (Plank et al., 1999).

Gene transfection in cell culture is a function of aggregation

The cationic lipid/DNA complex may enter cells in tissue culture by either phagocytosis or endocytosis. Phagocytosis of particles in the tissue culture media takes place when the size of the particle is an excess of a 300–500 nm diameter (Jahraus et al., 1998). The efficiency of transfection of the transgene in cell culture is directly proportional to the aggregation properties of the cationic lipid/DNA complex (Niidome et al., 1997). Owing to the large size of the complex that is formed in the saline environment of cell culture media, the principal mode of uptake of the cationic lipid/DNA complex in cell culture is phagocytosis and not endocytosis (Matsui et al., 1997). The absence of phagocytic pathways in certain cells in culture explains why some cells are relatively resistant to transfection in tissue culture. Electron microscopy and confocal microscopy of cultured cells exposed to cationic lipid/DNA complexes shows that these complexes remain confined to vesicles within the cells (Zabner et al., 1995). These vesicles coalesce into multivesicular organelles with diameters >1 μm, which are prelysosomal structures. Cationic lipid/DNA complexes that are multilamellar vesicles of 300–700 nm in diameter are more effective in cell culture with respect to gene transfection than are small unilamellar vesicles of 50–100 nm in size (Felgner et al., 1994).

Intravenously administered cationic liposomes are selectively sequestered within the lung

If cationic liposome/DNA structures must be formulated in water to eliminate the aggregation of these structures, it is possible that the aggregation will occur immediately upon injection into the blood stream (Mahato et al., 1997). Not only would the complex be made electrically neutral by the physiological saline, but the highly charged complex is coated by serum proteins, which promotes further the formation of structures of neutral charge that aggregate (Huang and Li, 1997). If the size of the aggregate approximates 1–2 μm, then it is possible the structure will embolize in the first capillary bed entered upon intravenous injection, and this capillary bed is the pulmonary microcirculation. In vivo studies with cationic liposome/DNA complexes uniformly show that >99% of the injected dose of a cationic liposome/DNA complex is sequestered in the lung (Zhu et al., 1993; Osaka et al., 1996; Hofland et al., 1997; Hong et al., 1997; Song et al., 1997; Mounkes et al., 1998; Barron et al., 1999). The level of gene expression in the lung is log orders of magnitude greater than the gene expression in liver or spleen (Zhu et al., 1993; Hong et al., 1997). An additional tendency of cationic liposomes to localize in the lung is the high affinity of these structures for the negatively charged heparan proteogly-cans such as syndecan-1 on plasma membranes (Mounkes et al., 1998). The cell in the lung that is specifically targeted by the cationic liposome/DNA complex is the pulmonary capillary endothelial cell (Hofland et al., 1997).

There is no expression of a transgene in the brain in vivo following the intrave-nous injection of a cationic liposome/DNA complex. There is some gene expres-sion in liver, spleen, and heart following the intravenous injection of cationic liposome/DNA complexes. However, the cationic liposome/DNA complexes are too large to cross the BBB, and there is no entry into the brain (Osaka et al., 1996). In addition to the negligible permeability at the BBB, the very low plasma area under the concentration curve (AUC) of these structures contributes to the lack of brain uptake. Because of the rapid sequestration of the cationic liposome/DNA complexes in lung, >90% of the injected dose is removed from blood in the first 2 min after intravenous injection in mice (Osaka et al., 1996). The low plasma AUC and negligible BBB permeability both contribute to the lack of brain uptake of cat-ionic liposome/DNA complexes following intravenous injection.

The limitations of either viral vectors or cationic liposomes have been recognized and several laboratories have developed methods of gene targeting to cells that utilize the endogenous receptor-mediated endocytosis systems that are expressed on the cell membrane. In this approach a naked plasmid DNA is conjugated to a receptor ligand. The asialoglycoprotein receptor on liver cells (Wu et al., 1991), the transferrin receptor (TfR) widely distributed on many cells (Wagner et al., 1992), and the folate receptor (Vogel et al., 1996; Leamon et al., 1999) have all been tar-geted with various soluble formulations of gene complexes. In all of these cases, the naked DNA is complexed to the targeting ligand with a polylysine bridge.

Receptor-mediated gene targeting of polylysine/naked DNA

The receptor ligand is conjugated to polylysine using a variety of approaches that include either chemical linkages or avidin-biotin technology, such as those reviewed in Chapter 6. The polycationic polylysine then binds to the polyanionic DNA to form a three-part structure comprised of receptor ligand/polyly-sine/plasmid DNA. While the soluble polylysine/DNA formulations have proven to be effective in cell culture, there have been few in vivo applications of these formu-lations.

Administration of soluble polylysine/DNA complexes in vivo

The polylysine bridge method, although active in cell culture, is apparently less effective in vivo (Service, 1995). In one study involving the conjugation of the receptor ligand, insulin, to the polylysine/DNA complex, it was necessary physically to inject the mixture directly into the target organ, the mammary gland (Sobolev et al., 1998). Apparently no mammary gland gene expression could be observed following intravenous injection of the complex. The complex of the polycationic polylysine and the polyanionic DNA may be rapidly neutralized by the absorption of serum proteins following intravenous injection, and this may cause a physical separation of the DNA and the polylysine, which are only joined together by electrostatic charge.

Soluble polylysine/DNA formulations have been targeted to the liver in vivo using ligands of the asialoglycoprotein receptor on the hepatocyte plasma membrane (Wu et al., 1991). This receptor is very active in vivo and removes on a single pass 99% of asialoglycoprotein injected into the portal vein (Pardridge et al., 1983). The efficiency of this targeting system was increased by the compaction of the polylysine/DNA complex into a structure as small as 10–30 nm (Perales et al., 1997). The addition of high salt to a polycation/DNA complex initially produces aggregation of the complex that is subsequently followed by DNA compaction into small spherical structures with diameters of 10–30 nm. These small spherical structures may be more diffusible within the cell subsequent to receptor-mediated endocytosis into hepatocytes. Expression in liver of a luciferase transgene in vivo was observed following the intravenous administration of 300 μg of plasmid DNA into the rat (Perales et al., 1997). The plasmid DNA was adsorbed to polylysine, which was conjugated with ligand to the asialoglycoprotein receptor, and the DNA was compacted with high salt prior to intravenous administration in rats. The level of expression of the luciferase transgene in liver was 10 000 relative light units (RLU) per mg protein at 48 h after injection (Perales et al., 1997).

Endosomal release

The targeting of a plasmid DNA to a cell via an endogenous receptor system will result in distribution of the plasmid DNA into endosomal structures of the target cell following receptor-mediated endocytosis at the plasma membrane (barrier 2, Figure 9.1). However, the plasmid DNA must then undergo transport across the third barrier, which is the endosomal membrane, prior to release into the cytoplasm (Figure 9.1). In order to promote endosomal release, various approaches have been developed to circumvent the endosomal membrane. Coat proteins from the adenovirus normally disrupt the endosomal membrane and conjugates of targeting ligand/adenovirus/polylysine/DNA have been developed to enable receptor-mediated endocytosis into a target cell followed by endosomal release (Cotton et al., 1992). A second approach relies not on endosomal membrane lysis, which is the case for adenovirus, but on endosomal membrane fusion using synthetic peptides derived from the amino terminus of the influenza virus hemagglutinin (HA-2). These highly amphipathic peptides cause membrane fusion at acid pH (Plank et al.,

1994). However, relatively high concentrations of the peptide, 25–250 μmol/l, must be used to cause membrane fusion. While such high concentrations may be achieved in tissue culture, it would not be possible to generate concentrations of the fusion peptide of 25–250 μmol/l in vivo.

Release from the endosome allows for diffusion through the cytoplasm and transport across the nuclear membrane (Figure 9.1). If there is no release of the structure from the endosome, then the plasmid DNA will invariably stay sequestered in lysosomal structures with subsequent degradation. The persistence of the transgene was no greater than 1–2 days in liver owing to degradation in the lysosomal system. However, when the transgene was administered to rats following partial hepatectomy, there was a persistence of the transgene in excess of 32 days (Perales et al., 1994). The partial hepatectomy caused division of the liver cells, which resulted in a depolymerization of the intracellular microtubules in association with cell mitosis. This loss of microtubular structures within the liver cell delayed entry into the lysosomal system, and this accounted for the persistence of the transgene (Chowdhury et al., 1993).

Nuclear membrane barrier

Following endosomal release into the cytoplasm, the therapeutic gene must diffuse through the cytoplasm and traverse the fourth barrier, the nuclear membrane (Figure 9.1). The nuclear membrane is freely porous to small molecules as there are thousands of pores in the nuclear membrane (Finlay et al., 1987). The diameter of the nuclear pore complex (NPC) is up to 28 nm (Wilson et al., 1999). The mechanisms by which nucleic acids are transported across the nuclear membrane are poorly understood. Active mechanisms exist because primary transcripts are exported from the nucleus to the cytoplasmic compartment. How plasmid DNA moves from the cytoplasm into the nuclear compartment is also poorly understood, but may involve a receptor-mediated mechanism, and be facilitated by specific sequences within the plasmid (Wilson et al., 1999).

Movement of the plasmid DNA into the nucleus may also be facilitated with compaction of the size of the nucleic acid. A 3.4 kb plasmid DNA has an overall length of 1400 nm (Monnard et al., 1997), but owing to supercoiling, the effective diameter of the plasmid DNA is much less. Nevertheless, the effective diameter of a supercoiled plasmid DNA is greater than the diameter of the NPC. Compaction of the plasmid DNA into a structure with a small diameter may have beneficial effects in promoting transgene movement through the cytoplasm and into the nuclear compartment. DNA can be compacted with cationic proteins such as polylysine, protamine, or histone. A formulation of compacted plasmid DNA and a polycationic protein would mimic the chromosomal structure in the nucleus.

Noninvasive gene targeting to the brain

The goal of noninvasive gene therapy of the brain is to administer a formulation that does not cause inflammation in the brain and does not require invasive delivery methods such as craniotomy or BBB disruption (Figure 9.2). The gene formulation should be made from natural, nonimmunogenic components, which are degraded by cells in vivo without causing an inflammatory response in the brain similar to adenovirus or HSV-1. The formulation should be soluble following intravenous injection into the blood stream, and not aggregate in the blood or sequester in the pulmonary microcirculation like cationic liposomes. The formulation must undergo both receptor-mediated transcytosis across the BBB and receptor-mediated endocytosis across the plasma membrane of target cells within the brain. By using endogenous transport systems localized within the brain microvasculature (Figure 9.2B), the therapeutic gene can be delivered throughout brain proper. Following targeting of the gene to brain cells, the tissue-specificity of gene expression in the brain in vivo can then be driven by the 5'- or 3'-promoter and enhancer elements inserted in the gene construct.

Molecular formulation

Exogenous genes are delivered to brain following intravenous injection using pegylated immunoliposomes (Shi and Pardridge, 2000), and the structure of the formulation is shown in Figure 9.3A. This formulation was developed with three goals in mind. First, the DNA must be packaged in the *interior* of liposomes to afford protection against the ubiquitous exo- and endo-nucleases present in the body in vivo. The packaging of the supercoiled double-stranded circular DNA in the interior of the liposomes also maintains the attachment of the DNA to the targeting moiety that extends from the liposome surface. Unlike conjugation strategies that use a DNA/polylysine bridge, there is no separation of the plasmid DNA from the targeting moiety in vivo when the DNA is packaged in the interior of immunoliposomes. The second goal is the optimization of the plasma pharmacokinetics, so that the formulation is not rapidly removed from blood. As discussed in Chapter 3, the pharmacokinetics of liposomes is optimized with the use of pegylation technology, and pegylated liposomes are slowly cleared from blood. Pegylation involves the covalent attachment of polyethylene glycol (PEG) to the surface of the liposome. The formulation used for brain gene targeting employs pegylated liposomes (Figure 9.3A). The third goal is the targeting of endogenous receptor systems within both the BBB and the brain cell membrane (BCM), and this requires the introduction of a targeting moiety that is tethered to the tips of the PEG strands (Figure 9.2B). Initial studies used a peptidomimetic monoclonal antibody (MAb) to the TfR, which is expressed both at the BBB and the BCM (Chapter 4).

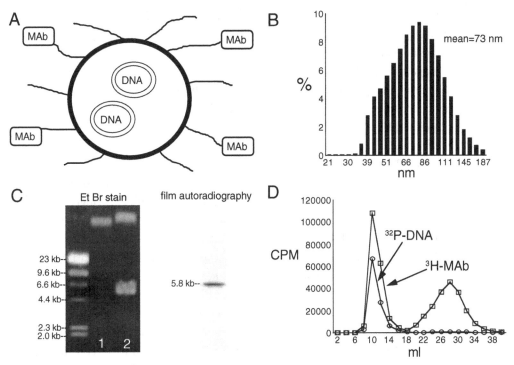

Figure 9.3   (A) Diagram showing the plasmid (DNA) encapsulated in pegylated immunoliposomes constructed from neutral lipids. There are approximately 3000 strands of polyethylene glycol of 2000 Da molecular weight, designated PEG^{2000}, attached to the liposome surface, and about 1% of the PEG strands are conjugated with a monoclonal antibody (MAb) that targets a blood–brain barrier (BBB) endogenous receptor. (B) The mean diameter of the pegylated liposomes encapsulating the pGL2 plasmid DNA is 73 nm. (C) Liposomes before (lane 2) and after (lane 1) DNAse I/exonuclease III treatment are resolved with 0.8% agarose gel electrophoresis followed by ethidium bromide (Et Br) staining. DNA molecular weight size standards are shown on the left side. Approximately 50% of the DNA associated with the pegylated liposome is bound to the exterior of the liposome (lane 2) and this was quantitatively removed by the nuclease treatment (lane 1). A trace amount of the pGL2 plasmid was radiolabeled with [^{32}P] and film autoradiography of the gel shows a single 5.8 kb band with no low molecular weight radiolabeled DNA. (D) The conjugation of the OX26 MAb to the pegylated liposomes carrying the encapsulated pGL2 plasmid DNA following nuclease digestion is demonstrated by Sepharose CL-4B gel filtration chromatography. A trace amount of the encapsulated pGL2 plasma DNA was radiolabeled with [^{32}P] and a trace amount of the OX26 MAb was radiolabeled with [^{3}H]. The study shows comigration of the conjugated OX26 MAb attached to the PEG strands and the encapsulated pGL2 plasmid DNA in the interior of the liposome. From Shi, N. and Pardridge, W.M. (2000). Antisense imaging of gene expression in the brain in vivo. *Proc. Natl Acad. Sci. USA*, **97**, 14709–14. Copyright (2000) National Academy of Sciences, USA.

Each liposome contains about 2000 strands of PEG. The PEG strands are each 2000 Da molecular weight, designated PEG^{2000}, and these are attached to the surface of the liposome (Huwyler et al., 1996). About 30–40 of these PEG^{2000} strands are conjugated with the MAb at the tip of the strand (Figure 9.3A). Since the gene formulation must be delivered to the cytoplasm of brain cells, the targeting MAb must not only cause the receptor-mediated transcytosis through the BBB in vivo, but also cause the receptor-mediated endocytosis of the pegylated immunoliposome into brain cells.

Two different plasmid DNAs were prepared, the 5.8 kb pGL2 luciferase reporter plasmid, and the 6.8 kb pSV-β-galactosidase expression plasmid, and both of these genes are under the influence of the SV40 promoter (Shi and Pardridge, 2000). The liposomes were synthesized with the following lipids: 1-palmitoyl-2-oleoyl-sn-glycero-3-phosphocholine (POPC), didodecyldimethyl ammonium bromide (DDAB), distearoylphosphatidylethanolamine (DSPE)-PEG^{2000}, and DSPE-PEG-MAL, where MAL equals maleimide. The POPC, the DDAB, the DSPE-PEG^{2000}, and the DSPE-PEG^{2000}-maleimide were dissolved in chloroform/methanol. Following evaporation, the lipids were dispersed in 0.05 mol/l Tris buffer and sonicated for 10 min. Supercoiled plasmid DNA (100 μg) and 1 μCi of [^{32}P]-labeled DNA were added to the lipids. This solution was subjected to several freeze/thaw cycles and was then extruded through two stacks each of 400 nm, 200 nm, 100 nm, and 50 nm pore size polycarbonate membranes using a hand-held extruder. The mean vesicle diameter was determined by quasielastic light scattering and this showed that the pegylated liposomes carrying the DNA in the interior of the liposomes had a mean diameter of 73 nm (Figure 9.3B).

The plasmid DNA that was not incorporated in the interior of the liposome, and remained absorbed to the exterior of the liposome, was removed by nuclease digestion using pancreatic endonuclease I and exonuclease III (Monnard et al., 1997). The extent to which the nuclease digestion removed the exteriorized plasmid DNA was determined by agarose gel electrophoresis and ethidium bromide (Et Br) staining, as shown in Figure 9.3C. This shows complete removal of any exterior bound plasmid DNA from the liposome. When the pGL2 plasmid DNA was radiolabeled with [^{32}P] prior to incorporation into the liposome, only the 5.8 kb pGL2 plasmid was detected and no low molecular weight forms of DNA were observed, as demonstrated by a film autoradiography (Figure 9.3C). Either the OX26 MAb or the mouse immunoglobulin G type 2a (IgG$_{2a}$) isotype control was conjugated to the tips of the PEG strands. These antibodies were purified by protein G affinity chromatography and radiolabeled with [^{3}H]-N-succinimidyl propionate (NSP), as described in Chapter 8. The OX26 or mouse IgG$_{2a}$ was thiolated using a 40:1 molar ratio of 2-iminothiolane (Traut's reagent), as described previously (Huwyler et al., 1996). The number of OX26 molecules conjugated per liposome was calculated from the total OX26 radioactivity in the liposome pool and the specific activity of the [^{3}H]OX26 MAb, assuming 100 000 lipid molecules per liposome (Huwyler et al., 1996). The final percentage entrapment of the plasmid DNA in the liposome was computed from the [^{32}P] radioactivity, and this was typically 30% or 30 μg plasmid DNA. Following covalent conjugation of the OX26 MAb to the tips of PEG strands on the liposome carrying the DNA, the unconjugated MAb was separated by Sepharose CL-4B gel filtration chromatography (Figure 9.3D). These studies show comigration of the [^{32}P]pGL2 plasmid incorporated in the interior of the liposome with the [^{3}H]OX26 MAb attached to the PEG strands. In this preparation, each pegylated immunoliposome contained 39 molecules of the OX26 MAb conjugated per liposome (Shi and Pardridge, 2000).

Plasma pharmacokinetics and organ clearance in vivo

Linearized luciferase plasmid DNA was [^{32}P]-radiolabeled at both the 5′- and 3′-ends with T4 polymerase and purified by gel filtration chromatography to a trichloroacetic acid (TCA) precipitability of 98%. For the pharmacokinetic experiments, the plasmid DNA was incorporated into liposomes in the linearized form. For the gene expression studies described below, the plasmid DNA was incorporated into the liposome in the supercoiled circular form. The [^{32}P]-labeled pGL2 plasmid DNA was injected intravenously into anesthetized rats in one of three formulations: (a) naked DNA, (b) DNA encapsulated in pegylated liposomes without antibody attached, or (c) DNA encapsulated in pegylated liposomes with OX26 MAb conjugated to the PEG strands. The naked DNA was rapidly removed from the plasma with a clearance (Cl) of 4.1 ± 0.5 ml/min per kg and a systemic volume of distribution of 514 ± 243 ml/kg (Figure 9.4). The naked DNA was rapidly taken up by tissues and converted to low molecular weight TCA soluble radioactivity, as shown in Figure 9.4 (right panel). The Cl of the DNA was reduced more than fourfold to 0.95 ± 0.05 ml/min per kg when the DNA was incorporated in the interior of pegylated liposomes carrying no OX26 MAb. The systemic clearance increased to 2.3 ± 0.2 ml/min per kg when the OX26 MAb was tethered to the tip of the PEG tail of the liposome (Figure 9.4), owing to uptake of the complex by TfR-bearing cells (Shi and Pardridge, 2000).

The attachment of the OX26 MAb to the tip of the pegylated liposome carrying the DNA exerted minor increases in tissue uptake in kidney or heart, moderate increases in liver, and a marked increase in the brain uptake of the pegylated immunoliposome (Figure 9.5). The brain uptake (percentage of injected dose per gram brain: %ID/g) of the pegylated immunoliposome carrying the plasmid DNA is comparable to the brain uptake of a neuroactive small molecule such as morphine (Wu et al., 1997a). The measurement of organ radioactivity (Figure 9.5) does not accurately reflect the organ targeting of the gene, because there is significant uptake

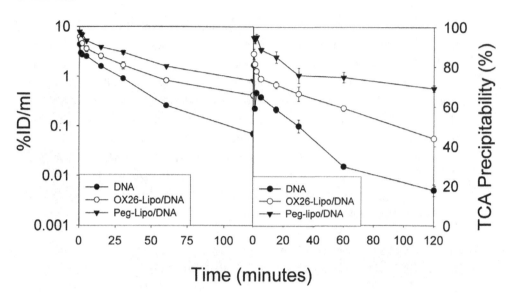

Figure 9.4   Left: The percentage of injected dose (ID) per milliliter of plasma that is precipitated by trichloroacetic acid (TCA) is plotted versus time after intravenous injection of the [^{32}P] DNA in anesthetized rats for up to 120 min. The DNA was injected in one of three formulations: (a) naked DNA (DNA), (b) pGL2 plasmid DNA encapsulated within the interior of nuclease-treated OX26 pegylated immunoliposomes (OX26–Lipo/DNA), and (c) pGL2 plasmid DNA encapsulated in the interior of nuclease-treated pegylated liposomes without OX26 MAb attached (Peg-Lipo/DNA). Right: The percentage of plasma radioactivity that is precipitable by TCA is shown. Data are mean±SE (n = 3 rats per group). From Shi, N. and Pardridge, W.M. (2000). Antisense imaging of gene expression in the brain in vivo. *Proc. Natl Acad. Sci. USA*, **97**, 14709–14. Copyright (2000) National Academy of Sciences, USA.

of [^{32}P]-labeled metabolites that are released following degradation of the radiolabeled plasmid DNA (Shi and Pardridge, 2000). As shown by the decrease in TCA precipitability of the plasma radioactivity (Figure 9.4), there is degradation of the plasmid DNA in vivo, which results in the release to blood of TCA-soluble metabolites such as [^{32}P]phosphate. A similar phenomenon is observed following the intravenous injection in rats of radiolabeled phosphodiester oligodeoxynucleotides, as reviewed in Chapter 8. The radiolabeled phosphate or other small molecular weight metabolites are rapidly taken up by tissues such as liver or kidney and much less so by organs such as brain. This uptake of metabolites accounts for the relatively high tissue radioactivity of the liver following administration of the labeled DNA packaged in pegylated liposomes without the OX26 MAb attached (Figure 9.5).

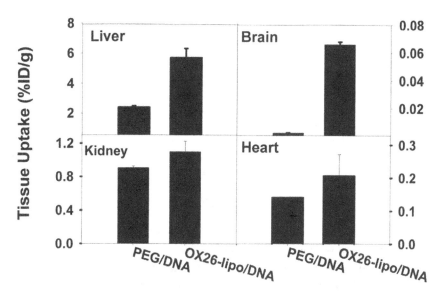

Figure 9.5   The tissue uptake, expressed as percentage of injected dose (ID) per gram tissue, for liver, brain, kidney, or heart is shown at 120 min after intravenous injection of the encapsulated [^{32}P]-labeled pGL2 plasmid DNA incorporated in either pegylated liposomes without antibody attached (polyethylene glycol (PEG)/DNA) or within the OX26 pegylated immunoliposomes (OX26–Lipo/DNA). Data are mean $\pm$ SE ($n = 3$ rats per group). From Shi, N. and Pardridge, W.M. (2000). Antisense imaging of gene expression in the brain in vivo. *Proc. Natl Acad. Sci. USA*, **97**, 14709–14. Copyright (2000) National Academy of Sciences, USA.

Expression of luciferase transgene in the brain

The luciferase gene expression in brain and peripheral tissues was examined in rats administered 10 μg of plasmid DNA per rat (Shi and Pardridge, 2000). Although there was minimal targeting of the luciferase gene in the heart or kidney, the luciferase gene expression in the brain was comparable to that of lung or spleen and peaked at 48 h after intravenous administration (Figure 9.6). The peak luciferase gene expression in liver was approximately sixfold higher than in brain, owing to the abundant expression of the TfR on the hepatocyte plasma membranes. Anti-TfR MAbs are also targeted to spleen and lung (Lee et al., 2000). For control studies, pegylated immunoliposomes were prepared, except the mouse IgG$_{2a}$ isotype control was conjugated to the pegylated liposomes instead of the OX26 MAb. These mouse IgG$_{2a}$ pegylated immunoliposomes carrying the pGL2 luciferase plasmid DNA were injected intravenously into anesthetized rats at a dose of 10 μg plasmid DNA per rat. However, there was no measurable luciferase expression in brain or any of the other peripheral organs at 48 h after intravenous administration (Shi and Pardridge, 2000). This control experiment demonstrates that the targeting

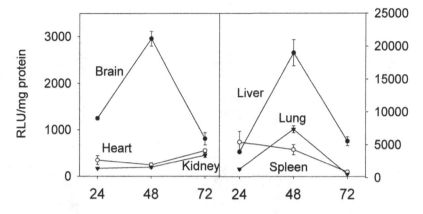

Figure 9.6   The organ luciferase activity, expressed as relative light units (RLU) per milligram tissue protein, is shown for brain, heart, kidney, liver, lung, and spleen at 24, 48, and 72 h after injection of the pGL2 plasmid DNA encapsulated in pegylated immunoliposomes that were conjugated with the OX26 monoclonal antibody (MAb). Data are mean $\pm$ SE ($n = 3$ rats per group). From Shi, N. and Pardridge, W.M. (2000). Antisense imaging of gene expression in the brain in vivo. *Proc. Natl Acad. Sci. USA*, **97**, 14709–14. Copyright (2000) National Academy of Sciences, USA.

specificity of the pegylated immunoliposomes is strictly a function of the targeting moiety attached to the tip of the PEG strands. The replacement of the TfR MAb with an IgG isotype control MAb results in no organ expression of the luciferase gene.

The level of the luciferase gene expression in liver that is obtained with the OX26 pegylated immunoliposomes following intravenous injection in rats is 15000–20000 RLU/mg protein at 48 h. This is comparable to the level of luciferase gene expression in rats injected with a luciferase plasmid DNA absorbed to polylysine and conjugated to carbohydrate moieties that target the asialoglycoprotein receptor on the hepatocyte plasma membrane (Perales et al., 1997). However, in this latter study, 300 µg of plasmid DNA was intravenously administered to adult rats. This dose is 30-fold higher than the dose used in the present studies, which was 10 µg of plasmid DNA per adult rat or 40 µg plasmid DNA per kg body weight (Shi and Pardridge, 2000). The dose of cationic liposome/DNA complex administered to mice in vivo to generate gene expression in the lung ranges from 1000 to 4000 µg plasmid DNA per kg body weight (Liu et al., 1995; Hofland et al., 1997; Song et al., 1997; Barron et al., 1999). These doses are up to 100-fold greater than the dose of plasmid DNA administered in the experiments reported in Figure 9.6.

Gene expression in the brain of a β-galactosidase gene

The studies with the luciferase transgene (Figure 9.6) demonstrate it is possible to target an exogenous gene to the brain with a noninvasive route of administration.

However, these experiments do not reveal where in the brain the luciferase transgene is expressed. Thus far, no evidence is provided that the transgene is actually transcytosed through the endothelial barrier. It is possible the pegylated immunoliposomes only target the exogenous gene to the microvasculature of brain. For example, gene expression in the lung induced by the intravenous administration of cationic liposome/DNA complexes is confined only to the endothelial cell in that organ (Hofland et al., 1997).

In order to localize the cellular origin of the transgene expression in brain, the luciferase plasmid was replaced with a plasmid encoding for β-galactosidase. This expression plasmid was incorporated in the interior of OX26 pegylated immunoliposomes and injected intravenously into anesthetized adult rats at a dose of 30 μg plasmid DNA per adult rat (Shi and Pardridge, 2000). At 48 h, the brain and liver were removed and rapidly frozen and 15 μm frozen sections were prepared on a cryostat. The sections were fixed at 5 min at room temperature in 0.5% glutaraldehyde and stored at -70 °C until β-galactosidase histochemistry was performed with 5-bromo-4-chloro-3-indoyl-β-D-galactoside (X-gal). Slides were developed overnight at 37 °C and some slides were counterstained with hematoxylin. The results of the β-galactosidase histochemistry are shown in Figure 9.7 (colour plate).

The β-galactosidase gene is widely expressed in brain, which can be seen at the low magnification in Figure 9.7A. There is no β-galactosidase gene expression in control animals (Figure 9.7B). Pyramidal neurons of the CA1–CA3 sectors of hippocampus are clearly visualized, as are the choroid plexi in both lateral ventricles and in both the dorsal horn and the mammillary recess of the third ventricle (Figure 9.7A). The paired supraoptic nuclei (son) of the hypothalamus at the base of the brain are viewed at low magnification (Figure 9.7A). At higher magnification, the microvasculature of brain parenchyma (Figure 9.7C), the choroid plexus epithelium (Figure 9.7D), and the thalamic nuclei (Figure 9.7E) all show β-galactosidase gene expression. Lower levels of gene expression in neurons throughout the brain are also visualized (Shi and Pardridge, 2000).

Gene expression was also detected histochemically throughout the liver, and the gene was expressed in a periportal pattern (Shi and Pardridge, 2000). The high magnification view of the liver histochemistry shows a punctate deposition of the enzyme product on a tubulovesicular network throughout the liver cell (Figure 9.8). This observation suggests the β-galactosidase protein has been targeted to endoplasmic reticulum of the hepatocyte.

The β-galactosidase brain histochemistry shows the exogenous gene is widely expressed throughout the brain, including neurons in the hippocampus (Figure 9.7A), and the thalamus (Figure 9.7E). For gene expression to occur in neurons, the pegylated immunoliposomes carrying the transgene must traverse both the BBB and the neuronal cell membrane. This occurs because the targeting moiety, a peptidomimetic MAb to the TfR, mediates both the transcytosis through the BBB and

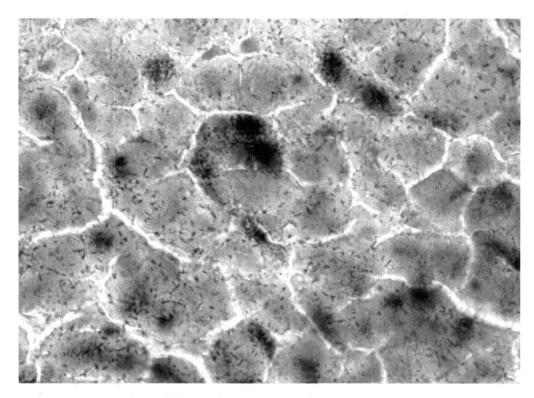

Figure 9.8   β-Galactosidase histochemistry in rat liver shows a speckled pattern suggesting localization of the β-galactosidase enzyme within the liver cell endoplasmic reticulum. From Shi, N. and Pardridge, W.M. (2000). Antisense imaging of gene expression in the brain in vivo. *Proc. Natl Acad. Sci. USA*, **97**, 14709–14. Copyright (2000) National Academy of Sciences, USA.

the endocytosis of the complex into brain cells. The exogenous gene must also escape the endosomal system within the brain cell. The release of the exogenous plasmid DNA to the cytosol may be facilitated by fusion of the lipid surface of the liposomes with the endosomal membrane within brain cells. Once inside the cytosol, the plasmid DNA can then diffuse to the nuclear space, as depicted in Figure 9.1.

Tissue-specific gene expression in the brain following noninvasive administration of exogenous genes

The results in Figures 9.6 and 9.7 demonstrate that it is possible to achieve widespread expression of an exogenous or therapeutic gene in brain following noninvasive intravenous administration. In future work, it will be desirable to cause gene expression in brain in a region- and cell-specific pattern. The plasmid carrying the luciferase transgene is shown in Figure 9.9, and includes SV40 elements at both the

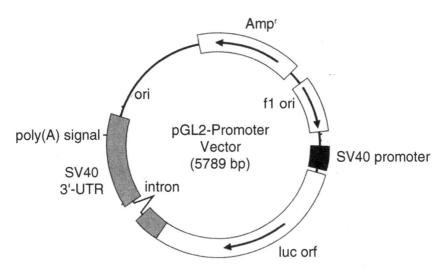

Figure 9.9   Structure of the luciferase (luc) expression plasmid used in the studies reported in Figure 9.6. orf, open reading frame.

5'- and 3'-ends of the luciferase (luc) open reading frame (orf). The SV40 promoter is at nucleotides 43–238, and the SV40 3'-untranslated region (UTR) is at nucleotides 2084–2935 with an SV40 intron incorporated at nucleotides 2160–2225 (Figure 9.9). In contrast, the pSV-β-galactosidase expression plasmid, which was used in the experiments reported in Figure 9.7, has a different 3'-UTR, which is comprised of 200 nucleotides from the lacY gene and only 110 nucleotides from the SV40 3'-UTR (Shi and Pardridge, 2000). The 3'-UTR of the β-galactosidase plasmid lacks the heterologous intron that is inserted in the luciferase plasmid (Figure 9.9). Liu et al. (1995) observed that the insertion of heterologous introns in the 3'-UTR of expression plasmids decreases gene expression in vivo. Therefore, the absence of the intron insert in the 3'-UTR of the β-galactosidase plasmid may account for the greater expression in the brain with this plasmid (Figure 9.7), as compared to the luciferase plasmid (Figure 9.6).

Cell-specific gene expression in the brain may be achieved with the replacement of the viral SV40 promoter with promoter elements from astrocyte or neuron-specific genes, such as the glial fibrillary acidic protein (GFAP) gene or neuron-specific enolase (NSE) gene, respectively (Segovia et al., 1998; Klein et al., 1999). Replacement of the SV40 promoter with the tissue- and gene-specific promoters may enable tissue-specific gene expression in the brain. For example, the lack of significant gene expression in the outer rim of the brain cortex (Figure 9.7A) suggests the SV40 promoter is not activated in this region. Alternatively, the elements in the 3'-UTR of the β-galactosidase expression plasmid may destabilize the β-galactosidase mRNA in this region. While there is much emphasis placed on the tissue- or gene-specificity of the promoter inserted in the 5'-position of the transgene, the elements inserted in the 3'-UTR of the transgene mRNA may also play an important role in regulating tissue-specific gene expression in brain cells. These 3'-UTR elements may determine the stability of the mRNA that is produced from transcription of the transgene. The 3'-UTR of the BBB *Glut1* glucose transporter mRNA (Chapter 3) contains cis sequences that react with cytosolic and polysome proteins that either stabilize or destabilize the *Glut1* mRNA (Tsukamoto et al., 1996). In addition, the 5'-UTR of the *Glut1* mRNA contains cis elements that promote translation of the mRNA (Boado et al., 1996). These cis elements from the 5'- or 3'-UTR of the BBB *Glut1* mRNA were inserted into the 5'- and 3'-UTR regions of the luciferase gene, and this chimeric plasmid was then used to transfect bovine brain capillary endothelial cells in culture (Boado and Pardridge, 1999). As shown in Figure 9.10, there is a synergistic interaction between the 5- and 3'-UTR elements and this results in a 60-fold increase in transgene expression. Other investigations have shown that the molecular basis of the increased gene expression is a stabilization of the mRNA caused by insertion of the cis elements derived from the *Glut1* mRNA 3'-UTR (Boado and Pardridge, 1998).

Persistence of gene expression in the brain

The goal of gene therapy of the brain is the cell-specific and persistent expression of the therapeutic gene following noninvasive administration. The frequency of administration of the gene medicine will be inversely related to the persistence of expression of the transgene in brain. The studies in Figure 9.6 show that luciferase transgene expression peaks at 48 h. However, this work used a transient transfection plasmid that only transcribes the DNA until the original plasmid is degraded. There is no episomal replication of the plasmid used in the studies shown in Figures 9.6–9.8. In contrast, the luciferase expression plasmid used in the gene-imaging studies described in Chapter 8 involved permanent transfection of the brain cells. The clone 790 plasmid contained the Epstein–Barr nuclear antigen (EBNA)-1 gene (Figure 8.9B). The EBNA-1 enables episomal replication in primate and canine cells (Makrides, 1999), and may facilitate persistent gene expression of plasmid DNA formulations in rodent cells (Tomiyasu et al., 1998). The pGL2 plasmid (Figure 9.9), which was used to generate the data shown in Figure 9.6, was replaced with the 790 plasmid (Figure 8.9B). The 790 plasmid is a 10.6 kb luciferase expression plasmid that contains both the EBNA-1, to promote episomal replication, and the *Glut1* mRNA 3'-UTR element, to promote mRNA stabilization. The brain luciferase activity at 48 h after intravenous injection of the 790 plasmid packaged in the OX26 pegylated immunoliposomes was increased 50-fold relative to the brain luciferase activity shown in Figure 9.6 (unpublished observations). These results indicate the persistence of the exogenous gene in brain can be prolonged for days after a single intravenous injection. For example, the β-galactosidase activity

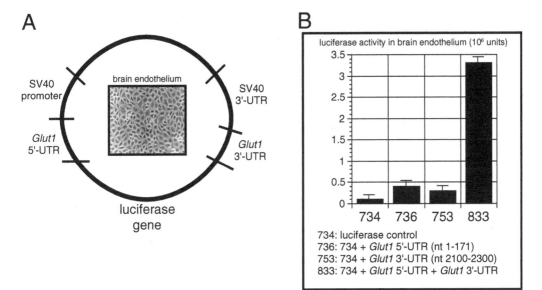

A

B

luciferase activity in brain endothelium (10⁶ units)

734: luciferase control
736: 734 + *Glut1* 5'-UTR (nt 1-171)
753: 734 + *Glut1* 3'-UTR (nt 2100-2300)
833: 734 + *Glut1* 5'-UTR + *Glut1* 3'-UTR

Figure 9.10   (A) Bovine brain capillary endothelial cells grown in tissue culture are shown in the inset. These cells were transiently transfected with a luciferase reporter plasmid, which is shown. The control luciferase plasmid is clone 734. A 171 nucleotide (nt) fragment, obtained from the 5'-untranslated region (UTR) of the BBB *Glut1* glucose transporter mRNA, was inserted at the 5'-end of the gene, and after the SV40 promoter, to generate clone 736. A 200 nt fragment, obtained from the 3'-UTR of the BBB *Glut1* glucose transporter mRNA, was inserted at the the 3'-end of the gene, and within the SV40 3'-UTR, to generate clone 753. Clone 833 contains both the 171 nt 5'-UTR and the 200 nt 3'-UTR fragments from the *Glut1* mRNA. (B) The luciferase enzyme activity in the brain endothelial cells is shown. The enzyme activity is expressed as relative light units per 20 μl lysate obtained from 65% confluent cells grown on 35 mm dishes. Cells were transfected with 0.7 μg plasmid DNA and 14 μg Lipofectamine for 16 h in media without serum. Fresh media (with 2.5% horse serum) was then added and the cells were harvested at 48 h. Reprinted from *Mol. Brain Res.*, **63**, Boado, R.J. and Pardridge, W.M., Amplification of gene expression using both 5'- and 3'-untranslated regions of GLUT1 glucose transporter mRNA, 371–4, copyright (1999), with permission from Elsevier Science.

in brain and liver shown in Figure 9.7 persists for at least 6 days after a single intravenous injection (unpublished observations).

Once a gene-targeting strategy has been developed that enables the expression of therapeutic genes in brain following noninvasive administration of nonviral gene formulations, then the limiting factor is the construct of the actual plasmid DNA (Makrides, 1999). Future studies may show that the cell-specificity that is required can be achieved with specific promoter elements inserted in the 5'-end of the gene. The persistence of the mRNA derived from the transgene may be increased with the insertion of mRNA stabilizing elements in the $3'$-end of the gene. The persistence of the transgene may be achieved by the addition of elements such as the EBNA-1, which enable episomal replication of the plasmid DNA without stable integration into the host genome.

Noninvasive gene therapy of the brain in humans

Gene therapy of the brain in humans can be accomplished by changing the targeting moiety of the formulation (Figure 9.3A) from a TfR MAb to a MAb that targets the human insulin receptor (HIR). As discussed in Chapter 5, the HIR MAb is nearly 10 times more active in primates as a BBB targeting vector than is an anti-TfR MAb. Chimeric forms of the HIR MAb have been produced and the genetically engineered chimeric HIR MAb has transport properties at the primate or human BBB that are identical to that of the original murine HIR MAb (Chapter 5). The insulin receptor is also widely distributed on brain cells (Zhao et al., 1999). Therefore, the HIR MAb could target the gene formulation through both barriers in brain, the BBB and the BCM.

Summary

Present-day gene therapy of the brain can be improved in two ways (Figure 9.2). Presently, therapeutic genes are administered by intracerebral implantation via craniotomy. The problem with intracerebral implantation of an exogenous gene is that the effective treatment volume is <1 mm^3 at the injection site, owing to the limited diffusion of the gene formulation in brain following injection into brain tissue. In addition, the exogenous transgene must be administered repeatedly, and repetitive craniotomy is not desirable. It would be advantageous to administer the therapeutic gene noninvasively so that patients are not subjected to multiple craniotomies or BBB disruptions. The second problem with present-day gene therapy of the brain is that the vectors that are employed involve viral gene formulations. Both adenovirus and herpes simplex virus cause extensive neuropathology, including demyelination following the intracerebral injection of single doses in rats, primate, or humans. The work reviewed in this chapter shows that it is possible to achieve widespread expression of an exogenous gene in the CNS following a simple intravenous administration. The gene formulation shown in Figure 9.3A requires the merger of recombinant DNA technology, liposome technology, pegylation technology, and the chimeric peptide technology (Shi and Pardridge, 2000). The availability of the human genome sequence makes future gene discovery much less difficult. Therefore, the future innovation in the development of gene medicines will be in the area of noninvasive gene targeting and tissue-specific gene expression.

10

Blood–brain barrier genomics

- Introduction
- Methodology
- Blood–brain barrier-specific gene expression
- Gene interactions
- Summary

Introduction

Blood–brain barrier (BBB) genomics involves an analysis of the tissue-specific expression of genes at the brain microvasculature, which forms the BBB in vivo. The application of genomics technology to BBB research is the single most powerful methodology ever applied to laboratory investigations of the BBB. Various physiologic, cell biological, and molecular biological methodologies have been adapted to BBB research, as reviewed previously (Pardridge, 1998d). The evolution of BBB methodology from the physiologic methods to molecular biological approaches led to incremental increases in knowledge as to how the BBB functions. However, with respect to the generation of new knowledge about BBB function that is acquired in a short time frame, the application of genomics is the most powerful new methodology ever applied to BBB research.

Purpose of BBB genomics

The discovery of genes specifically expressed at the BBB has at least two goals. First, the finding of a novel gene or a group of genes that is selectively expressed at the BBB will provide new insights into the role the microvasculature plays in brain physiology and pathology, as illustrated by the examples discussed below. Second, with respect to brain drug targeting, BBB genomics will lead to the identification of novel transporters selectively expressed at the BBB, and these discoveries will offer new targets for drug transport through the BBB in vivo. As reviewed in prior chapters of this book, and as shown in Figure 10.1, there are three general types of BBB transport processes for either large or small molecules. Carrier-mediated transport (CMT) systems are responsible for the uptake of circulating nutrients

BLOOD-BRAIN BARRIER ENDOGENOUS TRANSPORT SYSTEMS

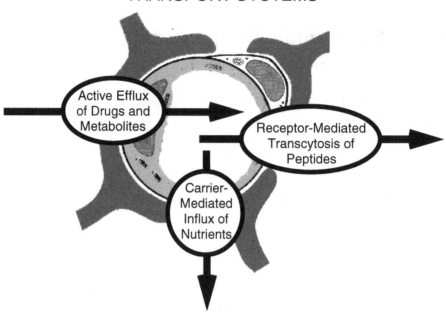

Figure 10.1   Three pathways of transport at the blood–brain barrier (BBB) include carrier-mediated transport (CMT) from blood to brain (Chapter 3), receptor-mediated transport (RMT) from blood to brain (Chapter 4), and active efflux transport (AET) from brain to blood (Chapter 3). BBB genomics programs may lead to the discovery of novel CMT, RMT, or AET systems. New CMT or RMT systems could be used to target drugs through the BBB. New AET systems could be used to develop codrugs, which inhibit the AET systems and thereby increase the brain uptake of drugs that are normally excluded from brain because of the efflux transporters at the BBB.

and vitamins by the brain from blood, as reviewed in Chapter 3. Receptor-mediated transcytosis (RMT) systems mediate the brain uptake from blood of circulating peptides or proteins, as reviewed in Chapter 4. A third class of BBB transport pathway is the active efflux transport (AET) systems, which are responsible for the selective transport from brain to blood of small molecules generated in brain metabolism. The AET systems are also responsible for the active efflux of numerous drugs from brain to blood. The classical active efflux system at the brain microvasculature is p-glycoprotein, as reviewed in Chapter 3. However, there may be dozens of active efflux systems other than p-glycoprotein that function at the brain microvasculature and are expressed at the endothelial plasma membrane, the per-

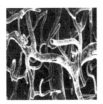

The volume of the brain capillary
endothelium is < 0.1% of brain, so most
BBB-specific targets are not detected by
screening whole-brain gene arrays.

Figure 10.2   Blood–brain barrier (BBB) genomics starts with an analysis of gene products from the
microvasculature of brain, not from whole brain. Since the sensitivity of current gene
microarrays is about 10^{-4} (Schena et al., 1995), and since the volume of the brain
endothelial compartment, relative to total brain volume, is 10^{-3}, only very abundant BBB-
specific gene products can be detected with gene microarrays from whole brain.
Conversely, BBB-specific genes are readily identified with a BBB genomics program,
which has as its starting point the isolation of brain capillaries. A vascular cast of the
human cerebellar cortex is shown. From Duvernoy et al. (1983) with permission.

icyte plasma membrane, or the astrocyte foot process plasma membrane. Drugs
that inhibit the BBB active efflux systems may act as "codrugs." In this setting,
a codrug is administered in conjunction with a drug that is normally actively
effluxed from brain to blood across the BBB. The inhibition of the active efflux
system by the codrug would allow for enhanced brain uptake of a drug that is
normally excluded from significant penetration into the brain from blood (Chapter
3).

Separation of BBB genomics from brain genomics

It might be assumed that BBB specific gene products may be routinely detected in
the microarray screening of tissue-specific gene expression within the brain.
However, the sensitivity of existing microarray gene detection systems is approximately 10^{-4} (Schena et al., 1995). Since the volume of the brain capillary endothelium is <1 µl/g brain, the volume of the endothelial cytoplasm in brain constitutes
$<0.1\%$ of the brain volume or a factor of 10^{-3} (Figure 10.2). Therefore, only transcripts that are highly expressed at the BBB will be detected in gene microarray
derived from RNA isolated from whole-brain homogenate. In contrast, a BBB
genomics program begins with the initial isolation of brain microvessels, as
depicted in Figure 10.3. The polyA+ RNA is then purified from isolated brain
microvessels to generate BBB cDNA containing highly enriched fractions of BBB-
specific gene products.

Methodology

Gene microarray methodologies

Genomic methodologies began with the isolation of expressed sequence tags (ESTs) which were originally identified in human brain (Adams et al., 1992). ESTs are small fragments of approximately 400 nucleotides and represent partial sequences of mRNAs. The majority of ESTs contain primarily sequence of the 3'-untranslated region (UTR) of the mRNA, which is not strongly conserved across species in many mRNAs. The simple identification of thousands of ESTs that are expressed in a given tissue has been refined into functional genomics programs. The goal of functional genomics is to identify fragments of genes that are selectively expressed in a given tissue relative to other tissues using "subtractive hybridization" methodologies (Liang and Pardee, 1992; Diatchenko et al., 1996; Welford et al., 1998). One such approach, subtractive suppressive hybridization (SSH) (Diatchenko et al., 1996), was used in initial evaluation of a BBB genomics program (Li et al., 2001). In this approach, brain capillary-derived cDNA was subtracted with cDNA obtained from rat liver or rat kidney (Figure 10.3).

Subtractive suppressive hybridization

The capillaries of rat brain were purified (Figure 10.4A), and rat brain capillary derived polyA + RNA was isolated (Boado and Pardridge, 1991) and used to produce "tester" cDNA. A subtraction procedure was completed using "driver" cDNA generated from rat liver and rat kidney mRNA. Double-stranded cDNA was synthesized from either tester or driver polyA + RNA (1 μg) and the reaction was followed with [^{32}P]deoxycytidine triphosphate. The tester or driver cDNA was digested with RsaI to obtain shorter, blunt-end molecules and two tester populations were created with either adapter 1 or adapter 2R, which were independently ligated to the tester cDNA (Diatchenko et al., 1996). The two populations of adapter-ligated tester cDNA were independently hybridized to the driver cDNA to enrich for differentially expressed sequences, and hybridized a second time to generate a polymerase chain reaction (PCR) template. A first-run PCR amplifies differentially expressed sequences and was performed for 30 cycles. A second-run PCR was performed for 15 cycles using nested PCR primers. This second PCR further enriches for differentially expressed sequences and suppresses the background.

Subtraction efficiency

The efficiency of the subtraction procedure was determined by PCR analysis of glyceraldehyde 3-phosphate dehydrogenase (G3PDH) expression in subtracted and

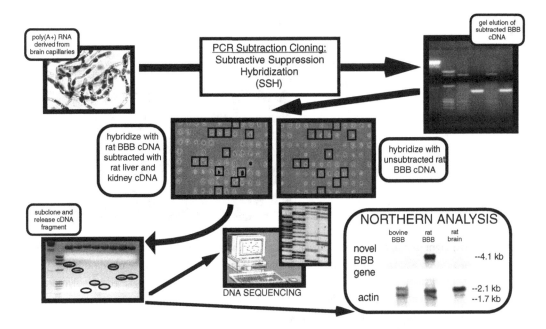

Figure 10.3 Outline of blood–brain barrier (BBB) genomics and cloning of differentially expressed genes at the brain microvasculature. The methodology starts with polyA + mRNA derived from brain capillaries, which provides the tester cDNA. A secondary source of mRNA provides the driver cDNA. In initial applications, the driver cDNA was derived from rat liver and rat kidney cDNA. The method uses a polymerase chain reaction (PCR) subtraction cloning methodology such as suppression subtractive hybridization (SSH). The SSH-PCR products were cloned into the pCR2.1 vector, and a cDNA library was prepared in *Escherichia coli* INVαF' cells. Positive clones were identified by differential hybridization. Colonies were individually blotted on to GeneScreen Plus membranes using a 96-well dot-blot system. Clones showing a strong hybridization signal with the subtracted probe compared to the unsubtracted one were selected for DNA sequencing. Northern analysis was done following release of the pCR2.1 insert with EcoRI. This insert was also subcloned into transcription plasmids for generation of antisense or sense RNA for in situ hybridization.

unsubtracted cDNA (Li et al., 2001). The cDNA products of the first- and second-cycle PCR ranged in size from 0.2 to 1.4 kb and the majority of the PCR products had sizes ranging from 0.3 to 0.7 kb. The efficiency of the subtraction procedure was analyzed by PCR amplification of cDNA for G3PDH, as shown in Figure 10.4B. Using the subtracted tester cDNA, no G3PDH PCR product was identified until 33 cycles of PCR (lane 5, Figure 10.4B). Conversely, the G3PDH cDNA was identified in PCR of the unsubtracted tester cDNA as early as 18 cycles (lane 8, Figure 10.4B).

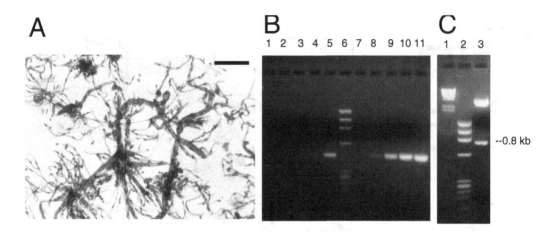

Figure 10.4 (A) Light micrograph of freshly isolated rat brain capillaries showing the microvessels are free of adjoining brain tissue. The capillaries were stained with ortho-toluidine blue. Magnification bar = 83 μm. (B) The subtraction efficiency is demonstrated by polymerase chain reaction (PCR) amplification of the cDNA for glyceraldehyde 3-phosphate dehydrogenase (G3PDH). Lanes 1, 2, 3, 4, and 5 are subtracted tester G3PDH PCR products at 13, 18, 23, 28, and 33 cycles, respectively. Lane 6 is DNA markers 1.4, 1.1, 0.87, 0.60, 0.31, 0.28, 0.23, and 0.19 kb. Lanes 7–11 are unsubtracted tester G3PDH PCR products at 13, 18, 23, 28, and 33 cycles respectively. (C) Agarose gel electrophoresis of the rat BBB organic anion transporting polypeptide type 2 (oatp2) cloned fragment after EcoRI digestion showing the insert size to be 0.8 kb (lane 3). High and low molecular weight DNA size standards are shown in lanes 1 and 2, respectively. From Li et al. (2001) with permission.

Subtractive cDNA screening

The SSH PCR products were cloned into the pCR2.1 vector and a cDNA library was prepared in *Escherichia coli* INVαF' cells (Li et al., 2001). Positive clones were identified by differential hybridization. *E. coli* was transformed and randomly selected bacterial colonies were cultured overnight in a 96-well plate followed by Southern dot blot hybridization with [^{32}P]-labeled subtracted and unsubtracted cDNA followed by film autoradiography, as shown in Figure 10.3. Clones showing a strong hybridization signal with a subtracted probe compared to the unsubtracted one were selected for DNA sequencing and Northern analysis, following release of the insert from the pCR2.1 vector with EcoRI (Figure 10.3). For example, the size of the gene product released from one clone was 0.8 kb, as shown in Figure 10.4C. This clone proved to be 100% identical to rat organic anion transporting polypeptide type 2 (oatp2), as described below.

Summary of initial screening of subtracted BBB library

The initial BBB library was generated from rat brain capillary mRNA-derived tester cDNA that was subtracted with driver cDNA derived from rat kidney and rat liver. A library was prepared from 5% of the subtracted tester cDNA, and screening of this initial library yielded the identification of 50 clones, which selectively hybridized with the subtracted cDNA (Li et al., 2001). All 50 clones were subjected to DNA sequence analysis and Northern analysis, as outlined in Figure 10.3; 49 of the 50 clones had cDNA inserts and multiple copies were detected for five of the gene products, as shown in Figure 10.5. The genes were designated LK1–LK50, indicating BBB clones 1–50 that were subtracted with liver (L) and kidney (K). Twelve of the clones, or 24%, have novel DNA sequence not found in current databases. One of the novel clones was LK3, and this partial cDNA was used to generate full-length cDNA, which was sequenced and named BBB-specific anion transporter type 1 (BSAT1), as described below. Fragments of the BSAT1 cDNA were found in eight different clones or 16% of the 50 clones. This high frequency was corroborated by Northern analysis which showed that the mRNA for LK3 or BSAT1 was very abundant at the rat brain microvasculature, as described below. Clones encoding the mRNA for carboxypeptidase E were found six times, or a frequency of 12%. Clones representing mRNAs for the vascular endothelial growth factor (VEGF) receptor type 2, also known as flt-1, were found four times, and clones encoding for myelin basic protein were found three times for a frequency of 6% (Figure 10.5). Sequences for several clones were found in the rat EST database. All but two of these ESTs were selectively expressed at the BBB, as shown in Figure 10.5. Indeed, 37 of the 50 clones, or 74%, were selectively expressed at the BBB as shown by Northern blot analysis, a finding that corroborates the efficiency of the subtraction procedure.

Blood–brain barrier-specific gene expression

BSAT1

The sequence of LK3 was novel and not found in any databases (Li et al., 2001). This clone was used to screen a rat brain capillary cDNA library in the pSPORT vector, which had been described previously (Boado et al., 1999), and a 2.6 kb full-length cDNA was identified and sequenced. The full sequence for BSAT1 encompassed the sequences of seven other clones found in the initial BBB library. Therefore, the BSAT1 clones represented 16% of the initial 50 clones identified. This suggests the mRNA for BSAT1 is highly enriched at the BBB and this was confirmed by Northern blot analysis, as shown in Figure 10.6A. The 2.6 kb

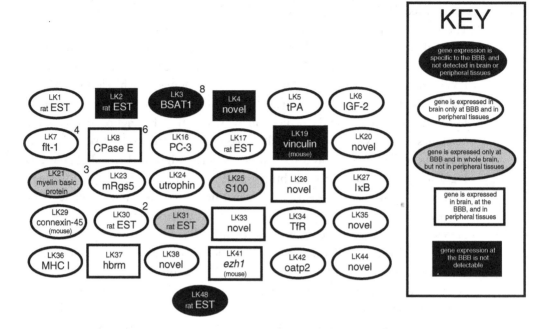

Figure 10.5 Summary of the results of analysis of the first 50 clones isolated from screening 5% of the rat blood–brain barrier (BBB) cDNA library described in Figure 10.3. The 50 clones are designated as LK1–LK50, since the BBB library was subtracted with rat liver (L) and kidney (K). Gene expression was analyzed with Northern blotting for each of the 50 clones. One clone out of the 50 had no insert. Five of the clones were represented by multiple copies in the 50 clones, and these include LK3, which is blood–brain barrier-specific anion transporter type 1 (BSAT1) (Figure 10.6); LK8, which is carboxypeptidase E; LK7, which is the flt-1 receptor for vascular endothelial growth factor (VEGF); LK21, which is myelin basic protein; and LK30, which is a rat expressed sequence tag (EST). The number of replicates of these clones in the library is shown as a numerical superscript beside the respective clone. The genes are classified into one of five categories depending on the BBB-specificity of the gene expression. From Li et al. (2001) with permission.

Abbreviations: tPA, tissue plasminogen activator; IGF-2, insulin-like growth factor2; CPase E, carboxypeptidase E; flt-1, vascular endothelial growth factor receptor; mRgs5, mouse regulator of G protein signaling; TfR, transferrin receptor; MHC, multiple histocompatibility complex; oatp, organic anion transporting polypeptide.

transcript for BSAT1 was identified in rat brain capillary mRNA with Northern analysis following only a 3-h exposure at room temperature of the blotted membrane to X-ray film, whereas no BSAT1 mRNA was found in total rat brain at this level of exposure (Figure 10.6A). The BSAT1 transcript could be found in brain at longer exposure, such as 24 h (Figure 10.6A), and this suggests that the signal for the BSAT1 mRNA in whole brain is derived solely from the brain microvasculature.

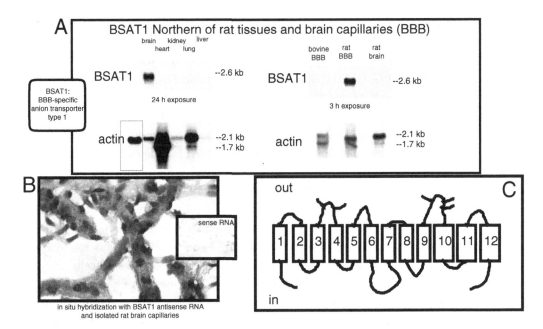

Figure 10.6   Cloning of blood–brain barrier (BBB) specific anion transporter type 1 (BSAT1). (A) Northern blot analysis shows BSAT1 is only expressed at the BBB and is not detected in whole rat brain, heart, kidney, lung, or liver. (B) In situ hybridization with the BSAT1 antisense RNA labeled with digoxigenin (DIG) and detected with an anti-DIG antibody conjugated to alkaline phosphatase. The study shows continuous immunostaining of the capillaries, which is indicative of an endothelial origin of the transporter. In situ hybridization with the BSAT1 sense RNA yields no immunostaining, as shown in the inset. (C) Secondary structure analysis of the predicted amino acid sequence of the BSAT1 protein indicates the protein is comprised of 12 transmembrane regions with five predicted N-linked glycosylation sites projecting into the extracellular space. This structure is typical of a membrane transporter, as shown for LAT1 in Figure 3.14. From Li et al. (2001) with permission.

The BSAT1 mRNA was not detected in rat heart, kidney, lung, or liver, as shown in the Northern analysis in Figure 10.6A, although all tissues contained actin transcript. These Northern studies were performed with a BSAT1 partial cDNA encoding for the 3'-UTR and there was no cross-hybridization between this clone and mRNA generated from bovine brain capillaries, as shown in Figure 10.6A. The failure to detect BSAT1 in the bovine brain capillary preparation suggests the 3'-UTR of the BSAT1 mRNA is not conserved across species. In situ hybridization (ISH) was performed on cytocentrifuged isolated rat brain capillaries, as shown in Figure 10.6B. The 0.8 kb insert for LK3 generated from the initial screening of the library was released from the pCR2.1 vector and cloned into pSPT19, which is a transcription plasmid (Li et al., 2001). This enabled the production of both antisense and sense RNA probes which were incorporated with digoxigenin-11-uridine triphosphate (DIG-11–UTP). The hybridization of the sense or antisense RNA labeled with DIG-11–UTP was detected with an anti-DIG antibody conjugated to alkaline phosphatase and the ISH studies showed no hybridization of the sense RNA for BSAT1 with isolated rat brain capillaries (inset, Figure 10.6B). In contrast, there was continuous immunostaining of isolated rat brain capillaries with the antisense RNA probe to BSAT1, indicating the BSAT1 at the rat brain microvasculature was expressed in the endothelial cell. Nucleotide sequencing of the full-length cDNA encoding for BSAT1 allowed for prediction of the deduced amino acid sequence of the BSAT1 protein. This predicted a transporter protein with 12 transmembrane regions and five N-linked glycosylation sites projecting into the extracellular compartment, as shown in Figure 10.6C. Both the amino terminal and the carboxyl terminal segments are predicted to project into the intracellular compartment. In summary, clone LK3 and seven other clones identified in the first 50 clones of the BBB subtracted library encoded for novel gene product, termed BSAT1, and the expression of this gene product is specific for the BBB. The amino acid sequence of BSAT1 has a distant homology with other anion transporter proteins (Abe et al., 1999). Therefore, BSAT1 may be a novel efflux system at the BBB similar to oatp2, as discussed below.

Tissue plasminogen activator

Clone LK5 was an 0.4 kb insert with a 99% identity with nucleotides 1550–1882 of rat tissue plasminogen activator (tPA) (Ny et al., 1988). Northern analysis showed the expression of a 2.5 kb transcript in rat brain microvessels that was detected after a 2-day exposure of the X-ray film. tPA transcripts were also found in rat heart and rat lung. These Northern studies suggested that, although tPA is expressed in the periphery, the expression of the tPA gene in brain is largely confined to the microvasculature. Since tPA plays a role in neurite outgrowth and learning in brain (Seeds et al., 1999), it is possible that BBB-derived tPA mediates neuronal migration, synaptic connections, and learning. Recent studies also suggest that tPA plays a role in excitotoxic death of neurons in cell culture (Kim et al., 1999). tPA converts plasminogen to plasmin, which plays a role in fibrinolysis, but may also accelerate excitotoxic brain damage. Kainate toxicity requires plasminogen and is lost in plasminogen knockout mice (Chen et al., 1999b). The secretion of tPA in excitotoxic brain damage may also result in BBB disruption as inhibitors of tPA result in diminished BBB disruption in experimental allergic encephalomyelitis (Paterson et al., 1987).

Insulin-like growth factor (IGF)2

A surprising finding was that the clone designated LK6 encoded for rat IGF2 transcript (Li et al., 2001). The mRNA for IGF2 is highest in adult rat brain compared to any other tissue (Murphy et al., 1987; Ueno et al., 1988). However, ISH showed IGF2 transcript only at the choroid plexus in brain (Hynes et al., 1988; Tseng et al., 1989; Couce et al., 1992), and this led to the hypothesis that choroid plexus is the site of origin of IGF2 production in brain. However, the IGF2 receptor is widely expressed on neurons throughout the brain (Valentino et al., 1988; Werner et al., 1992), and cerebrospinal fluid (CSF)-derived IGF2 would only have access to those receptors by diffusion, which is a limited means of distribution within the brain (Chapter 2). This suggests that there may be an additional source of IGF2 in brain. One source could be transcytosis of IGF2 from blood via the BBB IGF2 receptor (Duffy et al., 1988), as discussed in Chapter 4. However, an additional source of IGF2 in brain may be local production at the brain microvasculature. The size of the IGF2 clone isolated from the BBB library was 0.5 kb and sequence analysis indicated this clone was 100% identical to rat IGF2 corresponding to nucleotides 2717–3170 of the 3′-UTR of the rat IGF2 mRNA including the polyA tail (accession no. X16703). In Northern analysis, the LK6 clone selectively hybridized to 3.3 and 1.5 kb IGF2 mRNAs in rat brain capillaries, as shown in Figure 10.7A and B. No detectable IGF2 transcript at this exposure was found in C6 glioma cells or in rat heart, kidney, lung, or liver. When rat brain microvasculature-derived RNA was compared to whole-rat brain RNA, the concentration of the IGF2 mRNA was much higher in the microvascular fraction, as shown in Figure 10.7B.

The quality of mRNA used in these studies was demonstrated by 4F2hc Northern blotting for rat tissues, as shown in Figure 10.7A, and actin blotting for bovine and rat brain microvessel preparations, as shown in Figure 10.7B. The cDNA for 4F2hc, which is the heavy chain of the large neutral amino acid transporter (Chapter 3), is widely expressed in tissues and was used as a control for rat tissue RNA. The actin mRNA production varies too widely in liver and heart. The processing of the IGF2 mRNA in tissues is complex and multiple transcripts of different sizes are found in Northern blotting and at least six transcripts have been reported, with the size ranging from 6.0 to 1.2 kb (Brown et al., 1986). These transcripts have different 5′-UTRs, owing to different transcription sites (Frunzio et al., 1986), and some of the transcripts have different 3′-UTRs, owing to different polyadenylation sites (Ueno et al., 1989). The sequence analysis showed that the clone LK6 corresponded to the most distal part of the 3′-UTR of the rat IGF2 mRNA. Prior work has shown that rat IGF2 cDNAs that contain only the 3′-UTR selectively hybridize to smaller-sized variant IGF2 transcripts (Chiariotti et al., 1988). The failure of the rat BBB IGF2 cDNA to hybridize to mRNA in bovine brain microvessels (Figure 10.7B) shows a

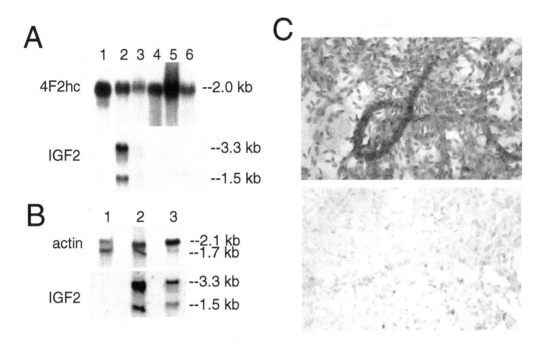

Figure 10.7 Northern hybridization of brain capillaries and rat tissues with the cloned insulin-growth factor-2 (IGF2) cDNA. (A) mRNA isolated from C6 rat glioma cells, rat brain, rat heart, rat kidney, rat lung, or rat liver was applied to lanes 1–6 of panel A, respectively, and was hybridized with either the cloned IGF2 or 4F2hc cDNA (top and lower panels, respectively). 2 μg of polyA+ RNA was applied to each lane and the 4F2hc or IGF2 X-ray film was exposed to the filter at −70 °C for 20 h or 5 days, respectively. (B) IGF2 or actin Northern blots are shown for mRNA isolated from bovine brain capillaries, rat brain capillaries, or whole rat brain in lanes 1, 2, and 3, respectively. 2 μg of polyA+ mRNA was applied to each lane. The IGF2 Northern blot was exposed for 20 h at −70 °C, and the actin Northern blot was exposed for 24 h at −70 °C. (C) In situ hybridization of isolated rat brain capillaries with either antisense (top) or sense (bottom) probes, respectively, for rat IGF2. The specimens were not counterstained. From Li et al. (2001) with permission.

lack of sequence conservation at this distal part of the 3′-UTR in rat and bovine IGF2 mRNA.

The sequence of the partial clone for bovine IGF2 present in the database (accession no. X53553) does not overlap with the 3′-UTR sequence of the rat IGF2 clone isolated in these studies, but does overlap with the open reading frame of the rat IGF2 mRNA (accession no. X16703). ISH studies were performed and demonstrated continuous immunostaining of isolated rat brain capillaries with the antisense probe, but minimal immunostaining with the sense probe, as shown in Figure 10.7C. In addition, the expression of the IGF2 mRNA was prominent in precapillary arterioles, as shown in the top panel of Figure 10.7C. These studies show that the IGF2 gene in brain is selectively expressed at the microvascular endothelium. In peripheral tissues, the expression of the IGF2 gene is regulated by growth hormone (Olney and Mougey, 1999). The brain is also an end organ for growth hormone action. Growth hormone-knockout mice have decreased myelin production and microencephaly (Beck et al., 1995). Growth hormone effects in brain may be mediated via interactions of circulating growth hormone with the brain microvasculature, since immunoreactive growth hormone receptor is expressed at the brain capillary in pathologic conditions and is upregulated in hypoxia (Scheepens et al., 1999). Since IGF2 is neuroprotective in cerebral ischemia (Guan et al., 1993), one source of endogenous neuroprotection of the brain may be mediated by circulating growth hormone and the release of IGF2 to the brain by the microvascular endothelium.

VEGF receptor

There are at least three receptors for VEGF and these are designated as flt-1, flk-2/kdr, and flt-4 (Stacker et al., 1999). VEGF biology is complex as there are multiple VEGF isoforms ranging from 121 to 206 amino acids in length (Ferrara and Davis-Smyth, 1997). In whole-body autoradiography, the organ with the highest binding of radiolabeled VEGF is the brain and this binding in brain was restricted to both the choroid plexus and to the microvasculature (Jakeman et al., 1992). In the initial BBB genomics investigation, four clones for the flt-1 receptor were identified; LK7, LK10, LK18, and LK43 (Li et al., 2001). Clones LK10 and LK18 were identical. LK7 was an 0.5 kb insert and LK10/LK18 was an 0.65 kb insert that corresponded to two different regions of the rat (Yamane et al., 1994) and mouse (Finnerty et al., 1993) flt-1 receptor, respectively. Clone LK7 was 97% identical to nucleotides 2191–2474 of rat flt-1, and clones LK10/LK18 were 87% identical to nucleotides 5499–5652 of mouse flt-1. Clone LK43 was 87% identical to nucleotides 5311–5733 of mouse flt-1. The LK7 clone hybridized to a 6.4 kb transcript that was selectively expressed at the microvasculature in brain with minimal expression in peripheral tissues, with the exception of rat lung. The LK10 clone hybridized to a series of transcripts ranging from 3.9 to 7.8 kb that were selectively expressed at the microvasculature in brain but were also detected in rat lung. VEGF, basic fibroblast growth factor (FGF), and hepatocyte growth factor are angiogenesis factors (Liu et al., 1999). The flt-1 VEGF receptor is overexpressed at the brain microvasculature in brain tumors, including hemangioblastoma (Wizigmann-Voos et al., 1995) and malignant gliomas (Plate and Risau, 1995).

PC-3 gene product

PC-3 is an immediate early gene isolated from rat PC-12 cells that is upregulated in parallel with PC-12 cell differentiation induced by nerve growth factor (NGF) (Montagnoli et al., 1996). Overexpression of the PC-3 gene product is associated with decreased cell division and a parallel increase in the production of the retino-blastoma (RB) gene product (Montagnoli et al., 1996). Clone LK16 was comprised of 0.8 and 0.45 kb inserts that were 99% identical to nucleotides 1859–2332 of rat PC-3 (Iacopetti et al., 1994). Northern analysis showed that PC-3 was expressed in rat brain, but the level of expression at the BBB was several-fold greater. The PC-3 gene product was also expressed in peripheral tissues such as rat heart and lung. BBB expression of the PC-3 gene product may be decreased in states of angiogenesis, and this expression may be mediated in concert with the gene expression of angiogenesis factors, angiogenesis factor receptors, such as flt-1, or transcription factors.

Myelin basic protein

Three identical clones encoding for rat myelin basic protein were identified in the initial screening of the BBB library. Clones LK21, LK28, and LK32 were 0.4 kb inserts that were 98% identical with nucleotides 308–652 of rat myelin basic protein (Roach et al., 1983). Northern analysis with the LK21 cDNA hybridized to a 2.1 kb transcript that was found only in brain and not in any peripheral tissues. The level of the transcript for myelin basic protein in whole rat brain was comparable to the level of myelin basic protein mRNA in isolated rat brain capillaries, as shown in Figure 10.8A. (The amount of mRNA from rat brain applied to lane 8 (2.0 µg) was fourfold greater than the amount of rat brain capillary mRNA applied to lane 7 (0.5 µg) in Figure 10.8A.) The finding of gene expression for myelin basic protein at the BBB was unexpected. The expression of the gene for myelin basic protein at the BBB is of interest, since both the formation of myelin and the BBB evolved in parallel in all vertebrates. To identify further the site of origin of the myelin basic protein transcript at the rat brain microvasculature, ISH studies were performed, and these are shown in Figure 10.8B. The ISH shows continuous immunostaining of the brain microvessels, which is indicative of an endothelial origin of the transcript encoding for myelin basic protein. Prominent hybridization was also found in precapillary arterioles.

The function of microvascular myelin basic protein is unknown at present. It is of interest that the earliest neuropathologic lesion in the brain of multiple sclerosis (MS) is a perivascular cuffing of lymphocytes around brain microvessels (Adams, 1977), and myelin basic protein is an autoantigen in MS (Bornstein et al., 1987). There is increased antigen presentation in microvessels of MS brain. As shown in Figure 10.9B and C, immunoreactivity for the DR antigen, which is the

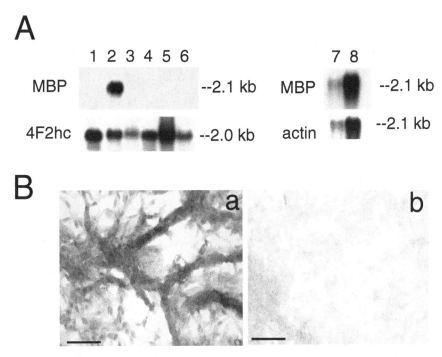

Figure 10.8 Northern hybridization of brain capillaries and rat tissues with the cloned myelin basic protein (MBP) cDNA. (A left panel) mRNA isolated from C6 rat glioma cells, rat brain, rat heart, rat kidney, rat lung, or rat liver was applied to lanes 1–6, respectively, and was hybridized with either the cloned MBP or 4F2hc cDNA (top and lower panels, respectively). 2 μg of polyA + RNA was applied to each lane and the 4F2hc or MBP X-ray film was exposed to the filter at −70 °C for 20 h or 1 day, respectively. (A right panel) MBP or actin Northern blots are shown for mRNA isolated from rat brain capillaries, or rat whole brain in lanes 7 and 8, respectively. Aliquots of 0.5 and 2.0 μg of polyA + mRNA were applied to lanes 7 and 8, respectively. The MBP Northern blot was exposed for 1 day at −70 °C, and the actin Northern blot was exposed for 24 h at −70 °C. Since the amount of whole rat brain mRNA applied in lane 8 is fourfold greater than the amount of rat brain capillary mRNA applied in lane 7, the MBP signal is comparable for both the rat brain capillary and whole rat brain fractions. (B) In situ hybridization with the MBP antisense RNA labeled with digoxigenin (DIG) and detected with an anti-DIG antibody conjugated to alkaline phosphatase is shown in Panel a. The study shows continuous immunostaining of the capillaries, which is indicative of an endothelial origin of the MBP mRNA at the brain microvasculature. In situ hybridization with the MBP sense RNA yields no immunostaining as shown in Panel b. The magnification bar in Panels a and b is 58 μm. From Li et al. (2001) with permission.

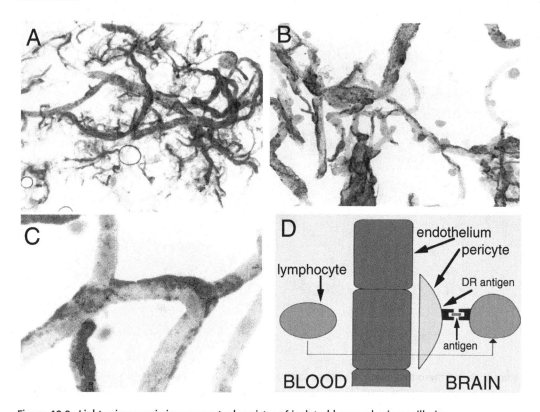

Figure 10.9 Light microscopic immunocytochemistry of isolated human brain capillaries cytocentrifuged to a glass slide and stained with a mouse monoclonal antibody to the human DR antigen. Microvessels were isolated from either control brain (A) or multiple sclerosis (MS) plaque tissue (B, C). The immunoreactive DR antigen is found on precapillary arteriolar smooth muscle cells in normal brain, and on pericytes in MS brain with little, if any, immunoreactivity on the capillary endothelium. Magnification: (A) ×25, (B) ×100, (C) ×250. (D) Model for antigen presentation in brain is shown. Antigen presentation to activated lymphocytes occurs on the brain side of the BBB, since the DR antigen is expressed on either smooth muscle cells or on pericytes. From Human brain microvascular DR antigen, Pardridge, W.M., Yang, J., Buciak, J. and Tourtellotte, W.W., *J. Neurosci. Res.*, copyright © 1989, Wiley-Liss, Inc., a subsidiary of John Wiley & Sons, Inc.

class II multiple histocompatibility complex (MHC), is specifically localized to the pericytes of human brain microvessels isolated from MS plaque lesions (Pardridge et al., 1989b). This suggests that microvascular antigen presentation in the brain in MS occurs on the brain side of the BBB at the pericyte plasma membrane, as outlined in Figure 10.9D. Antigen presentation at the brain microvasculature may also be mediated via the class I MHC, as discussed below for clone LK36.

Regulator of G protein signaling

Clone LK23 was an 0.28 kb insert that was 91% identical with 135 nucleotides of mouse regulator of G protein signaling (Rgs)5 (accession no. NM_009063). This sequence is part of the 3′-UTR of the mouse Rgs5 mRNA, and is repeated at three different regions of the 3′-UTR: nucleotides 640–774, 1439–1573, and 2238–2372. The LK23 clone hybridized with a 4.0 kb transcript that was selectively expressed at the rat brain microvasculature compared to total rat brain and was also expressed in rat heart and lung. Rgs5 acts as a guanosine triphosphatase (GTPase)-activating protein for subunits of heterotrimeric G proteins (Chen et al., 1999a), and these proteins play a role in the regulation of caveolin and endothelial cell transcytosis (Schnitzer et al., 1995), as reviewed in Chapter 4.

Utrophin

Clone LK24 was an 0.35 kb insert that was 99% identical with nucleotides 8721–9009 of the rat utrophin cDNA (accession no. AJ002967). Utrophin is also called dystrophin-related protein (DRP) and is a 395 amino acid protein that is 73% identical to dystrophin (Galvagni and Oliviero, 2000), which is the product of the gene that is mutated in Duchenne's muscular dystrophy (Khurana et al., 1991). Dystrophin is a large cytoskeletal protein related to spectrin and links the actin/cytoskeleton complex to extracellular matrix. The LK24 clone hybridized to a 9.0 kb transcript that was selectively expressed in the rat brain capillary preparation and was not detected with RNA preparations isolated from rat brain, heart, kidney, lung, or liver. This suggests that utrophin is selectively expressed in the brain microvascular endothelium, which parallels prior observations that utrophin is also expressed in the endothelial cell in skeletal muscle (Khurana et al., 1991).

S100

Clone LK25 was a 1.0 kb insert that was 96% identical to nucleotides 340–913 of rat S100 protein (Kuwano et al., 1984). Northern analysis detected a 1.5 kb transcript at the BBB, which was less abundant than the S100 mRNA concentration in whole rat brain. No S100 mRNA was detected in peripheral tissues, similar to myelin basic protein and LK31, a rat EST (Figure 10.5). The S100 family of proteins are 6–14 kDa acidic proteins that bind calcium (Shapiro et al., 1999). Plasma S100 concentrations increase in preterm infants as an early indicator of intraventricular hemorrhage (Gazzolo et al., 1999). It is not known if this S100 protein released to blood is primarily derived from brain cells or the brain microvasculature.

Inhibitor-κB

Clone LK27 was an 0.15 kb insert that was 100% identical with nucleotides 834–1035 of rat inhibitor (I) κB (Tewari et al., 1992). This protein is an inhibitor of the transcription factor NFκB. The IκB binds NFκB and retains the transcription factor in the cytoplasm (Wu and Ghosh, 1999). NFκB is activated by the degradation of IκB which is increased by either basic FGF or tumor necrosis factor α (TNFα) (Hoshi et al., 2000). Northern analysis with the LK27 clone showed that a 1.8 kb transcript encoding IκB was selectively expressed in brain at the microvasculature and was also expressed in rat heart and lung.

Connexin-45

Clone LK29 was an 0.7 kb insert that was 94% identical with nucleotides 1432–1947 of mouse connexin-45 (Hennemann et al., 1992). Connexins are plasma membrane proteins that form hemichannels and when hemichannels of apposed plasma membranes are joined, a gap junction is formed (Quist et al., 2000). Although gap junctions are not prominent at the BBB, the connexins may form hemichannels of physiologic function. The role of nongap junction hemichannels comprised of the connexins is unknown, but may regulate the cell volume in response to changes in extracellular calcium (Quist et al., 2000). There are several connexin mRNAs in brain, but few immunoreactive connexin proteins (Kunzelmann et al., 1997). This suggests that the mRNAs of the connexins may be translated under pathologic states. Northern analysis with the LK29 clone showed selective hybridization to a 2.0 kb transcript in rat brain microvessels (Li et al., 2001). There was also connexin-45 mRNA at lower levels in rat heart or lung as well as C6 glial cells (Figure 10.10A). However, the expression of the connexin-45 mRNA in rat brain capillaries was many-fold greater than the expression for this gene product in total rat brain homogenate. ISH with the connexin-45 clone was performed and this showed continuous immunostaining of the microvessel, indicating the connexin-45 was localized in the endothelial cell. There was also increased immunostaining in precapillary arterioles (Figure 10.10B).

Transferrin receptor

Clone LK34 was comprised of 0.28 and 0.15 kb inserts that were 100% identical to nucleotides 3349–3413 of the rat TfR (Roberts and Griswold, 1990). Northern analysis with this clone demonstrated selective expression of 5.0 and 6.6 kb transcripts in isolated rat brain capillaries, as shown in Figure 10.11A. The expression of the 6.6 kb TfR transcript was specific for rat brain capillaries and the 5.0 kb transcript was also found in total rat brain, although at much reduced levels compared to isolated rat brain capillaries. The 5.0 kb TfR transcript was also detected in C6 glial cells and rat heart and there was no detectable transcript in rat liver. Recent studies have identified a second form of the TfR, designated TfR2, which is encoded by mRNAs of 2.9 and 2.5 kb (Kawabata et al., 1999). The TfR2 is a type 2 membrane protein and is 45% identical in the extracellular domain to the

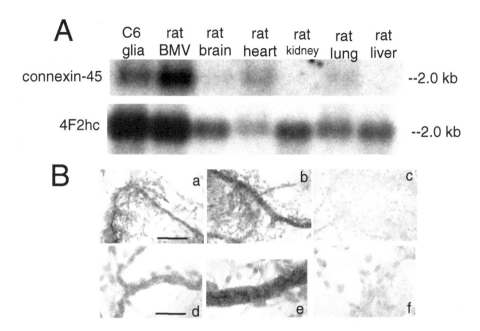

Figure 10.10 Northern hybridization of brain capillaries and rat tissues with the cloned connexin-45 cDNA. (A) mRNA (2 μg/lane) isolated from C6 rat glioma cells, rat brain microvessels (BMV), rat brain, rat heart, rat kidney, rat lung, or rat liver was hybridized with either the cloned connexin-45 cDNA or 4F2hc cDNA (top and lower panels, respectively). The 4F2hc or connexin-45 X-ray film was exposed to the filter at −70 °C for 20 h or 5 days, respectively. (B) In situ hybridization with the connexin-45 antisense RNA labeled with digoxigenin (DIG) and detected with an anti-DIG antibody conjugated to alkaline phosphatase is shown in Panels a, b, d, and e. The study shows continuous immunostaining of the capillaries, which is indicative of an endothelial origin of the connexin-45 at the brain microvasculature. There is also prominent immunostaining of the precapillary arteriolar smooth muscle cells. In situ hybridization with the connexin-45 sense RNA yields no immunostaining, as shown in Panels c and f. The magnification bar in Panels a and d is 100 μm and 40 μm, respectively. The magnifications in Panels a, b, and c are the same and the magnification in Panels d, e, and f are the same. From Li et al. (2001) with permission.

TfR1 (Kawabata et al., 1999). The TfR2 expression is selective for liver. The selective expression of TfR2 in liver may explain the failure to detect the mRNA for TfR1 in rat liver, as shown in Figure 10.11A. The TfR1 transcript is 5.0 kb (Kuhn et al., 1984), and the finding of significant levels of the transcript for the TfR1 for total brain is consistent with previous studies showing the TfR is expressed on both neuronal and glial cells in brain (Moos et al., 1999). Neuronal TfR1 expression is prominent in Ammon's horn of the hippocampus (Moos et al., 1999), and

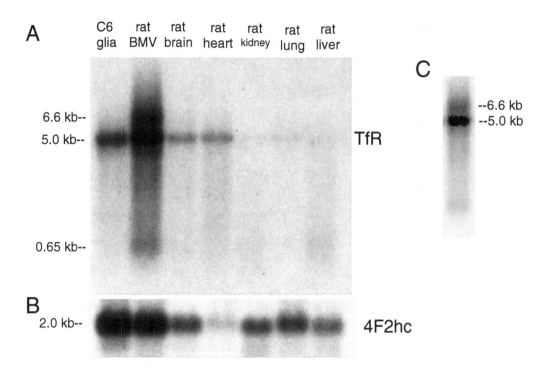

Figure 10.11 Northern hybridization of brain capillaries and rat tissues with the cloned transferrin receptor (TfR) cDNA. mRNA (2 μg/lane) isolated from C6 rat glioma cells, rat brain microvessels (BMV), rat brain, rat heart, rat kidney, rat lung, or rat liver was hybridized with either the cloned rat blood–brain barrier (BBB) TfR cDNA (A) or 4F2hc cDNA (B). The 4F2hc or TfR X-ray film was exposed to the filter at −70 °C for 20 h or 5 days, respectively. (C) The rat BMV Northern blot was underexposed to reveal the double TfR transcripts of 6.6 and 5.0 kb. Only the rat BMV preparation contained the 6.6 kb TfR mRNA. From Li et al. (2001) with permission.

the TfR is overexpressed in brain tumors relative to normal brain (Wen et al., 1995).

The finding of a novel 6.6 kb transcript encoding TfR1 that is selective for the rat brain capillary has not been reported previously and suggests there may be differential processing of the primary transcript for the TfR1 at the BBB. As discussed in Chapter 4, the BBB TfR1 is a prominent transcytotic pathway mediating the brain uptake of circulating transferrin. The expression of the TfR on both brain cells and at the BBB in brain enabled the targeting of plasmid-based gene formulations to neurons using pegylated immunoliposomes, as discussed in Chapter 9.

Multiple histocompatibility complex-I

Clone LK36 was an 0.4 kb insert that was 99% identical with nucleotides 33–415 of the rat MHC class I (Salgar et al., 1995). Northern analysis showed the expression of the MHC class I transcript was many-fold greater in rat brain capillary as compared to total rat brain or rat peripheral tissues. This high abundance of the mRNA encoding the MHC class I cell surface glycoprotein parallels previous studies showing a selective expression of β_2-microglobulin at the rat brain microvasculature (Whelan et al., 1986). β_2-Microglobulin is the light chain of the heterodimer comprising the MHC class I complex. These findings of extensive expression of the MHC class I at the brain microvasculature under normal conditions and the MHC class II at the pericyte in pathologic conditions (Figure 10.9) do not corroborate the long-held notion that the brain is an immune-privileged site (Pollack and Lund, 1990). Rather, active antigen presentation may occur in the central nervous system and this antigen presentation appears to be most prominent at the brain microvasculature (Pardridge et al., 1989b).

hbrm transcription factor

The hbrm gene product is the human homolog of yeast SW12/NSF2 protein and is an activator of transcription factors (Trouche et al., 1997). For example, the RB gene product requires hbrm to enable an inhibition of cell proliferation, and most human cancer is associated with an inactivation of the RB gene product (Kaelin, 1999). The hbrm has an RB-binding domain (Trouche et al., 1997). The hbrm can itself act as a transcription factor, but this function is lost upon binding to the RB gene product protein. Clone LK37 was an 0.2 kb transcript that was 96% identical to nucleotides 5736–5813 of the human hbrm protein (Muchardt and Yaniv, 1993). Northern analysis with clone LK37 showed hybridization to a 6.0 kb transcript present in the rat brain capillary at levels comparable to that in total rat brain. These results indicate clone LK37 is the rat analog of hbrm.

EZH1

The human homolog of the *Drosophila* gene, Enhancer of zeste [E(z)], is designated EZH1. E(z) is a member of the Polycomb group of genes that encode chromosomal proteins and act as negative regulators of the segment identity genes of the Antennapedia complex of *Drosophila* (Abel et al., 1996). Clone LK41 was 79% identical to 479 nucleotides in the 3′-UTR of the mouse homolog of EZH1 (Ogawa et al., 1998). Northern blot analysis with clone LK41 indicated the transcript encoding EZH1 was selectively expressed in the rat brain capillary at a level that was approximately two- to three-fold higher than that found in total brain or other tissues and the size of this transcript was 4.5 kb. The finding that several transcription factors such as PC-3, IκB, hbrm, or EZH1, are selectively expressed at the BBB suggests these proteins may regulate cell division at the brain microvasculature in states of angiogenesis.

Oatp2

Clone LK42 was an 0.7 kb transcript that was 99% identical with nucleotides 1648–2161 of the rat oatp2. Another clone encoding for oatp2 was also detected with this methodology in pilot studies involving preparation of a BBB cDNA library subtracted with rat kidney cDNA (Li et al., 2001). This clone, designated K2, was an 0.8 kb transcript that was 98% identical with nucleotides 2573–3230 of the rat oatp2 mRNA, which corresponds to the 3'-UTR of the oatp2 mRNA (Noe et al., 1997). The K2 clone was used in Northern analysis, as shown in Figure 10.12A, and this cDNA hybridized to 4.1 kb transcripts in brain and liver as well as a 1.2 kb transcript in liver following a 24-h exposure of the film. The oatp2 mRNA was not detected in rat liver after 4-h exposure of the film. Similarly, no oatp2 mRNA was detected with this cDNA in C6 rat glioma cells, rat heart, rat kidney, or rat lung after 24-h exposure. Northern analysis of mRNA isolated from rat brain capillaries is shown in Figure 10.12A and a 4.1 kb oatp2 transcript was detected in this preparation after only a brief 3-h film exposure time, indicating the oatp2 mRNA at the BBB is more abundant than in whole rat liver. The K2 clone was also used in ISH and shows continuous immunostaining of isolated rat brain capillaries, indicating an endothelial origin of the oatp2 transcript (Figure 10.12C). Conversely, no significant immunostaining of the capillaries was detected with the sense oatp2 probe. oatp2 transports digoxin, bile acids, and sex steroid glucuronate or sulfate conjugates, and oatp2 mRNA was originally reported for brain, liver, and kidney (Noe et al., 1997). Subsequent studies showed that, while oatp3 is expressed in rat kidney, oatp2 is not expressed in kidney (Abe et al., 1998). Western blotting with an antipeptide antiserum specific for the carboxyl terminus of rat oatp2 shows immunoreactive oatp2 protein in rat liver is at least 10-fold more abundant than immunoreactive oatp2 in rat brain (Kakyo et al., 1999), which is opposite from the results obtained with Northern blotting (Figure 10.12A). However, the small amount of immunoreactive oatp2 in the total rat brain homogenate is due to selective expression of the oatp2 protein at the microvasculature in brain and to the 1000-fold dilution of the microvascular fraction in whole-brain homogenate. The oatp2 mRNA signal in a Northern blot of rat brain capillary-derived mRNA following exposure to film for only 3 h is greater than the signal detected for rat brain following a 24-h film exposure. By comparison, a *Glut1* glucose transporter Northern blot of bovine brain capillary polyA + mRNA must be developed several days at −70 °C to yield a signal comparable to that shown for oatp2 with only a 3-h exposure (Boado and Pardridge, 1990a). Therefore, the level of the oatp2 mRNA at the rat BBB is comparable to the high level of mRNA found at the BBB for the large neutral amino acid transporter type 1, LAT1 (Boado et al., 1999), discussed in Chapter 3.

There is little conservation between the 3'-UTR of the rat and bovine LAT1

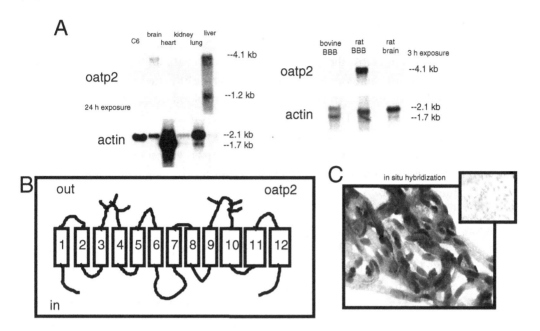

Figure 10.12 Cloning of the blood–brain barrier (BBB) organic anion transporting polypeptide type 2 (oatp2). (A) Northern blot analysis shows oatp2 is selectively expressed at the BBB in brain and can be detected with only a 3-h exposure of the blot to the X-ray film (right). At longer exposure times (24 h) the oatp2 mRNA can be detected in brain (left) and this is probably due to the oatp2 mRNA localized in the capillary fraction of whole brain. The oatp2 mRNA is not detected in C6 glial cells, rat heart, rat kidney, or rat lung. The oatp2 transcripts are detected in rat liver at the 24-h exposure (left). (B) Secondary structure analysis of the predicted amino acid sequence of the oatp2 protein indicates the protein is comprised of 12 transmembrane regions with six predicted N-linked glycosylation sites projecting into the extracellular space. This structure is highly homologous to BBB-specific anion transporter type 1 (BSAT1), as shown in Figure 10.6C. (C) In situ hybridization with the oatp2 antisense RNA labeled with digoxigenin (DIG) and detected with an anti-DIG antibody conjugated to alkaline phosphatase. The study shows continuous immunostaining of the capillaries, which is indicative of an endothelial origin of the transporter. In situ hybridization with the BSAT1 sense RNA yields no immunostaining as shown in the inset. Data in panels A and C are from Li et al. (2001) with permission.

mRNA such that a cDNA corresponding only to a region of the 3′-UTR of rat LAT1 would not hybridize to bovine LAT1 (Boado et al., 1999). The situation may be similar for oatp2 mRNA and this explains why the K2 oatp2 clone, which corresponds only to the 3′-UTR, does not hybridize to mRNA in isolated bovine brain capillaries (Figure 10.12B). The functional role of oatp2 at the BBB is not clear, but this protein may participate as an active efflux system at the BBB. For example, a principal substrate of oatp2 is estrone sulfate (Noe et al., 1997). However, estrone sulfate does not cross the BBB in vivo (Steingold et al., 1986), which suggests that oatp2 may function as an active efflux system at the BBB. Recent studies have shown that bile acids are actively effluxed from brain to blood (Kitazawa et al., 1998), possibly via BBB oatp2. The structure of the oatp2 protein is shown in Figure 10.12B and is comprised of 12 transmembrane regions with six predicted extracellular sites of N-linked glycosylation. The structure of oatp2 is very similar to that of BSAT1, as shown in Figure 10.6, and both oatp2 and BSAT1 may represent active efflux systems at the BBB.

TNFα-inducible EST

Clone LK44 is an 0.45 kb insert with a novel DNA sequence. Part of this sequence is 84% identical with nucleotides 129–320 of an EST identified in human aortic endothelium exposed to TNFα (Adams et al., 1995). Northern analysis with LK44 shows a selective expression of 5.1 and 3.5 kb transcripts at the rat BBB that are present at levels many-fold higher than in total rat brain, heart, kidney, lung, or liver. The finding of a TNFα-inducible gene product at the BBB parallels prior studies showing that the receptors for TNFα, designated TNFR1 and TNFR2, which are members of the NGF receptor family, are both expressed at the BBB (Nadeau and Rivest, 1999). The intracerebral injection of TNFα causes BBB disruption, and this is mediated by serine proteases (Megyeri et al., 1999). The role that the gene product corresponding to clone LK44 plays in mediating TNFα-induced BBB disruption is at present not known. TNFα also increases antigen presentation in brain (Vidovic et al., 1990) and promotes cell division by increasing transcription factors such as NF-κB (Hohmann et al., 1990).

Gene interactions

A genomics approach to BBB research leads to the identification of multiple genes of common function. A given phenotype is often the result of multiple genes operating as a group, rather than the action of a single gene. From just the preliminary analysis of the clones shown in Figure 10.5, it is possible to consider grouping BBB-specific genes. For example, angiogenesis involves the VEGF receptor, flt-1, but must also be dependent on the action of certain transcription factors, such as the PC-3 gene product, IκB, hbrm, or EZH1 (Figure 10.5). Signal transduction phenomena at the BBB may require the coordinate actions of connexin-45, a calcium hemichannel, S100 calcium-binding proteins, or Rgs5 and the regulation of G proteins. Changes in brain capillary endothelial function caused by either angiogenesis or alterations in signal transduction may affect the endothelial cytoskeleton and proteins such as utrophin, which is highly enriched at the BBB (Figure 10.5). The action of endothelial transporters at the BBB includes the transferrin receptor, which is responsible for the receptor-mediated transport of transferrin, or active efflux transporters, such as oatp2 or BSAT1 (Figure 10.5). Cytokines promote inflammation at the BBB, and LK44 is a novel gene related to a human gene that is upregulated with TNFα, and this cytokine also regulates the transcription factor, IκB, and the expression of human leukocyte antigens (HLAs). Both class I and II HLAs are expressed at the BBB, as is myelin basic protein, which may be an auto-antigen in MS. Many of these gene groupings are hypothetical at this early stage. However, the elucidation of genes that are selectively expressed at the BBB can lead to the grouping of genes of common function that regulate BBB physiology and pathophysiology.

Summary

This chapter describes the initial results of a BBB genomics program (Li et al., 2001), and the numerous gene products that are selectively expressed at the BBB compared to whole brain. The initial library was prepared from rat brain capillary-derived polyA + mRNA following subtraction with cDNA derived from rat liver and rat kidney. Screening just 5% of the subtracted tester cDNA resulted in identification of 50 gene products and over 80% of these were selectively expressed at the BBB. Numerous ESTs or genes with novel sequences of unknown function were selectively expressed at the BBB and the availability of these partial cDNAs will enable cloning of the full-length gene products for subsequent elucidation of the function of these unknown genes. These initial applications of a BBB genomics program led to the identification of a novel transporter, designated BSAT1, that is selectively expressed at the BBB relative to other tissues in the body (Li et al., 2001). Other genes that are selectively expressed at the BBB include LK20, which hybridizes to a 5.0 kb mRNA, LK35, which hybridizes to a 4.0 mRNA, LK38, which hybridizes to a 5.8 kb mRNA, and LK44, which hybridizes to 3.5 and 5.1 kb mRNAs (Li et al., 2001). Like LK3, which led to the cloning of BSAT1, LK20, LK35, LK38, and LK44 are all partial cDNAs that contain sequences that are novel and not found in the GenBank or rat EST databases (Figure 10.5). In addition to these BBB-selective clones, LK26 and LK33 are partial cDNAs that encode novel sequences, although the mRNAs targeted by these cDNAs are widely expressed in peripheral tissues in addition to the BBB (Li et al., 2001).

The initial results with the BBB genomics program suggest that known gene products may play important roles in mediating BBB function, since the transcripts of these gene products are selectively expressed at the BBB compared to brain. These brain capillary-enriched genes include tPA, IGF2, flt-1, PC-3, myelin basic protein, Rgs5, utrophin, IκB, connexin-45, the MHC class I, and transcription factors, such as EZH1 or hbrm. The subtracted BBB library was prepared from just 5% of the subtracted tester cDNA (Li et al., 2001), and this initial evaluation led to the elucidation of the tissue-specific gene expression at the BBB shown in Figure 10.5. Based on these findings, it is clear that the application of genomics technology to BBB research will accelerate the pace of discovery in the future. The discovery of novel BBB gene products will yield new pathways of drug targeting to the brain via endogenous BBB transporters.

References

Aasmundstad, T.A., Morg, J. and Paleness, R.E. (1995). Distribution of morphine 6-glucuronide and morphine across the blood–brain barrier in awake, freely moving rats investigated by in vivo microdialysis sampling. *J. Pharmacol. Exp. Ther.*, **275**, 435–41.

Abe, T., Kakyo, M., Sakagami, H. et al. (1998). Molecular characterization and tissue distribution of a new organic anion transporter subtype (oatp3) that transports thyroid hormones and taurocholate and comparison with oatp2. *J. Biol. Chem.*, **273**, 22395–401.

Abe, T., Kakyo, M., Tokui, T. et al. (1999). Identification of a novel gene family encoding human liver-specific organic anion transporter LST-1. *J. Biol. Chem.*, **274**, 17159–63.

Abel, K.J., Brody, L.C., Valdes, J.M. et al. (1996). Characterization of EZH1, a human homolog of *Drosophila* enhancer of zeste near BRCA1. *Genomics*, **37**, 161–71.

Abuchowski, A., McCoy, J.R., Palczuk, N.C., van Es, T. and Davis, F.F. (1977a). Effect of covalent attachment of polyethylene glycol on immunogenicity and circulating life of bovine liver catalase. *J. Biol. Chem.*, **252**, 3582–6.

Abuchowski, A., van Es, T., Palczuk, N.C. and Davis, F.F. (1977b). Alteration of immunological properties of bovine serum albumin by covalent attachment of polyethylene glycol. *J. Biol. Chem.*, **252**, 3578–81.

Adams, C.W.M. (1977). Pathology of multiple sclerosis: progression of the lesion. *Br. Med. Bull.*, **33**, 15–20.

Adams, M.D., Dubnick, M., Kerlavage, A.R. et al.(1992). Sequence identification of 2375 human brain genes. *Nature*, **355**, 632–4.

Adams, M.D., Kerlavage, A.R., Fleischmann, R.D. et al. (1995). Initial assessment of human gene diversity and expression patterns based upon 83 million nucleotides of cDNA sequence. *Nature*, **377**, 3–174.

Agrawal, S. (1991). Antisense oligonucleotides: a possible approach for chemotherapy of AIDS. In *Prospects for Antisense Nucleic Acid Therapy of Cancer and AIDS*, ed. E. Wickstrom, pp. 143–58. New York: Wiley-Liss.

Agrawal, S., Jiang, Z., Zhao, Q. et al. (1997). Mixed-backbone oligonucleotides as second generation antisense oligonucleotides: in vitro and in vivo studies. *Proc. Natl Acad. Sci. USA*, **94**, 2620–5.

Agus, D.B., Ghambir, S.S., Pardridge, W.M. et al. (1997). Vitamin C crosses the blood–brain barrier in the oxidized form through the glucose transporters. *J. Clin. Invest.*, **100**, 2842–8.

Ahmed, A.E., Jacob, S., Loh, J.-P. et al. (1991). Comparative disposition and whole-body auto-radiographic distribution of [2-^{14}C] azidothymidine in mice. *J. Pharmacol. Exp. Ther.*, **257**, 479–86.

Aird, R.B. (1984). A study of intrathecal, cerebrospinal fluid-to-brain exchange. *Exp. Neurol.*, **86**, 342–58.

Allinquant, B., Hantraye, P., Mailleux, P. et al. (1995). Downregulation of amyloid precursor protein inhibits neurite outgrowth in vitro. *J. Cell Biol.*, **128**, 919–27.

Almers, W. (1990). Exocytosis. *Annu. Rev. Physiol.*, **52**, 607–24.

Alyautdin, R.N., Petrov, V.E., Langer, K. et al. (1997). Delivery of loperamide across the blood–brain barrier with polysorbate 80-coated polybutylcyanoacrylate nanoparticles. *Pharm. Res.*, **14**, 325–8.

Andersson, L. and Lundahl, P. (1988). C-terminal specific monoclonal antibodies against the human red cell glucose transporter. Epitope localization with synthetic peptides. *J. Biol. Chem.*, **263**, 11414–20.

Andersson, M., Marie, J.-C., Carlquist, M. and Mutt, V. (1991). The preparation of biotinyl-ε-aminocaproylated forms of the vasoactive intestinal polypeptide (VIP) as probes for the VIP receptor. *FEBS Lett.*, **282**, 35–40.

Anthony, D., Dempster, R., Fearn, S. et al. (1998a). CXC chemokines generate age-related increases in neutrophil-mediated brain inflammation and blood–brain barrier breakdown. *Curr. Biol.*, **8**, 923–6.

Anthony, D.C., Miller, K.M., Fearn, S. et al. (1998b). Matrix metalloproteinase expression in an experimentally-induced DTH model of multiple sclerosis in the rat CNS. *J. Neuroimmunol.*, **87**, 62–72.

Apfel, S. (1997). *Clinical Applications of Neurotrophic Factors*, p. 5. New York: Lippincott-Raven.

Aquilonius, S.M., Ceder, G., Lying-Tunell, U., Malmlund, H.O. and Schuberth, J. (1975). The arteriovenous differences of choline across the brain of man. *Brain Res.*, **99**, 430–3.

Arboix, M., Paz, O.G., Colombo, T. and D'incalci, M. (1997). Multidrug resistance-reversing agents increase vinblastine distribution in normal tissues expressing the p-glycoprotein but do not enhance drug penetration in brain and testis. *J. Pharmacol. Exp. Ther.*, **281**, 1226–30.

Aschner, M. and Aschner, J.L. (1990). Manganese transport across the blood–brain barrier: relationship to iron homeostasis. *Brain Res. Bull.*, **24**, 857–60.

Azmin, M.N., Stuart, J.F.B. and Florence, A.T. (1985). The distribution and elimination of methotrexate in mouse blood and brain after concurrent administration of polysorbate-80. *Cancer Chemother. Pharmacol.*, **14**, 238–42.

Banks, W.A. and Kastin, A.J. (1990). Peptide transport systems for opiates across the blood–brain barrier. *Am. J. Physiol.*, **259**, E1–10.

Banks, W.A., Kastin, A.J. and Barrera, C.M. (1991). Delivering peptides to the central nervous system: dilemmas and strategies. *Pharm. Res.*, **8**, 1345–50.

Banks, W.A., Kastin, A.J., Huang, W., Jaspan, J.B. and Maness, L.M. (1996). Leptin enters the brain by a saturable system independent of insulin. *Peptides*, **17**, 305–11.

Barron, L.G., Uyechi, L.S. and Szoka, F.C. (1999). Cationic lipids are essential for gene delivery mediated by intravenous administration of lipoplexes. *Gene Ther.*, **6**, 1179–83.

Baskin, D.G., Porte, D., Guest, K. and Dorsa, D.M. (1983a). Regional concentrations of insulin in the rat brain. *Endocrinol.*, **112**, 898–903.

Baskin, D.G., Woods, S.C., West, D.B. et al. (1983b). Immunocytochemical detection of insulin in rat hypothalamus and its possible uptake from cerebrospinal fluid. *Endocrinol.*, **113**, 1818–25.

Basu, S.K, Goldstein, J.L., Anderson, R.G.W. and Brown, M.S. (1976). Degradation of cationized low density lipoprotein and regulation of cholesterol metabolism in homozygous familial hypercholesterolemia fibroblasts. *Proc. Natl Acad. Sci. USA*, **73**, 3178–82.

Beck, T., Lindholm, D., Castren, E. and Wree, A. (1994). Brain-derived neurotrophic factor protects against ischemic cell damage in rat hippocampus. *J. Cereb. Blood Flow Metab.*, **14**, 689–92.

Beck, K.D., Powellbraxton, L., Widmer, H.R., Valverde, J. and Hefti, F. (1995). IGF-I gene disruption results in reduced brain sizes, CNS hypomyelination, and loss of hippocampal granule and striatal parvalbumin containing neurons. *Neuron*, **14**, 717–30.

Begley, D.J. (1996). The blood–brain barrier: principles for targeting peptides and drugs to the central nervous system. *J. Pharm. Pharmacol.*, **48**, 136–46.

Beisiegel, U., Schneider, W.J., Goldstein, J.L., Anderson, R.G. and Brown, M.S. (1981). Monoclonal antibodies to the low density lipoprotein receptor as probes for study of receptor-mediated endocytosis and the genetics of familial hypercholesterolemia. *J. Biol. Chem.*, **256**, 11923–31.

Belayev, L., Busto, R., Watson, B.D. and Ginsberg, M.D. (1995). Post-ischemic administration of HU-211, a novel non-competitive NMDA antagonist, protects against blood–brain barrier disruption in photochemical cortical infarction in rats: a quantitative study. *Brain Res.*, **702**, 266–70.

Beltinger, C., Saragovi, H.U., Smith, R.M. et al. (1995). Binding, uptake, and intracellular trafficking of phosphorothioate-modified oligodeoxynucleotides. *J. Clin. Invest.*, **95**, 1814–23.

Bemelmans, A.-P., Horellou, P., Pradier, L. et al. (1999). Brain-derived neurotrophic factor-mediated protection of striatal neurons in an excitotoxic rat model of Huntington's disease, as demonstrated by adenoviral gene transfer. *Hum. Gene Ther.*, **10**, 2987–97.

Bergmann, P., Kacenelenbogen, R. and Vizet, A. (1984). Plasma clearance, tissue distribution of catabolism of cationized albumins with increasing isoelectric points in the rat. *Clin. Sci.*, **67**, 35–43.

Berne, R.M., Knabb, R.M., Ely, S.W. and Rubio R. (1983). Adenosine in the local regulation of blood flow: a brief overview. *Fed. Proc.*, **42**, 3136–42.

Bickel, U., Yoshikawa, T., Landaw, E.M., Faull, K.F. and Pardridge, W.M. (1993a). Pharmacologic effects in vivo in brain by vector-mediated peptide drug delivery. *Proc. Natl Acad. Sci. USA*, **90**, 2618–22.

Bickel, U., Yoshikawa, T. and Pardridge, W.M. (1993b). Delivery of peptides and proteins through the blood–brain barrier. *Adv. Drug Del. Rev.*, **10**, 205–45.

Bickel, U., Kang, Y.-S., Yoshikawa, T. and Pardridge, W.M. (1994a). In vivo demonstration of subcellular localization of anti-transferrin receptor monoclonal antibody-colloidal gold conjugate within brain capillary endothelium. *J. Histochem. Cytochem.*, **42**, 1493–7.

Bickel, U., Lee, V.M.Y., Trojanowski, J.Q. and Pardridge, W.M. (1994b). Development and in vitro characterization of a cationized monoclonal antibody against βA4 protein: a potential probe for Alzheimer's disease. *Bioconj. Chem.*, **5**, 119–25.

Bickel, U., Yamada, S. and Pardridge, W.M. (1994c). Synthesis and bioactivity of monobiotinylated DALDA: a mu-specific opioid peptide designed for targeted brain delivery. *J. Pharmacol. Exp. Ther.*, **269**, 344–50.

Bickel, U., Kang, Y.-S. and Pardridge, W.M. (1995a). In vivo cleavage of a disulfide-based chimeric opioid peptide in rat brain. *Bioconj. Chem.*, **6**, 211–18.

Bickel, U., Lee, V.M.Y. and Pardridge, W.M. (1995b). Pharmacokinetic differences between ^{111}In and ^{125}I-labeled cationized monoclonal antibody against β-amyloid in mouse and dog. *Drug Delivery*, **2**, 128–35.

Bickel, U., Schumacher, O., Kang, Y.-S. and Voigt, K. (1996). Poor permeability of morphine-3-glucuronide and morphine-6-glucuronide through the blood–brain barrier in the rat. *J. Pharmacol. Exp. Ther.*, **278**, 107–13.

Billiau, A., Heremans, H., Ververken, D. et al. (1981). Tissue distribution of human interferons after exogenous administration in rabbits, monkeys, and mice. *Arch. Virol.*, **68**, 19–25.

Birkenmeier, E.H., Barker, J.E., Vogler, C.A. et al. (1991). Increased life span and correction of metabolic defects in murine mucopolysaccharidosis type VII after syngeneic bone marrow transplantation. *Blood*, **78**, 3081–92.

Birnbaum, M.J., Haspel, H.C. and Rosen, O.M. (1986). Cloning and characterization of a cDNA encoding the rat brain glucose-transporter protein. *Proc. Natl Acad. Sci. USA*, **83**, 5784–8.

Bishop, J.S., Guy-Caffey, J.K., Ojwang, J.O. et al. (1996). Intramolecular G-quartet motifs confer nuclease resistance to a potent anti-HIV oligonucleotide. *J. Biol. Chem.*, **271**, 5698–703.

Black, K.L., Cloughesy, T., Huang, S.-C. et al. (1997). Intracarotid infusion of RMP-7, a bradykinin analog, and transport of gallium-68 ethylenediamine tetraacetic acid into human gliomas. *J. Neurosurg.*, **86**, 603–9.

Blasberg, R.G. and Groothuis, D.R. (1991). Blood–tumor barrier disruption controversies. *J. Cereb. Blood Flow Metab.*, **11**, 165–6.

Blasberg, R.G., Patlak, C. and Fenstermacher, J.D. (1975). Intrathecal chemotherapy: brain tissue profiles after ventriculocisternal perfusion. *J. Pharmacol. Exp. Ther.*, **195**, 73–83.

Blumcke, I., Eggli, P. and Celio, M.R. (1995). Relationship between astrocyte processes and "perioneuronal nets" in rat neocortex. *Glia*, **15**, 131–40.

Boado, R.J. and Pardridge, W.M. (1990a). Molecular cloning of the bovine blood–brain barrier glucose transporter cDNA and demonstration of phylogenetic conservation of the 5′-untranslated region. *Mol. Cell. Neurosci.*, **1**, 224–32.

Boado, R.J. and Pardridge, W.M. (1990b). The brain-type glucose transporter mRNA is specifically expressed at the blood–brain barrier. *Biochem. Biophys. Res. Commun.*, **166**, 174–9.

Boado, R.J. and Pardridge, W.M. (1991). A one-step procedure for isolation of poly A+ mRNA from isolated brain capillaries and endothelial cells in culture. *J. Neurochem.*, **57**, 2136–9.

Boado, R.J. and Pardridge, W.M. (1992). Complete protection of antisense oligonucleotides against serum nuclease degradation by an avidin-biotin system. *Bioconj. Chem.*, **3**, 519–23.

Boado, R.J. and Pardridge, W.M. (1994). Complete inactivation of target mRNA by biotinylated antisense oligodeoxynucleotide-avidin conjugates. *Bioconj. Chem.*, **5**, 406–10.

Boado, R.J. and Pardridge, W.M. (1998). Ten nucleotide cis element in the 3′-untranslated region of the GLUT1 glucose transporter mRNA increases gene expression via mRNA stabilization. *Mol. Brain Res.*, **59**, 109–13.

Boado, R.J. and Pardridge, W.M. (1999). Amplification of gene expression using both 5′- and 3′-untranslated regions of GLUT1 glucose transporter mRNA. *Mol. Brain. Res.*, **63**, 371–4.

Boado, R.J., Kang, Y.-S., Wu, D. and Pardridge, W.M. (1995). Rapid plasma clearance and metabolism in vivo of a phosphorothioate oligodeoxynucleotide with a single, internal phospho-diester bond. *Drug Metab. Disp.*, **23**, 1297–300.

Boado, R.J., Tsukamoto, H. and Pardridge, W.M. (1996). Evidence for translational control elements within the 5'-untranslated region of GLUT1 glucose transporter mRNA. *J. Neurochem.*, **67**, 1335–43.

Boado, R.J., Golden, P.L., Levin, N. and Pardridge, W.M. (1998a). Upregulation of blood–brain barrier short form leptin receptor gene products in rats fed a high fat diet. *J. Neurochem.*, **71**, 1761–4.

Boado, R.J., Tsukamoto, H. and Pardridge, W.M. (1998b). Drug delivery of antisense molecules to the brain for treatment of Alzheimer's disease and cerebral AIDS. *J. Pharm. Sci.*, **87**, 1308–15.

Boado, R.J., Li, J.Y., Nagaya, M., Zhang, C. and Pardridge, W.M. (1999). Selective expression of the large neutral amino acid transporter (LAT) at the blood–brain barrier. *Proc. Natl Acad. Sci. USA*, **96**, 12049–84.

Bodor, N. and Simpkins, J. (1983). Redox delivery system for brain-specific, sustained release of dopamine. *Science*, **221**, 65–7.

Bodor, N., Prokai, L., Wu, W.-M. et al. (1992). A strategy for delivering peptides into the central nervous system by sequential metabolism. *Science*, **257**, 1698–700.

Bolton, S.J., Anthony, D.C. and Perry, V.H. (1998). Loss of the tight junction proteins occludin and zonula occludens-1 from cerebral vascular endothelium during neutrophil-induced blood–brain barrier breakdown in vivo. *Neurosci.*, **86**, 1245–57.

Bondy, C.A., Werner, H., Roberts, C.T. and LeRoith, D. (1990). Cellular pattern of insulin-like growth factor-I (IGF-I) and type I IGF receptor gene expression in early organogenesis: comparison with IGF-II gene expression. *Mol. Endocrinol.*, **4**, 1386–98.

Borison, H.L., Borison, R. and McCarthy, L.E. (1984). Role of the area postrema in vomiting and related functions. *Fed.Proc.*, **43**, 2955–8.

Bornstein, M.B., Miller, A., Slagle, S. et al. (1987). A pilot trial of COP 1 in exacerbating–remitting multiple sclerosis. *N. Engl. J. Med.*, **317**, 408–14.

Bottjer, S.W., Miesner, E.A. and Arnold, A.P. (1984). Vasoactive intestinal polypeptide-like substance: the potential transmitter for cerebral vasodilation. *Science*, **224**, 898–902.

Bourne, G.H. (1975). *The Rhesus Monkey*, vol. 1, *Anatomy and Physiology*, pp. 6–10. New York: Academic Press.

Bradbury, M.W.B. (1997). Transport of iron in the blood–brain–cerebrospinal fluid system. *J. Neurochem.*, **69**, 443–54.

Brandli, A.W., Adamson, E.D. and Simons, K. (1991). Transcytosis of epidermal growth factor. *J. Biol. Chem.*, **266**, 8560–6.

Braulke, T., Tippmer, S., Chao, H.-J. and Figura, K.V. (1990). Insulin-like growth factors I and II stimulate endocytosis but do not affect sorting of lysosomal enzymes in human fibroblasts. *J. Biol. Chem.*, **265**, 6650–5.

Brendel, K., Meezan, E. and Carlson, E.C. (1974). Isolated brain microvessels: a purified, metabolically active preparation from bovine cerebral cortex. *Science*, **185**, 953–5.

Brightman, M.W. (1977). Morphology of blood–brain interfaces. *Exp. Eye Res.*, **25** (Suppl.), 1–25.

Brightman, M.W. and Reese, T.S. (1969). Junctions between intimately apposed cell membranes in the vertebrate brain. *J. Cell. Biol.*, **40**, 648–77.

Brightman, M.W., Reese, T.S. and Feder, N. (1970). Assessment with the electron microscope of the permeability to peroxidase of cerebral endothelium and epithelium in mice and sharks. In *Capillary Permeability*, ed. C. Crone and N.A. Lassen, p. 463. Copenhagen: Munksgaard.

Brink, J.J. and Stein, D.G. (1967). Pemoline levels in brain: enhancement by dimethyl sulfoxide. *Science*, **158**, 1479–80.

Broadwell, R.D., Balin, B.J. and Salcman, M. (1988). Transcytotic pathway for blood-borne protein through the blood–brain barrier. *Proc. Natl Acad. Sci. USA*, **85**, 632–6.

Broadwell, R.D., Baker-Cairns, B.J., Friden, P.M., Oliver, C. and Villegas, J.C. (1996). Transcytosis of protein through the mammalian cerebral epithelium and endothelium. *Exp. Neurol.*, **142**, 47–65.

Broman, T. (1949). *The Permeability of the Cerebrospinal Vessels in Normal and Pathological Conditions*, pp. 1–92. Copenhagen: Ejnar Munksgaard.

Brown, J.R. (1977). Serum albumin: amino acid sequence. In *Albumin Structure, Function, and Uses*, ed. V.M. Rosehoer, M. Oratz and M.A. Rothschild, pp. 27–51. New York: Pergamon.

Brown, A.L., Graham, D.E., Nissley, S.P. et al. (1986). Developmental regulation of insulin-like growth factor II mRNA in different rat tissues. *J. Biol. Chem.*, **261**, 13144–50.

Brown, D.A., Kang, S.-H., Gryaznov, S.M. et al. (1994). Effect of phosphorothioate modification of oligodeoxynucleotides on specific protein binding. *J. Biol. Chem.*, **269**, 26801–5.

Brownlees, J. and Williams, C.H. (1993). Peptidases, peptides, and the mammalian blood–brain barrier. *J. Neurochem.*, **60**, 793–803.

Bruggemann, M., Winter, G., Waldmann, H. and Neuverger, M.S. (1989). The immunogenicity of chimeric antibodies. *J. Exp. Med.*, **170**, 2153–7.

Burgess, T.L., Fisher, E.F., Ross, S.L. et al. (1995). The antiproliferative activity of c-myb and c-myc antisense oligonucleotides in smooth muscle cells is caused by a nonantisense mechanism. *Proc. Natl Acad. Sci. USA*, **92**, 4051–5.

Burke, J.R., Enchild, J.J., Martin, J.E. et al. (1996). Huntingtin and DRPLA proteins selectively interact with the enzyme GAPDH. *Nat. Med.*, **2**, 347–50.

Capala, J., Barth, R.F., Bailey, M.Q. et al. (1997). Radiolabeling of epidermal growth factor with ^{99m}Tc and in vivo localization following intracerebral injection into normal and glioma-bearing rats. *Bioconj. Chem.*, **8**, 289–95.

Capon, D.J., Chamow, S.M., Mordenti, J. et al. (1989). Designing CD4 immunoadhesions for AIDS therapy. *Nature*, **337**, 525–31.

Cardone, M.H., Smith, B.L., Mennitt, P.A. et al. (1996). Signal transduction by the polymeric immunoglobulin receptor suggests a role in regulation of receptor transcytosis. *J. Cell. Biol.*, **133**, 997–1005.

Carter, D.C. and He, J.X. (1994). Structure of serum albumin. *Adv. Protein Chem.*, **45**, 153–203.

Casanova, J.E., Breitfeld, P.P., Ross, S.A. and Mostov, K.E. (1990). Phosphorylation of the polymeric immunoglobulin receptor required for its efficient transcytosis. *Science*, **248**, 742–6.

Catalan, R.E., Martinez, A.M., Aragones, M.D. and Fernandez, I. (1989). Substance P stimulates translocation of protein kinase C in brain microvessels. *Biochem. Biophys. Res. Comm.*, **164**, 595–600.

Catalan, R.E., Martinez, A.M., Aragones, M.D. and Hernandez, F. (1996). Protein phosphorylation in the blood–brain barrier, possible presence of marcks in brain microvessels. *Neurochem. Int.*, **28**, 59–65.

Chabrier, P.E., Roubert, P. and Braquet, P. (1987). Specific binding of atrial natriuretic factor in brain microvessels. *Proc. Natl Acad. Sci. USA*, **84**, 2078–81.

Chamberlain, M.C., Kormanik, P.A. and Barba, D. (1997). Complications associated with intraventricular chemotherapy in patients with leptomeningeal metastases. *J. Neurosurg.*, **87**, 694–9.

Chamow, S.M., Kogan, T.P., Venuti, M. et al. (1994). Modification of CD4 immunoadhesin with monomethoxypoly(ethylene glycol) aldehyde via reductive alkylation. *Bioconj. Chem.*, **5**, 133–40.

Chan, P.H., Longar, S. and Fishman, R.A. (1987). Protective effects of liposome-entrapped superoxide dismutase on posttraumatic brain edema. *Ann. Neurol.*, **21**, 540–7.

Chem, T.-L., Miller, P.S., Ts'o, P.O.P. and Colvin, O.M. (1990). Disposition and metabolism of oligodeoxynucleoside methylphosphonate following a single iv injection in mice. *Drug Metab. Disp.*, **18**, 815–18.

Chen, D., Li, Q.-T. and Lee, K.H. (1993). Antinociceptive activity of liposome-entrapped calcitonin by systemic administration in mice. *Brain Res.*, **603**, 139–42.

Chen, S.-H., Shine, H.D., Goodman, J.C., Grossman, R.G. and Woo, S.L.C. (1994). Gene therapy for brain tumors: regression for experimental gliomas by adenovirus-mediated gene transfer in vivo. *Proc. Natl Acad. Sci. USA*, **91**, 3054–7.

Chen, L.L., Frankel, A.D., Harder, J.L. et al. (1995). Increased cellular uuptake of the human immunodeficiency virus-1 tat protein after modification with biotin. *Anal. Biochem.*, **227**, 168–75.

Chen, C., Seow, K.T., Guo, K., Yaw, L.P. and Lin, S.C. (1999a). The membrane association domain of RGS16 contains unique amphipathic features that are conserved in RGS4 and RGS5. *J. Biol. Chem.*, **274**, 19799–806.

Chen, Z.-L., Indyk, J.A., Bugge, T.H. et al. (1999b). Neuronal death and blood–brain barrier breakdown after excitotoxic injury are independent processes. *J. Neurosci.*, **19**, 9813–20.

Chi, O.Z., Chang, Q., Wang, G. and Weiss, H.R. (1997). Effects of nitric oxide on blood–brain barrier disruption caused by intracarotid injection of hyperosmolar mannitol in rats. *Anesth. Analg.*, **84**, 370–5.

Chiariotti, L., Brown, A.L., Frunzio, R. et al. (1988). Structure of the rat insulin-like growth factor II transcriptional unit: heterogeneous transcripts are generated from two promoters by use of multiple polyadenylation sites and differential ribonucleic acid splicing. *Mol. Endocrinol.*, **2**, 1115–26.

Chikhale, E.G., Burton, P.S. and Borchardt, R.T. (1995). The effect of verapamil on the transport of peptides across the blood–brain barrier in rats: kinetic evidence for an apically polarized efflux mechanism. *J. Pharmacol. Exp. Ther.*, **273**, 298–303.

Choi, T. and Pardridge, W.M. (1986). Phenylalanine transport at the human blood–brain barrier: studies in isolated human brain capillaries. *J. Biol. Chem.*, **261**, 6536–41.

Choi-Lundberg, D.L., Lin, Q., Chang, Y.-N. et al. (1997). Dopaminergic neurons protected from degeneration by GDNF gene therapy. *Science*, **275**, 838–42.

Chonn, A., Semple, S.C. and Cullis, P.R. (1992). Association of blood proteins with large unilamellar liposomes in vivo. *J. Biol. Chem.*, **267**, 18759–65.

Chowdhury, N.R., Wu, C.H., Wu, G.Y. et al. (1993). Fate of DNA targeted to the liver by asialoglycoprotein receptor-mediated endocytosis in vivo. *J. Biol. Chem.*, **268**, 11265–71.

Clark, R., Olson, K., Fuh, G. et al. (1996). Long-acting growth hormones produced by conjugation with polyethylene glycol. *J. Biol. Chem.*, **271**, 21969–77.

Clark, W.G. (1973). Blood–brain barrier to carbidopa (MK-486) and Ro 4–4602, peripheral dopa decarboxylase inhibitors. *J. Pharm. Pharmacol.*, **25**, 416–18.

Clemmons, D.R. (1990). Insulinlike growth factor binding proteins. *Trends Endocrinol. Metab.*, **1**, 412–17.

Cole, H., Reynolds, T.R., Lockyer, J.M. et al. (1994). Human serum biotinidase. cDNA cloning, sequence, and characterization. *J. Biol. Chem.*, **269**, 6566–70.

Coleman, D.L. (1978). Obesity and diabetes: two mutant genes causing diabetes-obesity syndrome in mice. *Diabetologia*, **14**, 141–8.

Coloma, M.J., Lee, H.J., Kurihara, A., Landaw, E.M., Boado, R.J., Morrison, S.L. and Pardridge, W.M. (2000). Transport across the primate blood–brain barrier of a genetically engineered chimeric monoclonal antibody to the human insulin receptor. *Pharm. Res.*, **17**, 266–74.

Cool, W.M., Kurtz, N.M. and Chu, G. (1990). Transnasal delivery of systemic drugs. *Adv. Pain Res. Ther.*, **14**, 241–58.

Cordon-Cardo, C., O'Brien, J.P., Casals, D. et al. (1989). Multi-drug resistance gene (p-glycoprotein) is expressed by endothelial cells at blood–brain barrier sites. *Proc. Natl Acad. Sci. USA*, **86**, 695–8.

Cornford, E.M. and Oldendorf, W.H. (1975). Independent blood–brain barrier transport systems for nucleic acid precursors. *Biochim. Biophys. Acta*, **394**, 211–19.

Cornford, E.M., Braun, L.D. and Oldendorf, W.H. (1978). Carrier mediated blood–brain barrier transport of choline and certain choline analogs. *J. Neurochem.*, **30**, 299–308.

Cornford, E.M., Hyman, S. and Pardridge, W.M. (1993). An electron microscopic immunogold analysis of developmental up-regulation of the blood–brain barrier GLUT1 glucose transporter. *J. Cereb. Blood Flow Metab.*, **13**, 841–54.

Cornford, E.M., Young, D., Paxton, J.W. et al. (1992). Melphalan penetration of the blood–brain barrier via the neutral amino acid transporter in tumor-bearing brain. *Cancer Res.*, **52**, 138–43.

Cosolo, W. and Christophidis, N. (1987). Blood–brain barrier disruption and methotrexate in the treatment of a readily transplantable intracerebral osteogenic sarcoma of rats. *Cancer Res.*, **47**, 6225–8.

Cossum, P.A., Sasmor, H., Dellinger, D. et al. (1993). Disposition of the ^{14}C-labeled phosphorothioate oligonucleotide ISIS 2105 after intravenous administration to rats. *J. Pharmacol. Exp. Ther.*, **267**, 1181–90.

Cotton, M., Wagner, E., Zatloukal, K. et al. (1992). High-efficiency receptor-mediated delivery of small and large (48 kilobase) gene constructs using the endosome-disruption activity of defective or chemically inactivated adenovirus particles. *Proc. Natl Acad. Sci. USA*, **89**, 6094–8.

Couce, M.E., Weatherington, A.J. and McGinty, J.F. (1992). Expression of insulin-like growth factor-II (IGF-II) and IGF-II/mannose-6-phosphate receptor in the rat hippocampus: an in situ hybridization and immunocytochemical study. *Endocrinol.*, **131**, 1636–42.

Covell, D.G., Narang, P.K. and Poplack, D.G. (1985). Kinetic model for disposition of 6-mercaptopurine in monkey plasma and cerebrospinal fluid. *Am. J. Physiol.*, **248**, R147–56.

Crawley, J.N., Fiske, S.M., Durieux, C., Derrien, M. and Roques, B.P. (1991). Centrally administered cholecystokinin suppresses feeding through peripheral-type receptor mechanism. *J. Pharmacol. Exp. Ther.*, **257**, 1076–80.

Cremer, J.E., Cunningham, V.J., Pardridge, W.M., Braun, L.D. and Oldendorf, W.H. (1979). Kinetics of blood–brain barrier transport of pyruvate, lactate and glucose in suckling, weanling and adults rats. *J. Neurochem.*, **33**, 439–45.

Crone, C. (1963). The permeability of capillaries in various organs as determined by use of the "indicator diffusion" method. *Acta Physiol. Scand.*, **58**, 292–305.

Crone, C. (1965). Facilitated transfer of glucose from blood into brain tissue. *J. Physiol.*, **181**, 103–13.

Crooke, R.M. (1991). In vitro toxicology and pharmacokinetics of antisense oligonucleotides. *Anti-Cancer Drug Design*, **6**, 609–46.

Crooke, S.T. (1993). Progress toward oligonucleotide therapeutics: pharmacodynamic properties. *Faseb J.*, **7**, 533–9.

Cserr, H.F., Cooper, D.N., Suri, P.K. and Patlak, C.S. (1981). Efflux of radiolabeled polyethylene glycols and albumin from rat brain. *Am. J. Physiol.*, **240** (*Renal Fluid Electrolyte Physiol.* **9**), F319–28.

Culver, K.W., Ram, Z., Wallbridge, S. et al. (1992). In vivo gene transfer with retroviral vector-producer cells for treatment of experimental brain tumors. *Science*, **256**, 1550–2.

Cummings, B.J. and Cotman, C.W. (1995). Image analysis of β-amyloid load in Alzheimer's disease and relation to dementia severity. *Lancet*, **346**, 1524–8.

Dadparvar, S., Krishna, L., Miyamoto, C. et al. (1994). Indium-111-labeled anti-EGFr-425 scintigraphy in the detection of malignant gliomas. *Cancer*, **73**, 884–9.

Dallaire, L., Giroux, S. and Beliveau, R. (1992). Regulation of phosphate transport by second messengers in capillaries of the blood–brain barrier. *Biochim. Biophys. Acta*, **1110**, 59–64.

Daly, T.M., Carole, V., Levy, B., Haskins, M.E. and Sands, M.S. (1999). Neonatal gene transfer leads to widespread correction of pathology in a murine model of lysosomal storage disease. *Proc. Natl Acad. Sci. USA*, **96**, 2296–300.

Davidson, H.W., McGowan, C.H. and Balch, W.E. (1992). Evidence for the regulation of exocytic transport by protein phosphorylation. *J. Cell Biol.*, **116**, 1343–55.

De Lange, E.C.M., Danhof, M., De Boer, A.G. and Breimer, D.D. (1994). Critical factors of intra-cerebral microdialysis as a technique to determine the pharmacokinetics of drugs in rat brain. *Brain Res.*, **666**, 1–8.

de Smidt, P.C., Doan, T.L., de Falco, S. and van Berkel, T.J.C. (1991). Association of antisense oligonucleotides with lipoproteins prolongs the plasma half-life and modifies the tissue distribution. *Nucl. Acids Res.*, **19**, 4695–400.

Deguchi, Y., Inabe, K., Tomiyasu, K., Yamada, S. and Kimura, R. (1995). Study on brain interstitial fluid distribution and blood–brain barrier transport of baclofen in rats by microdialysis. *Pharm. Res.*, **12**, 1838–43.

Deguchi, Y., Kurihara, A. and Pardridge, W.M. (1999). Retention of biologic activity of human epidermal growth factor following conjugation to a blood–brain barrier drug delivery vector via an extended polyethyleneglycol linker. *Bionconj. Chem.*, **10**, 32–7.

Dehouck, B., Fenart, L., Dehouck, M.-P. et al. (1997). A new function for the LDL receptor: transcytosis of LDL across the blood–brain barrier. *J. Cell. Biol.*, **138**, 1–13.

Demidov, V.V., Potaman, V.N., Frank-Kamenetski, M.D. et al. (1994). Stability of peptide nucleic acids in human serum and cellular extracts. *Biochem. Pharmacol.*, **48**, 1310–13.

Dermietzel, R., Krause, D., Kremer, M., Wang, C. and Stevenson, B. (1992). Pattern of glucose transporter (Glut1) expression in embryonic brains is related to maturation of blood–brain barrier tightness. *Dev. Dynamics*, **193**, 152–63.

Derossi, D., Joliot, A.H., Chassaing, G. and Prochiantz, A. (1994). The third helix of the antennapedia homeodomain translocates through biological membranes. *J. Biol. Chem.*, **269**, 10444–50.

Dewey, R.A., Morrissey, G., Cowsill, C.M. et al. (1999). Chronic brain inflammation and persistent herpes simplex virus 1 thymidine kinase expression in survivors of syngeneic glioma treated by adenovirus-mediated gene therapy: implications for clinical trials. *Nat. Med.*, **5**, 1256–63.

Diamond, J.M. and Wright, E.M. (1969). Molecular forces governing non-electrolytic permeation through cell membranes. *Proc. R. Soc.*, **172**, 273–316.

Diatchenko, L., Lau, Y.-F.C., Campbell, A.P. et al. (1996). Suppression subtractive hybridization: a method for generating differentially regulated or tissue-specific cDNA probes and libraries. *Proc. Natl Acad. Sci. USA*, **93**, 6025–30.

Dobrogowska, D.H., Lossinsky, A.S., Tarnawski, M. and Vorbrodt, A.W. (1998). Increased blood–brain barrier permeability and endothelial abnormalities induced by vascular endothelial growth factor. *J. Neurocytol.*, **27**, 163–73.

Dohrmann, G.J. (1970). The choroid plexus: a historical review. *Brain Res.*, **18**, 197–218.

Domingo, D.L. and Trowbridge, I.S. (1985). Transferrin receptor as a target for antibody–drug conjugates. *Methods Enzymol.*, **112**, 238–47.

Drews, J. (2000). Drug discovery: a historical perspective. *Science*, **287**, 1960–4.

Driesse, M.J., Vincent, A.J.P.E., Sillevis, P.A.E. et al. (1998). Intracerebral injection of adenovirus harboring the HSVtk gene combined with ganciclovir administration: toxicity study in non-human primates. *Gene Ther.*, **5**, 1122–9.

Dubel, S., Breitling, F., Kontermann, R. et al. (1995). Bifunctional and multimeric complexes of streptavidin fused to single chain antibodies (scFv) *J. Immunol. Methods*, **178**, 201–9.

Duffy, K.R. and Pardridge, W.M. (1987). Blood–brain barrier transcytosis of insulin in developing rabbits. *Brain Res.*, **420**, 32–8.

Duffy, K.R., Pardridge, W.M. and Rosenfeld, R.G. (1988). Human blood–brain barrier insulin-like growth factor receptor. *Metabolism*, **37**, 136–40.

During, M.J., Naegele, J.R., O'Malley, K.L. and Geller, A.I. (1994). Long-term behavioral recovery in Parkinsonian rats by an HSV vector expressing tyrosine hydroxylase. *Science*, **266**, 1399–403.

Duvernoy, H., Delon, S. and Vannson, J.L. (1983). The vascularization of the human cerebellar cortex. *Brain Res. Bull.*, **11**, 419–80.

Dwyer, K.J. and Pardridge, W.M. (1993). Developmental modulation of blood–brain barrier and choroid plexus GLUT1 glucose transporter mRNA and immunoreactive protein in rabbits. *Endocrinol.*, **132**, 558–65.

Dykstra, K.H., Arya, A., Arriola, D.M. et al. (1993). Microdialysis study of zidovudine (AZT) transport in rat brain. *J. Pharmacol. Exp. Ther.*, **267**, 1227–36.

Egholm, M., Buchardt, O., Christensen, L. et al. (1993). PNA hybridizes to complementary oligonucleotides obeying the Watson–Crick hydrogen-bonding rules. *Nature*, **365**, 566–8.

Eibl, H. (1984). Phospholipids as functional constituents of biomembranes. *Angew. Chem. Int. Ed. Engl.*, **23**, 257–71.

Elliger, E. E., Elliger, C.A., Aguilar, C.P., Raju, N.R. and Watson, G.L. (1999). Elimination of lysosomal storage in brains of MPS VII mice treated by intrathecal administration of an adeno-associated virus vector. *Gene Ther.*, **6**, 1175–8.

Ellison, M.D., Krieg, R.J. and Povlishock, J.T. (1990). Differential central nervous system responses following single and multiple recombinant interleukin-2 infusions. *J. Neuroimmunol.*, **28**, 249–60.

Elo, H.A. (1980). Occurrence of avidin-like biotin-binding capacity in various vertebrate tissues and its induction by tissue injury. *Comp. Biochem. Physiol.*, **67**B, 221–4.

Emmanuel, N., Kedar, E., Bolotin, E.M., Smorodinsky, N.I. and Barenholz, Y. (1996). Targeted delivery of doxorubicin via sterically stabilized immunoliposomes: pharmacokinetics and biodistribution in tumor-bearing mice. *Pharm. Res.*, **13**, 861–8.

Ermisch, A., Brust, P., Kretzschmar, R. and Ruhle, H.-J. (1993). Peptides and blood–brain barrier transport. *Physiol. Rev.*, **73**, 489–527.

Fabian, R.H. and Hulsebosch, C.E. (1993). Plasma nerve growth factor access to the postnatal central nervous system. *Brain Res.*, **611**, 46–52.

Farrell, C.L. and Pardridge, W.M. (1991a). Blood–brain barrier glucose transporter is asymmetrically distributed on brain capillary endothelial luminal and abluminal plasma membranes; an electron microscopic immunogold study. *Proc. Natl Acad. Sci. USA*, **88**, 5779–83.

Farrell, C.L., and Pardridge, W.M. (1991b). Ultrastructural localization of blood–brain specific antibodies using immunogold-silver enhancement techniques. *J. Neurosci. Meth.*, **37**, 103–10.

Farrell, C.L., Yang, J. and Pardridge, W.M. (1992). GLUT1 glucose transporter is present within apical and basolateral membranes of brain epithelial interfaces and in microvascular endothelia barriers with and without tight junctions. *J. Histochem. Cytochem.*, **40**, 193–9.

Fawell, S., Seery, J., Daikh, Y. et al. (1994). Tat-mediated delivery of heterologous proteins into cells. *Proc. Natl Acad. Sci. USA*, **91**, 664–8.

Feener, E.P., Shen, W.-C. and Ryser, H.J.-P. (1990). Cleavage of disulfide bonds in endocytosed macromolecules. *J. Biol. Chem.*, **265**, 18780–5.

Felgner, P.L. and Ringold, G.M. (1989). Cationic liposome-mediated transfection. *Nature*, **337**, 387–9.

Felgner, J.H., Kumar, R., Sridhar, C.N. et al. (1994). Enhanced gene delivery and mechanism studies with a novel series of cationic lipid formulations. *J. Biol. Chem.*, **269**, 2550–61.

Fennewald, S.M. and Rando, R.F. (1995). Inhibition of high affinity basic fibroblast growth factor binding by oligonucleotides. *J. Biol. Chem.*, **270**, 21718–21.

Fenstermacher, J. and Kaye, T. (1988). Drug "diffusion" within the brain. *Ann. N.Y. Acad. Sci.*, **531**, 29–39.

Fenstermaker, R.A., Capala, J., Barth, R.F. et al. (1995). The effect of epidermal growth factor receptor (EGFR) expression on in vivo growth of rat 6C glioma cells. *Leukemia*, **9**, S106–12.

Ferguson, I.A. and Johnson, E.M. (1991). Fibroblast growth factor receptor-bearing neurons in the CNS: identification by receptor-mediated retrograde transport. *J. Comp. Neurol.*, **313**, 693–706.

Ferguson, I.A., Schweitzer, J.B., Bartlett, P.F. and Johnson, E.M. (1991). Receptor-mediated retrograde transport in CNS neurons after intraventricular administration of NGF and growth factors. *J. Comp. Neurol.*, **313**, 680–92.

Ferrara, N. and Davis-Smyth, T. (1997). The biology of vascular endothelial growth factor. *Endocrine Rev.*, **18**, 4–25.

Finlay, D.R., Newmeyer, D.D., Price, T.M. and Forbes, D.J. (1987). Inhibition of in vitro nuclear transport by a lectin that binds to nuclear pores. *J. Cell. Biol.*, **104**, 189–200.

Finnerty, H., Kelleher, K., Morris, G.E. et al. (1993). Molecular cloning of murine FLT and FLT4. *Oncogene*, **8**, 2293–8.

Fishman, R.A. (1980). *Cerebrospinal Fluid in Disease of the Nervous System*, pp. 1–384. Philadelphia: W.B. Saunders.

Fishman, R.A. and Christy, N.P. (1965). Fate of adrenal cortical steroids following intrathecal injections. *Neurol.*, **15**, 1–6.

Fishman, J.B., Rubin, J.B., Handrahan, J.V., Connor, J.R. and Fine, R.E. (1987). Receptor-mediated transcytosis of transferrin across the blood–brain barrier. *J. Neurosci. Res.*, **18**, 299–304.

Flier, J.S., Mueckler, M., McCall, A.L. and Lodish, H.F. (1987). Distribution of glucose transporter messenger RNA transcripts in tissues of rat and man. *J. Clin. Invest.*, **79**, 657–61.

Foote, J. and Winter, G. (1992). Antibody framework residues affecting the conformation of the hypervariable loops. *J. Mol. Biol.*, **224**, 487–99.

Foulon, C.F., Alston, K.L. and Zalutsky, M.R. (1998). Astatine-211-labeled biotin conjugates resistant to biotinidase for use in pretargeted radioimmunotherapy. *Nucl. Med. Biol.*, **25**, 81–8.

Frank, H.J.L. and Pardridge, W.M. (1981). A direct in vitro demonstration of insulin binding to isolated brain microvessels. *Diabetes*, **30**, 757–61.

Frank, H.J.L., Jankovic-Vokes, T., Pardridge, W.M. and Morris, W.L. (1985). Enhanced insulin binding to blood–brain barrier in vivo and to brain microvessels in vitro in newborn rabbits. *Diabetes*, **34**, 728–33.

Frank, H.J.L., Pardridge, W.M., Jankovic-Vokes, T., Vinters, H.V. and Morris, W.L. (1986). Insulin binding to the blood–brain barrier in the streptozotocin diabetic rat. *J. Neurochem.*, **47**, 405–11.

Freese, A., Geller, A.I. and Neve, R. (1990). HSV-1 vector mediated neuronal gene delivery. *Biochem. Pharmacol.*, **40**, 2189–99.

French, A.R., Tadaki, D.K., Niyogi, S.K. and Lauffenburger, D.A. (1995). Intracellular trafficking of epidermal growth factor family ligands is directly influenced by the pH sensitivity of the receptor/ligand interaction. *J. Biol. Chem.*, **270**, 4334–40.

Friden, P.M., Walus, L.R., Musso, G.F. et al. (1991). Anti-transferrin receptor antibody and antibody–drug conjugates cross the blood–brain barrier. *Proc. Natl Acad. Sci. USA*, **88**, 4771–5.

Friden, P.M., Olson, T.S., Obar, R., Walus, L.R. and Putney, S.D. (1996). Characterization, receptor mapping, and blood–brain barrier transcytosis of antibodies to the human transferrin receptor. *J. Pharmacol. Exp. Ther.*, **278**, 1491–8.

Frunzio, R., Chiariotti, L., Brown, A.L. et al. (1986). Structure and expression of the rat insulin-like growth factor II (rIGF-II) gene. *J. Biol. Chem.*, **261**, 17138–49.

Fukuta, M., Okada, H., Iinuma, S., Yanai, S. and Toguchi, H. (1994). Insulin fragments as a carrier for peptide delivery across the blood–brain barrier. *Pharm. Res.*, **11**, 1681–8.

Fung, L.K., Shin, M., Tyler, B., Brem, H. and Saltzman, W.M. (1996). Chemotherapeutic drugs released from polymers: distribution of 1,3-bis(2-chloroethyl)-1-nitrosourea in the rat brain. *Pharm. Res.*, **13**, 671–82.

Galinsky, R.E., Hoesterey, B.L. and Anderson, B.D. (1990). Brain and cerebrospinal fluid uptake of zidovudine (AZT) in rats after intravenous injection. *Life Sci.*, **47**, 781–8.

Galvagni, F. and Oliviero, S. (2000). Utrophin transcription is activated by an intronic enhancer. *J. Biol. Chem.*, **275**, 3168–72.

Gambhir, S.S., Barrier, J.R., Phelps, M.E. et al. (1999a). Imaging adenoviral-directed reporter gene expression in living animals with positron emission tomography. *Proc. Natl Acad. Sci. USA*, **96**, 2333–8.

Gambhir, S.S., Barrio, J.R., Herschman, H.R. and Phelps, M.E. (1999b). Assays for noninvasive imaging of reporter gene expression. *Nucl. Med. Biol.*, **26**, 481–90.

Gamper, H.B., Reed, M.W., Cox, T. et al. (1992). Facile preparation of nuclease resistant 3′ modified oligodeoxynucleotides. *Nucl. Acids Res.*, **21**, 145–50.

Gao, W.-Y., Han, F.-S., Storm, C., Egan, W. and Cheng, Y.-C. (1992). Phosphorothioate oligonucleotides are inhibitors of human DNA polymerases and RNAse H: implications for antisense technology. *Mol. Pharmacol.*, **41**, 223–9.

Gao, M., Yamazaki, M., Loe, D.W. et al. (1998). Multidrug resistance protein. Identification of regions required for active transport of leukotriene C_4. *J. Biol. Chem.*, **273**, 10733–40.

Gao, B., Stieger, B., Noe, B., Fritschy, J.-M. and Meier, P.J. (1999). Localization of the organic anion transporting polypeptide 2 (oatp2) in capillary endothelium and choroid plexus epithelium of rat brain. *J. Histochem. Cytochem.*, **47**, 1225–63.

Gauthier, V.J., Mannik, M. and Striker, G.E. (1982). Effect of cationized antibodies in preformed immune complexes on deposition and persistence in renal glomeruli. *J. Exp. Med.*, **156**, 766–77.

Gazzolo, D., Vinesi, P., Bartocci, M. et al. (1999). Elevated S100 blood level as an early indicator of intraventricular hemorrhage in preterm infants: correlation with cerebral Doppler velocimetry. *J. Neurol. Sci.*, **170**, 32–5.

Gearing, M., Rebeck, G.W., Hyman, B.T., Tigges, J. and Mirra, S.S. (1994). Neuropathology and apolipoprotein E profile of aged chimpanzees: implications for Alzheimer disease. *Proc. Natl Acad. Sci. USA*, **91**, 9382–6.

Gennuso, R., Spigelman, M.K., Chinol, M. et al. (1993). Effect of blood–brain barrier and blood–tumor barrier modification on central nervous system liposomal uptake. *Cancer Invest.*, **11**, 118–28.

Georges, E., Tsuruo, T. and Ling, V. (1993). Topology of p-glycoprotein as determined by epitope mapping of MRK-16 monoclonal antibody. *J. Biol. Chem.*, **268**, 1792–8.

Gerhart, D.Z. and Drewes, L.R. (1987). Butyrylcholinesterase in pericytes associated with canine brain capillaries. *Cell Tissue Res.*, **247**, 533–6.

Gerhart, D.Z., Leino, R.L. and Drewes, L.R. (1999). Distribution of monocarboxylate transporters MCT1 and MCT2 in rat retina. *Neurosci.*, **92**, 367–75.

Gidda, J.S., Evans, D.C., Cohen, M.L. et al. (1995). Antagonism of serotonin$_3$ (5-HT$_3$) receptors within the blood–brain barrier prevents cisplatin-induced emesis in dogs. *J. Pharmacol. Exp. Ther.*, **273**, 695–701.

Giddings, S.J., Chirgwin, J. and Permutt, M.A. (1985). Evaluation of rat insulin messenger RNA in pancreatic and extrapancreatic tissues. *Diabetologia*, **28**, 343–7.

Gitlin, G., Bayer, E.A. and Wilchek, M. (1990). Studies on the biotin-binding sites of avidin and streptavidin. Tyrosine residues are involved in the binding site. *Biochem. J.*, **269**, 527–30.

Gizurarson, S., Thorvaldsson, T., Sigurdsson, P. and Gunnarsson, E. (1997). Selective delivery of insulin into the brain: intraolfactory absorption. *Int. J. Pharm.*, **146**, 135–41.

Glenner, G.G. and Wong, C.W. (1984). Alzheimer's disease: initial report of the purification and characterization of a novel cerebrovascular amyloid protein. *Biochem. Biophys. Res. Commun.*, **120**, 885–80.

Golden, P.L. and Pardridge, W.M. (1999). P-glycoprotein on astrocyte foot processes of unfixed isolated human brain capillaries. *Brain Res.*, **819**, 143–6.

Golden, M.P. and Shelly, C. (1987). Modulation of alveolar macrophage-derived 5-lipoxygenase products by the sulfhydryl reactant, N-ethylmaleimide. *J. Biol. Chem.*, **262**, 10594–600.

Golden, P.L., Maccagnan, T.J. and Pardridge, W.M. (1997). Human blood–brain barrier leptin receptor. Binding and endocytosis in isolated human brain microvessels. *J. Clin. Invest.*, **99**, 14–18.

Goldfine, I.D. (1987). The insulin receptor: molecular biology and transmembrane signaling. *Endocr. Rev.*, **8**, 235–55.

Goldman, M., Dratman, M.B., Crutchfield, F.L. et al. (1985). Intrathecal triiodothyronine administration causes greater heart rate stimulation in hypothyroid rats than intravenously delivered hormone. Evidence for a central nervous system site of thyroid hormone action. *J. Clin. Invest.*, **76**, 1622–5.

Goldstein, G.W., Wolinsky, J.S., Csejtey, J. and Diamond, I. (1975). Isolation of metabolically active capillaries from rat brain. *J. Neurochem.*, **25**, 715–17.

Grant, C.W.M. and Peters, M.W. (1984). Lectin–membrane interactions. Information from model systems. *Biochim. Biophys. Acta*, **779**, 403–22.

Gravina, S.A., Ho, L., Eckman, C.B. et al. (1995). Amyloid β protein (Aβ) in Alzheimer's disease brain. *J. Biol. Chem.*, **270**, 7013–16.

Green, N.M. (1975). Avidin. *Adv. Prot. Chem.*, **29**, 85–133.

Greenwood, J. and Pratt, O.E. (1983). Inhibition of thiamine transport across the blood–brain barrier in the rat by a chemical analogue of the vitamin. *J. Physiol.*, **336**, 479–86.

Gref, R., Minamitake, Y., Peracchia, M.T. et al. (1994). Biodegradable long-circulating polymeric nanospheres. *Science*, **263**, 1600–3.

Gregoriadis, G. (1976). The carrier potential of liposomes in biology and medicine. *N. Engl. J. Med.*, **295**, 704–10.

Greig, N.H., Fredericks, W.R., Holloway, H.W., Soncrant, T.T. and Rapoport, S.I. (1988). Delivery of human interferon-alpha to brain by transient osmotic blood–brain barrier modification in the rat. *J. Pharmacol. Exp. Ther.*, **245**, 581–6.

Greig, N.H., Daly, E.M., Sweeney, D.J. and Rapoport, S.I. (1990a). Pharmacokinetics of chlorambucil-tertiary butyl ester, a lipophilic chlorambucil derivative that achieves and maintains high concentrations in brain. *Cancer Chemother. Pharmacol.*, **25**, 320–5.

Greig, N.H., Soncrant, T.T., Shetty, H.U. et al. (1990b). Brain uptake and anticancer activities of vincristine and vinblastine are restricted by their low cerebrovascular permeability and binding to plasma constituents in rat. *Cancer Chemother. Pharmacol.*, **26**, 263–8.

Griffiths, D.A., Hall, S.D. and Sokol, P.P. (1991). Interaction of $3'$-azido-$3'$-deoxythymidine with organic ion transport in rat renal basolateral membrane vesicles. *J. Pharmacol. Exp. Ther.*, **257**, 149–55.

Gross, P.M., Teasdale, G.M., Angerson, W.J. and Harper, A.M. (1981). H_2-receptors mediate increases in permeability of the blood–brain barrier during arterial histamine infusion. *Brain Res.*, **210**, 396–400.

Gruber, H.J., Marek, M., Schindler, H. and Kaiser, K. (1997). Biotin-fluorophore conjugates with poly (ethylene glycol) spacers retain intense fluorescence after binding to avidin and streptavidin. *Bioconj. Chem.*, **8**, 552–9.

Grzanna, R., Dubin, J.R., Dent, G.W. et al. (1998). Intrastriatal and intraventricular injections of oligodeoxynucleotides in the rat brain: tissue penetration, intracellular distribution and c-fos antisense effects. *Mol. Brain Res.*, **63**, 35–52.

Guan, J., Williams, C., Gunning, M., Mallard, C. and Gluckman, P. (1993). The effects of IGF1 treatment after hypoxic–ischemic brain injury in adult rats. *J. Cereb. Blood Flow Metab.*, **13**, 609–16.

Gutekunst, C.-A., Levey, A.I., Heilman, C.J. et al. (1995). Identification and localization of huntington in brain and human lymphoblastoid cell lines with an anti-fusion protein antibodies. *Proc. Natl Acad. Sci. USA*, **92**, 8710–14.

Hanig, J.P., Morrison, J.M. and Krop, S. (1972). Ethanol enhancement of blood–brain barrier permeability to catecholamines in chicks. *Eur. J. Pharmacol.*, **18**, 79–82.

Hansch, C. and Steward, A.R. (1964). The use of substituent constants in the analysis of the structure–activity relationship in penicillin derivatives. *J. Med. Chem.*, **7**, 691–4.

Hanvey, J.C., Pfeffer, N.J., Bisi, J.E. et al. (1992). Antisense and antigene properties of peptide nucleic acids. *Science*, **258**, 1481–6.

Haque, N. and Isacson, O. (1997). Antisense gene therapy for neurodegenerative disease. *Exp. Neurol.*, **144**, 139–45.

Hargreaves, K.M. and Pardridge, W.M. (1988). Neutral amino acid transport at the human blood–brain barrier. *J. Biol. Chem.*, **263**, 19392–7.

Haselbacher, G.K., Schwab, M.E., Pasi, A. and Humbel, R.E. (1984). Insulin-like growth factor II (IGF II) in human brain: regional distribution of IGF II and of higher molecular mass forms. *Proc. Natl Acad. Sci. USA*, **82**, 2153–7.

Hashimoto, M., Ishikawa, Y., Yokota, S. et al. (1991). Action site of circulating interleukin-1 on the rabbit brain. *Brain Res.*, **540**, 217–23.

Hashmi, M. and Rosebrough, S.F. (1995). Synthesis, pharmacokinetics, and biodistribution of [67]GA deferoxamineacetyl-cysteinylbiotin. *Drug Metab. Disp.*, **23**, 1362–7.

Haskell, J.F., Meezan, E. and Pillion, D.J. (1985). Identification of the insulin receptor of cerebral microvessels. *Am. J. Physiol.*, **248**, E115–25.

Hauser, M., Donhardt, A.M., Barnes, D., Naider, F. and Becker, J.M. (2000). Enkephalins are transported by a novel eukaryotic peptide uptake system. *J. Biol. Chem.*, **275**, 3037–41.

Havrankova, J. and Roth, J. (1979). Concentrations of insulin and of insulin receptors in the brain are independent of peripheral insulin levels. *J. Clin. Invest.*, **64**, 636–42.

Hawkins, R.A., Mans, A.M. and Davis, D.W. (1986). Regional ketone body utilization by rat brain in starvation and diabetes. *Am. J. Physiol.*, **250**, E169.

Hayashi, T., Abe, K. and Itoyama, Y. (1998). Reduction of ischemic damage by application of vascular endothelial growth factor in rat brain after transient ischemia. *J. Cereb. Blood Flow Metab.*, **18**, 887–95.

Heffetz, D., Fridkin, M. and Zick, Y. (1989). Antibodies directed against phosphothreonine residues as potent tools for studying protein phosphorylation. *Eur. J. Biochem.*, **182**, 343–8.

Hefti, F. (1997). Pharmacology of neurotrophic factors. *Ann. Rev. Pharmacol. Toxicol.*, **37**, 239–67.

Henderson, G.B. and Strauss, B.P. (1991). Evidence for cAMP and cholate extrusion in C6 rat glioma cells by a common anion efflux pump. *J. Biol. Chem.*, **266**, 1641–5.

Hendricks, S.A., Agardh, C.-D., Taylor, S.I. and Roth, J. (1984). Unique features of the insulin receptor in rat brain. *J. Neurochem.*, **43**, 1302–9.

Hengge, U.R., Brockmeyer, N.H., Malessa, R., Ravens, U. and Goos, M. (1993). Foscarnet penetrates the blood–brain barrier: rationale for therapy of cytomegalovirus encephalitis. *Antimicrob. Agents Chemother.*, **37**, 1010–14.

Hennemann, H., Schwarz, H.J. and Willecke, K. (1992). Characterization of gap junction genes expressed in F9 embryonic carcinoma cells: molecular cloning of mouse connexin 31 and 45 cDNAs. *Eur. J. Cell. Biol.*, **57**, 51–8.

Herrlinger, U., Kramm, C.M., Aboody-Guterman, K.S. et al. (1998). Pre-existing herpes simplex virus 1 (HSV-1) immunity decreases, but does not abolish, gene transfer to experimental brain tumors by a HSV-1 vector. *Gene Ther.*, **5**, 809–19.

Hertz, M.M. and Bolwig, T.G. (1976). Blood brain barrier studies in the rat: an indicator dilution technique with tracer sodium as an internal standard for estimation of extracerebral contamination. *Brain Res.*, **107**, 333–43.

Herz, A., Albus, K., Metys, J., Schubert, P. and Teschemacher, H.J. (1970). On the central sites for the antinociceptive action of morphine and fentanyl. *Neuropharmacol.*, **9**, 539–51.

Hiesiger, E.M., Voorhies, R.M., Basler, G.A. et al. (1986). Opening the blood–brain and blood–tumor barriers in experimental rat brain tumors: the effect of intracarotid hyperosmolar mannitol on capillary permeability and blood flow. *Ann. Neurol.*, **19**, 50–9.

Hirohashi, T., Terasaki, T., Shigetoshi, M. and Sugiyama, Y. (1997). In vivo and in vitro evidence for nonrestricted transport of 2′,7′-bis(2-carboxyethyl)-5(6)-carboxyfluorescein tetraacetoxymethyl ester at the blood–brain barrier. *J. Pharmacol. Exp. Ther.*, **280**, 813–19.

Hnatowich, D.J., Virzi, F. and Rusckowski, M. (1987). Investigations of avidin and biotin for imaging applications. *J. Nucl. Med.*, **28**, 1294–302.

Hobbs, S.M. and Jackson, L.E. (1987). Binding of subclasses of rat immunoglobulin G to detergent-isolated Fc receptor from neonatal rat intestine. *J. Biol. Chem.*, **262**, 8041–6.

Hodgkinson, S.C., Spencer, G.S.G., Bass, J.J., Davis, S.R. and Gluckman, P.D. (1991). Distribution of circulating insulin-like growth factor I (IGF1) into tissues. *Endocrinol.*, **129**, 2085–93.

Hofland, H.E.J., Nagy, D., Liu, J.-J. et al. (1997). In vivo gene transfer by intravenous administration of stable cationic lipid/DNA complex. *Pharm. Res.*, **14**, 742–9.

Hogg, R.S., Heath, K.V., Yip, B. et al. (1998). Improved survival among HIV-infected individuals following initiation of antiretroviral therapy. *JAMA*, **279**, 450–4.

Hohmann, H.-P., Brockhaus, M., Baeuerle, P.A. et al. (1990). Expression of the types A and B tumor necrosis factor (TNF) receptors is independently regulated, and both receptor mediate activation of the transcription factor NF-κB. *J. Biol. Chem.*, **265**, 22409–17.

Homayoun, P. and Harik, S.I. (1991). Bradykinin receptors of cerebral microvessels stimulate phosphoinositide turnover. *J. Cereb. Blood Flow Metab.*, **11**, 557–66.

Hommel, U., Harvey, T.S., Driscoll, P.C. and Campbell, I.D. (1992). Human epidermal growth factor. High resolution solution structure and comparison with human transforming growth factor α. *J. Mol. Biol.*, **227**, 271–82.

Hong, K., Zheng, W., Baker, A. and Papahadjopoulos, D. (1997). Stabilization of cationic liposome-plasmid DNA complexes by polyamines and poly(ethylene glycol)-phospholipid conjugates for efficient in vivo gene delivery. *FEBS Lett.*, **400**, 233–7.

Honig, B. and Nicholls, A. (1995). Classical electrostatics in biology and chemistry. *Science*, **268**, 1144–9.

Horie, T., Mizuma, T., Kasai, S. and Awazu, S. (1988). Conformational change in plasma albumin due to interaction with isolated rat hepatocyte. *Am. J. Physiol.*, **254**, G465–70.

Horton, R.M., Hunt, H.D., Ho, S.N., Pullen, J.K. and Pease, L.R. (1989). Engineering hybrid genes without the use of restriction enzymes: gene splicing by overlap extension. *Gene*, **7**, 61–8.

Hoshi, S., Goto, M., Koyama, N., Nomoto, K. and Tanaka, H. (2000). Regulation of vascular smooth muscle cell proliferation by nuclear factor-κB and its inhibitor, I-κB. *J. Biol. Chem.*, **275**, 883–9.

Hsiao, K., Chapman, P., Nilsen, S. et al. (1996). Correlative memory deficits, Aβ elevation, and amyloid plaques in transgenic mice. *Science*, **274**, 99–102.

Huang, L. and Li, S. (1997). Liposomal gene delivery: a complex package. *Nat. Biotechnol.*, **15**, 620–1.

Huang, M. and Rorstad, O.P. (1984). Cerebral vascular adenylate cyclase: evidence for coupling to receptors for vasoactive intestinal peptide and parathyroid hormone. *J. Neurochem.*, **43**, 849–54.

Huang, H.J., Nagane, M., Klingbeil, C.K. et al. (1997). The enhanced tumorigenic activity of a mutant epidermal growth factor receptor common in human cancers is mediated by threshold levels of constitutive tyrosine phosphorylation and unattenuated signaling. *J. Biol. Chem.*, **272**, 2927–35.

Huffman, L.J., Connors, J.M. and Hedge, G.A. (1988). VIP and its homologues increase vascular conductance in certain endocrine and exocrine glands. *Am. J. Physiol.*, **254**, E435–42.

Huntington's Disease Collaborative Research Group (1993). A novel gene containing a trinucleotide repeat that is expanded and unstable on Huntington's disease chromosomes. *Cell*, **72**, 971–83.

Huwyler, J. and Pardridge, W.M. (1998). Examination of blood–brain barrier transferrin receptor by confocal fluorescent microscopy of unfixed isolated rat brain capillaries. *J. Neurochem.*, **70**, 883–6.

Huwyler, J., Wu, D. and Pardridge, W.M. (1996). Brain drug delivery of small molecules using immunoliposomes. *Proc. Natl Acad. Sci. USA*, **93**, 14164–9.

Huwyler, J., Yang, J. and Pardridge, W.M. (1997). Targeted delivery of daunomycin using immunoliposomes: pharmacokinetics and tissue distribution in the rat. *J. Pharmacol. Exp. Ther.*, **282**, 1541–6.

Hynes, M.A., Brooks, P.J., Van Wyk, J.J. and Lund, P.K. (1988). Insulin-like growth factor II messenger ribonucleic acids are synthesized in the choroid plexus of the rat brain. *Mol. Endocrinol.*, **2**, 47–54.

Iacopetti, P., Barsacchi, G., Tirone, F. and Cremisi, F. (1994). Developmental expression of PC-3 gene is correlated with neuronal cell birthday. *Mech. Dev.*, **47**, 127–37.

Ibáñez, C.F., Ebendal, T., Barbany, G. et al. (1992). Disruption of the low affinity receptor-binding site in NGF allows neuronal survival and differentiation by binding to the trk gene product. *Cell*, **69**, 329–41.

Imaoka, T., Date, I., Ohmoto, T. and Nagatsu, T. (1998). Significant behavioral recovery in Parkinson's disease model by direct intracerebral gene transfer using continuous injection of a plasmid DNA–liposome complex. *Hum. Gene Ther.*, **9**, 1093–102.

Inamura, T. and Black, K.L. (1994). Bradykinin selectively opens blood–tumor barrier in experimental brain tumors. *J. Cereb. Blood Flow Metab.*, **14**, 862–70.

Isaacson, L.G., Saffran, B.N. and Crutcher, K.A. (1990). Intracerebral NGF infusion induces hyperinnervation of cerebral blood vessels. *Neurobiol. Aging*, **11**, 51–5.

Itakura, T., Okuno, T., Nakakita, N. et al. (1984). A light and electron microscopic immunohistochemical study of vasoactive intestinal polypeptide- and substance P-containing nerve fibers along the cerebral blood vessels: comparison with aminergic and cholinergic nerve fibers. *J. Cereb. Flow Metab.*, **4**, 407–14.

Iwatsubo, T., Mann, D.M.A., Odaka, A., Suzuki, N. and Ihara, Y. (1995). Amyloid β (Aβ) disposition: Aβ42(43) precedes Aβ40 in Down syndrome. *Ann. Neurol.*, **37**, 294–9.

Jaehde, U., Masereeuw, R., De Boer, A.G. et al. (1994). Quantification and visualization of the transport of octreotide, a somatostatin analogue, across monolayers of cerebrovascular endothelial cells. *Pharm. Res.*, **11**, 442–8.

Jahraus, A., Tjelle, T.E., Berg, T. et al. (1998). In vitro fusion of phagosomes with different endocytic organelles from J774 macrophages. *J. Biol. Chem.*, **273**, 30379–90.

Jakeman, L.B., Winer, J., Bennett, G.L., Altar, C.A. and Ferrara, N. (1992). Binding sites for vascular endothelial growth factor are localized on endothelial cells in adult rat tissues. *J. Clin. Invest.*, **89**, 244–53.

Jarrett, J.T. and Lansbury, P.T. Jr. (1993). Seeing "one-dimensional crystallization" of amyloid: a pathogenic mechanism in Alzheimer's disease and scrapie? *Cell*, **73**, 1055–8.

Jefferies, W.A., Brandon, M.R., Hunt, S.V. et al. (1984). Transferrin receptor on endothelium of brain capillaries. *Nature*, **312**, 162–3.

Jefferies, W.A., Brandon, M.R., Williams, A.F. and Hunt, S.V. (1985). Analysis of lymphopoietic stem cells with a monoclonal antibody to the rat transferrin receptor. *Immunol.*, **54**, 333–41.

Jette, L., Tetu, B. and Beliveau, R. (1993). High levels of P-glycoprotein detected in isolated brain capillaries. *Biochim. Biophys. Acta*, **1150**, 147–54.

Jones, P.T., Dear, P.H., Foote, J., Neuberger, M.S. and Winter, G. (1986). Replacing the complementarity-determining regions in a human antibody with those from a mouse. *Nature*, 321, 522–5.

Joo, F. (1985). The blood–brain barrier in vitro: ten years of research on microvessels isolated from the brain. *Neurochem. Int.*, 7, 1–25.

Joo, F., Temesvari, P. and Dux, E. (1983). Regulation of the macromolecular transport in the brain microvessels: the role of cyclic GMP. *Brain Res.*, 278, 165–74.

Justicia, C. and Planas, A.M. (1999). Transforming growth factor-α acting at the epidermal growth factor receptor reduces infarct volume after permanent middle cerebral artery occlusion in rats. *J. Cereb. Blood Flow Metab.*, 19, 128–32.

Kabat, E.A., Wu, T.T., Perry, H.M., Gottesman, K.S. and Foeller, C. (1991). *Sequences of Proteins of Immunological Interests*, 5th edn. Bethesda, MD: National Institutes of Health.

Kacem, K., Lacombe, P., Seylaz, J. and Bonvento, G. (1998). Structural organization of the perivascular astrocyte endfeet and their relationship with the endothelial glucose transporter: a confocal study. *Glia*, 23, 1–10.

Kaelin, W.G. (1999). Choosing anticancer drug targets in the postgenomic era. *J. Clin. Invest.*, 104, 1503–6.

Kahn, J.O., Allan, J.D., Hodges, T.L. et al. (1990). The safety and pharmacokinetics of recombinant soluble CD4 (rCD4) in subjects with the acquired immunodeficiency syndrome (AIDS) and AIDS-related complex. *Ann. Intern. Med.*, 112, 254–61.

Kajiwara, K., Byrnes, A.P., Ohmoto, Y. et al. (2000). Humoral immune responses to adenovirus vectors in the brain. *J. Neuroimmunol.*, 103, 8–15.

Kakee, A., Terasaki, T. and Sugiyama, Y. (1996). Brain efflux index as a novel method of analyzing efflux transport at the blood–brain barrier. *J. Pharmacol. Exp. Ther.*, 277, 1550–9.

Kakyo, M., Sakagami, H., Nishio, T. et al. (1999). Immunohistochemical distribution and functional characterization of an organic anion transporting polypeptide 2 (oatp2). *FEBS Lett.*, 445, 343–6.

Kalaria, R.N. and Harik, S.I. (1988). Adenosine receptors and the nucleotide transporter in human brain vasculature. *J. Cereb. Blood Flow Metab.*, 8, 32–9.

Kalofonos, H.P., Pawlikowska, T.R., Hemingway, A. et al. (1989). Antibody guided diagnosis and therapy of brain gliomas using radiolabeled monoclonal antibodies against epidermal growth factor receptor and placental alkaline phosphatase. *J. Nucl. Med.*, 30, 1636–45.

Kanai, Y., Segawa, H., Miyamoto, K. et al. (1998). Expression cloning and characterization of a transporter for large neutral amino acids activated by the heavy chain of 4F2 antigen. *J. Biol. Chem.*, 273, 23629–32.

Kang, J., Lemaire, H.G., Unterbeck, A. et al. (1987). The precursor of Alzheimer disease amyloid A4 protein resembles a cell-surface receptor. *Nature*, 325, 733–6.

Kang, Y.-S. and Pardridge, W.M. (1994a). Brain delivery of biotin bound to a conjugate of neutral avidin and cationized human albumin. *Pharm. Res.*, 11, 1257–64.

Kang, Y.-S. and Pardridge, W.M. (1994b). Use of neutral-avidin improves pharmacokinetics and brain delivery of biotin bound to an avidin-monoclonal antibody conjugate. *J. Pharmacol. Exp. Ther.*, 269, 344–50.

Kang, Y.S., Terasaki, T., Ohnishi, T. and Tsuji, A. (1990). In vivo and in vitro evidence for a common carrier mediated transport of choline and basic drugs through the blood–brain barrier. *J. Pharmacobia-Dyn.*, **13**, 353–60.

Kang, Y.-S., Boado, R.J. and Pardridge, W.M. (1995a). Pharmacokinetics and organ clearance or a 3′-biotinylated internally [^{32}P]labeled phosphodiester oligodeoxynucleotide coupled to a neutral avidin/monoclonal antibody conjugate. *Drug Metab. Disp.*, **23**, 55–9.

Kang, Y.-S., Saito, Y. and Pardridge, W.M. (1995b). Pharmacokinetics of [^{3}H]biotin bound to different avidin analogues. *J. Drug Targeting*, **3**, 156–65.

Kang, Y.-S., Voigt, K. and Bickel, U. (2000). Stability of the disulfide bond in an avidin-biotin linked chimeric peptide during in vivo transcytosis through brain endothelial cells. *J. Drug Targeting*, **8**, 425–34.

Kartner, N., Evernden-Porelle, D., Bradley, G. and Ling, V. (1985). Detection of P-glycoprotein in multidrug-resistant cell lines by monoclonal antibodies. *Nature*, **316**, 820–3.

Kastin, A.J., Nissen, C., Schally, A.V. and Coy, D.H. (1976). Blood–brain barrier, half-time disappearance and brain distribution for labeled enkephalin and a potent analog. *Brain Res. Bull.*, **1**, 583–9.

Kawabata, H., Yang, R., Hirama, T. et al. (1999). Molecular cloning of transferrin receptor 2. *J. Biol. Chem.*, **274**, 20826–32.

Kety, S.S. (1951). The theory and applications of the exchange in inert gas at the lungs and tissues. *Pharmacol. Rev.*, **3**, 1–41.

Khurana, T.S., Watkins, S.C., Chafey, P. et al. (1991). Immunolocalization and developmental expression of dystrophin related protein in skeletal muscle. *Neuromuscular Disorders*, **1**, 185–94.

Kim, D.C., Sugiyama, Y., Fuwa, T. et al. (1989). Kinetic analysis of the elimination process of human epidermal growth factor (hEGF) in rats. *Biochem. Pharmacol.*, **38**, 241–9.

Kim, Y.-H., Park, J.-H., Hong, S.H. and Koh, J.-Y. (1999). Nonproteolytic neuroprotection by human recombinant tissue plasminogen activator. *Science*, **284**, 647–50.

Kipriyanov, S.M., Little, M., Kropshofer, H. et al. (1996). Affinity enhancement of a recombinant antibody: formation of complexes with multiple valency by a single-chain Fv fragment-core streptavidin fusion. *Protein Engineer*, **9**, 203–11.

Kissel, K., Hamm, S., Schulz, M. et al. (1998). Immunohistochemical localization of the murine transferrin receptor (TfR) on blood–tissue barriers using a novel anti-TfR monoclonal antibody. *Histochem. Cell Biol.*, **110**, 63–72.

Kitazawa, T., Terasaki, T., Suzuki, H., Kakee, A. and Sugiyama, Y. (1998). Efflux of taurocholic acid across the blood–brain barrier: interaction with cyclic peptides. *J. Pharmacol. Exp. Ther.*, **286**, 890–5.

Klecker, R.W., Collins, J.M., Yarchoan, R. et al. (1987). Plasma and cerebrospinal fluid pharmacokinetics of 3′-azido-3′-deoxythymidine: a novel pyrimidine analog with potential application for the treatment of patients with AIDS and related diseases. *Clin. Pharmacol. Ther.*, **41**, 407–12.

Klein, R.L., Lewis, M.H., Muzyczka, N. and Meyer, E.M. (1999). Prevention of 6-hydroxy-dopamine-induced rotational behavior by BDNF somatic gene transfer. *Brain Res.*, **847**, 314–20.

Klibanov, A.L., Martynov, A.V., Slinkin, M.A. et al. (1988). Blood clearance of radiolabeled antibody: enhancement by lactosamination and treatment with biotin-avidin or anti-mouse IgG antibodies. *J. Nucl. Med.*, **29**, 1951–6.

Klibanov, A.L., Maruyama, K., Beckerleg, A.M., Torchilin, V.P. and Huang, L. (1991). Activity of amphipathic poly(ethylene glycol) 5000 to prolong the circulation time of liposomes depends on the liposome size and is unfavorable for immunoliposome binding to target. *Biochim. Biophys. Acta*, **1062**, 142–8.

Kobiler, D., Lustig, S., Gozes, Y., Ben-Nathan, D. and Akov, Y. (1989). Sodium dodecylsulphate induces a breach in the blood–brain barrier and enables a West Nile virus variant to penetrate into mouse brain. *Brain Res.*, **496**, 314–16.

Kobori, N., Imahori, Y., Mineura, K., Ueda, S. and Fujii, R. (1999). Visualization of mRNA expression in CNS using ^{11}C-labeled phosphorothioate oligodeoxynucleotide. *NeuroReport*, **10**, 2971–4.

Kordower, J.H., Palfi, S., Chen, E.Y. et al. (1999). Clinicopathological findings following intraventricular glial-derived neurotrophic factor treatment in a patient with Parkinson's disease. *Ann. Neurol.*, **46**, 419–24.

Kragh-Hansen, U. (1981). Molecular aspects of ligand binding to serum albumin. *Pharmacol. Rev.*, **33**, 17–53.

Kramm, C.M., Rainov, N.G., Sena-Esteves, M. et al. (1996). Herpes vector-mediated delivery of marker genes to disseminated central nervous system tumors. *Hum. Gene Ther.*, **7**, 291–300.

Kreuter, J., Alyautdin, R.N., Kharkevich, D.A. and Ivanov, A.A. (1995). Passage of peptides through the blood–brain barrier with colloidal polymer particles (nanoparticles). *Brain Res.*, **674**, 171–4.

Krewson, C.E. and Saltzman, W.M. (1996). Transport and elimination of recombinant human NGF during long-term delivery to the brain. *Brain Res.*, **727**, 169–81.

Krewson, C.E., Klarman, M.L. and Saltzman, W.M. (1995). Distribution of nerve growth factor following direct delivery to brain interstitium. *Brain Res.*, **680**, 196–206.

Krieg, A.M., Tonkinson, J., Matson, S. et al. (1993). Modification of antisense phosphodiester oligodeoxynucleotides by a 5′ cholesterol moiety increases cellular association and improves efficacy. *Proc. Natl Acad. Sci. USA*, **90**, 1048–52.

Kristensson, K. and Olsson, Y. (1971). Uptake of exogenous proteins in mouse olfactory cells. *Acta Neuropathol.*, **19**, 145–54.

Kruman, I.I., Nath, A. and Mattson, M.P. (1998). HIV-1 protein Tat induces apoptosis of hippocampal neurons by a mechanism involving caspase activation, calcium overload, and oxidative stress. *Exp. Neurol.*, **154**, 276–88.

Kuhn, L.C., McClelland, A. and Ruddle, F.H. (1984). Gene transfer, expression, and molecular cloning of the human transferrin receptor gene. *Cell*, **37**, 95–103.

Kumagai, A.K., Eisenberg, J. and Pardridge, W.M. (1987). Absorptive-mediated endocytosis of cationized albumin and a β-endorphin-cationized albumin chimeric peptide by isolated brain capillaries. Model system of blood–barrier transport. *J. Biol. Chem.*, **262**, 15214–19.

Kuntz, I.D. (1992). Structure-based strategies for drug design and discovery. *Science*, **257**, 1078–82.

Kunz, J., Krause, D., Kremer, M. and Dermietzel, R. (1994). The 140 kDa protein of blood–brain barrier associated pericytes is identical to aminopeptidase N. *J. Neurochem.*, **62**, 2375–86.

Kunzelmann, P., Blumcke, I., Traub, O., Dermietzel, R. and Willecke, K. (1997). Coexpression of connexin45 and 32 in oligodendrocytes of rat brain. *J. Neurocytol.*, **26**, 17–22.

Kurihara, A. and Pardridge, W.M. (1999). Imaging brain tumors by targeting peptide radiopharmaceuticals through the blood–brain barrier. *Cancer Res.*, **54**, 6159–63.

Kurihara, A. and Pardridge, W.M. (2000). Aβ^{1-40} peptide radiopharmaceuticals for brain amyloid imaging, ^{111}In chelation, conjugation to polyethyleneglycol-biotin linkers, and autoradiography with Alzheimer's disease brain sections. *Bioconj. Chem.*, **11**, 380–6.

Kurihara, A., Deguchi, Y. and Pardridge, W.M. (1999). Epidermal growth factor radiopharmaceuticals: [111]In chelation, conjugation to a blood–brain barrier delivery vector via a biotin-polyethylene linker, pharmacokinetics, and in vivo imaging of experimental brain tumors. *Bionconj. Chem.*, **10**, 502–11.

Kuwano, R., Usui, H., Maeda, T. et al. (1984). Molecular cloning and the complete nucleotide sequence of cDNA to mRNA for S-100 protein of rat brain. *Nucl. Acid Res.*, **12**, 7455–65.

Lai, M.M., Hong, J.J., Ruggiero, A.M. et al. (1999). The calcineurin-dynamin 1 complex as a calcium sensor for synaptic vesicle endocytosis. *J. Biol. Chem.*, **274**, 25963–6.

Lambert, P.P., Doriauz, M., Sennesael, J., Vanholder, R. and Lammens-Verslijpe, M. (1983). The pathogenicity of cationized albumin in the dog. In *The Pathogenecity of Cationic Proteins*, ed. P.P. Lambert, P. Bergmann and R. Beauwens, pp. 307–17. New York: Raven Press.

Lane, H.A. and Nigg, E.A. (1996). Antibody microinjection reveals an essential role for human polo-like kinase 1 (Plk1) in the functional maturation of mitotic centrosomes. *J. Cell. Biol.*, **135**, 1701–13.

La Salle, G.L.G., Robert, J.J., Berrard, S. et al. (1993). An adenovirus vector for gene transfer into neurons and glia in the brain. *Science*, **259**, 988–90.

Lasbennes, R. and Gayet, J. (1983). Capacity for energy metabolism in microvessels isolated from rat brain. *Neurochem. Res.*, **9**, 1–9.

Laske, D.W., Youle, R.J. and Oldfield, E.H. (1997). Tumor regression with regional distribution of the targeted toxin TF-CRM 107 in patients with malignant brain tumors. *Nat. Med.*, **3**, 1362–8.

Lawrence, M.S., Foellmer, H.G., Elsworth, J.D. et al. (1999). Inflammatory responses and their impact on β-galactosidase transgene expression following adenovirus vector delivery to the primate caudate nucleus. *Gene Ther.*, **6**, 1368–79.

Leamon, C.P., Weigl, D. and Hendren, R.W. (1999). Folate copolymer-mediated transfection of cultured cells. *Bioconj. Chem.*, **10**, 947–57.

Lee, W.-H. and Bondy, C.A. (1993). Ischemic injury induces brain glucose transporter gene expression. *Endocrinol.*, **133**, 2540–4.

Lee, C.G., Gottesman, M.M., Cardarelli, C.O. et al. (1998). HIV-1 protease inhibitors are substrates for the MDR1 multidrug transporter. *Biochem.*, **37**, 3594–601.

Lee, H.J., Engelhardt, B., Lesley, J., Bickel, U. and Pardridge, W.M. (2000). Targeting rat antimouse transferrin receptor monoclonal antibodies through the blood–brain barrier in the mouse. *J. Pharmacol. Exp. Ther.*, **292**, 1048–52.

Leff, S.E., Spratt, S.K., Snyder, R.O. and Mandel, R.J. (1999). Long-term restoration of striatal L-aromatic amino acid decarboxylase activity using recombinant adeno-associated viral vector gene transfer in a rodent model of Parkinson's disease. *Neurosci.*, **92**, 185–96.

Leibrock, J., Lottspeich, F., Hohn, A. et al. (1989). Molecular cloning and expression of brain-derived neurotrophic factor. *Nature*, **341**, 149–52.

Leininger, B., Ghersi-Egea, J.-F., Siest, G. and Minn, A. (1991). In vivo study of the elimination from rat brain of an intracerebrally formed xenobiotic metabolite, 1-naphthyl-β-D-glucuronide. *J. Neurochem.*, **56**, 1163–8.

Leino, R.L., Gerhart, D.Z. and Drewes, L.R. (1999). Monocarboxylate transporter (MCT1). abundance in brains of suckling and adult rats: a quantitative electron microscopic immuno-gold study. *Dev. Brain Res.*, **113**, 47–54.

Lesley, J., Hyman, R., Schulte, R. and Trotter, J. (1984). Expression of transferrin receptor on murine hematopoietic progenitors. *Cell. Immunol.*, **83**, 14–25.

Levin, V.A. (1980). Relationship of octanol/water partition coefficient and molecular weight to rat brain capillary permeability. *J. Med. Chem.*, **23**, 682–4.

Li, J.Y., Sugimura, K., Boado, R.J. et al. (1999). Genetically engineered brain drug delivery vectors – cloning, expression, and in vivo application of an anti-transferrin receptor single chain anti-body-streptavidin fusion gene and protein. *Protein Engineer*, **12**, 787–96.

Li, J.Y., Boado, R.J. and Pardridge, W.M. (2001). Blood–brain barrier genomics. *J. Cereb. Blood Flow Metab.*, **21**, 61–8.

Liang, P. and Pardee, A.B. (1992). Differential display of eukaryotic messenger RNA by means of the polymerase chain reaction. *Science*, **257**, 967–71.

Lierse, W. and Horstmann, E. (1959). Quantitative anatomy of the cerebral vascular bed with especial emphasis on homogeneity and inhomogeneity in small parts of the gray and white matter. *Acta Neurol.*, **14**, 15–19.

Lin, J.H., Chen, I.-W. and Lin, T.-H. (1994). Blood–brain barrier permeability and in vivo activity of partial agonists of benzodiazepine receptor: a study of L-663,581 and its metabolites in rats. *J. Pharmacol. Exp. Ther.*, **271**, 1197–202.

Lindvall, M. and Owan, C. (1981). Autonomic nerves in the mammalian choroid plexus and their influence on the formation of cerbrospinal fluid. *J. Cereb. Blood Flow Metab.*, **1**, 245–66.

Liu, Y., Liggitt, D., Zhong, W. et al. (1995). Cationic liposome-mediated intravenous gene delivery. *J. Biol. Chem.*, **270**, 24864–70.

Liu, L, Karkanias, G.B., Morales, J.C. et al. (1998). Intracerebroventricular leptin regulates hepatic but not peripheral glucose fluxes. *J. Biol. Chem.*, **273**, 31160–7.

Liu, J., Razani, B., Tang, S. et al. (1999). Angiogenesis activators and inhibitors differentially regulate caveolin-1 expression and caveolae formation in vascular endothelial cells. *J. Biol. Chem.*, **274**, 15781–5.

Lodish, H.F. and Kong, N. (1993). The secretory pathway is normal in dithiothreitol-treated cells, but disulfide-bonded proteins are reduced and reversibly retained in the endoplasmic reticulum. *J. Biol. Chem.*, **268**, 20598–605.

Lossinsky, A.S., Vorbrodt, A.W. and Wisniewski, H.M. (1995). Scanning and transmission electron microscopic studies of microvascular pathology in the osmotically impaired blood–brain barrier. *J. Neurocytol.*, **24**, 795–806.

Lucia, M.B., Cauda, R., Landay, A.L. et al. (1995). Transmembrane p-glycoprotein (P-gp/P-170) in HIV infection: analysis of lymphocyte surface expression and drug-unrelated function. *Aids Res. Hum. Retroviruses*, **11**, 893–901.

Lynn, R.B., Cao, G.-Y., Considine, R.V., Hyde, T.M. and Caro, J.F. (1996). Autoradiographic localization of leptin binding in the choroid plexus of ob/ob and db/db mice. *Biochem. Biophys. Res. Commun.*, **219**, 884–9.

Maggio, J.E., Stimson, E.R., Ghilardi, J.R. et al. (1992). Reversible in vitro growth of Alzheimer disease β-amyloid plaques by deposition of labeled amyloid peptide. *Proc. Natl Acad. Sci. USA*, **89**, 5462–6.

Mahato, R.I., Rolland, A. and Tomlinson, E. (1997). Cationic lipid-based gene delivery systems: pharmaceutical perspective. *Pharm. Res.*, **14**, 853–9.

Maher, F., Vannucci, S.J. and Simpson, I.A. (1994). Glucose transporter proteins in brain. *FASEB J.*, **8**, 1003–11.

Mak, M., Fung, L., Strasser, J.F. and Saltzman, W.M. (1995). Distribution of drugs following controlled delivery to the brain interstitium. *J. Neuro-Oncol.*, **26**, 91–102.

Makrides, S.C. (1999). Components of vectors for gene transfer and expression in mammalian cells. *Protein Exp. Purif.*, **17**, 183–202.

Maness, L.M., Banks, W.A., Podlisny, M.B., Selkoe, D.J. and Kastin, A.J. (1994). Passage of human amyloid β-protein 1–40 across the murine blood–brain barrier. *Life Sci.*, **55**, 1643–50.

Mangiapane, M.L. and Simpson, J.B. (1980). Subfornical organ: forebrain site of pressor and dipsogenic action of angiotensin II. *Am. J. Physiol.*, **239**, R382–9.

Marasco, W.A., Haseltine, W.A. and Chen, S. (1993). Design, intracellular expression and activity of a human anti-human immunodeficiency virus type 1 gp120 single-chain antibody. *Proc. Natl Acad. Sci. USA*, **90**, 7889–93.

Markovitz, D.C. and Fernstrom, J.D. (1977). Diet and uptake of aldomet by the brain: competition with natural large neutral amino acids. *Nature*, **197**, 1014–15.

Martin, J.B. (1995). Gene therapy and pharmacological treatment of inherited neurological disorders. *Trends Biotechnol.*, **13**, 28–35.

Martin, L.J., Sangram, S.S., Koo, E.H. et al. (1991). Amyloid precursor protein in aged nonhuman primates. *Proc. Natl Acad. Sci. USA*, **88**, 1461–5.

Mash, D.C., Pablo, J., Flynn, D.D., Efange, S.M.N. and Weiner, W.J. (1990). Characterization and distribution of transferrin receptors in the rat brain. *J. Neurochem.*, **55**, 1972–9.

Masters, C.L., Simms, G., Weinman, N.A. et al. (1985). Amyloid plaque core protein in Alzheimer's disease and Down's syndrome. *Proc. Natl Acad. Sci. USA*, **82**, 4245–9.

Mastroberardino, L., Spindler, B., Pfeiffer, R. et al. (1998). Amino acid transport by heterodimers of 4F2hc/CD98 and members of a permease family. *Nature*, **395**, 288–91.

Masuzaki, H., Ogawa, Y., Isse, N., Satoh, N. et al. (1995). Human obese gene expression. Adipocyte-specific expression and regional differences in the adipose tissue. *Diabetes*, **44**, 855–8.

Matsui, H., Johnson, L.G., Randell, S.H. and Boucher, R.C. (1997). Loss of binding and entry of liposome-DNA complexes decreases transfection efficiency in differentiated airway epithelial cells. *J. Biol. Chem.*, **272**, 1117–26.

Matsukura, M., Mitsuya, H. and Broder, S. (1991). A new concept in AIDS treatment: an antisense approach and its current status towards clinical application. In *Prospects for Antisense Nucleic Acid Therapy of Cancer and AIDS*, ed. E. Wickstrom, pp. 159–78. New York: Wiley-Liss.

Mattila, K.M., Pirttila, T., Blennow, K. et al. (1994). Altered blood–brain barrier function in Alzheimer's disease? *Acta Neurol. Scand.*, **89**, 192–8.

Mayer, L.D., Tai, L.C.L., Ko, D.S.C. et al. (1989). Influence of vesicle size, lipid composition, and drug-to-lipid ratio on the biological activity of liposomal doxorubicin in mice. *Cancer Res.*, **49**, 5922–30.

Mayhan, W.G. (1996). Role of nitric oxide in histamine-induced increases in permeability of the blood–brain barrier. *Brain Res.*, **743**, 70–6.

Mayhan, W.G. and Didion, S.P. (1996). Glutamate-induced disruption of the blood–brain barrier in rats. *Stroke*, **27**, 965–70.

McCulloch, J. and Edvinsson, L. (1980). Cerebral circulatory and metabolic effects of vasoactive intestinal polypeptide. *Am. J. Physiol.*, **238**, H449–56.

McMenamin, M.M., Byrnes, A.P., Charlton, H.M. et al. (1998). A γ34.5 mutant of herpes simplex 1 causes severe inflammation in the brain. *Neurosci.*, **83**, 1225–37.

Megyeri, P., Nemeth, L., Pabst, K.M., Pabst, M.J. et al. (1999). 4-(2-aminoethyl)Benzenesulfonyl fluoride attenuates tumor-necrosis-factor-α-induced blood–brain barrier opening. *Eur. J. Pharmacol.*, **374**, 207–11.

Mena, I. and Cotzias, G.C. (1975). Protein intake and treatment of Parkinson's disease with levodopa. *N. Engl. J. Med.*, **292**, 181–4.

Menzies, S.A., Lorris Betz, A. and Hoff, J.T. (1993). Contributions of ions and albumin to the formation and resolution of ischemic brain edema. *J. Neurosurg.*, **78**, 257–66.

Meresse, S., Delbart, C., Fruchart, J.-C. and Cecchelli, R. (1989). Low-density lipoprotein receptor on endothelium of brain capillaries. *J. Neurochem.*, **53**, 340–5.

Merrill, M.J. and Edwards, N.A. (1990). Insulin-like growth factor I receptors in human glial tumors. *J. Clin. Endocrinol. Metab.*, **71**, 199–209.

Mesnil, M., Piccoli, C., Tiraby, G., Willecke, K. and Yamasaki, H. (1996). Bystander killing of cancer cells by herpes simplex virus thymidine kinase gene is mediated by connexins. *Proc. Natl Acad. Sci. USA*, **93**, 1831–5.

Milenic, D.E., Yokota, T., Filpula, D.R. et al. (1991). Construction, binding properties, metabolism, and tumor targeting of a single chain Fv derived from pancarcinoma monoclonal antibody CC49. *Cancer Res.*, **51**, 6363–71.

Mirabelli, C.K., Bennett, C.F., Anderson, K. and Crooke, S.T. (1991). In vitro and in vivo pharmacologic activities of antisense oligonucleotides. *Anti-Cancer Drug Des.*, **6**, 647–61.

Mistry, G. and Drummond, G.I. (1986). Adenosine metabolism in microvessels from heart and brain. *J. Mol. Cell. Cardiol.*, **18**, 13–22.

Miyazawa, T., Matsumoto, K., Ohmichi, H. et al. (1998). Protection of hippocampal neurons from ischemia-induced delayed neuronal death by a hepatocyte growth factor: a novel neurotrophic factor. *J. Cereb. Blood Flow Metab.*, **18**, 345–8.

Mollegaard, N.E., Buchardt, O., Egholm, M. and Nielsen, P.E. (1994). Peptide nucleic acid DNA strand displacement loops as artificial transcription promoters. *Proc. Natl Acad. Sci. USA*, **91**, 3892–5.

Mollgard, K. and Saunders, N.R. (1975). Complex tight junctions of epithelial and of endothelial cells in early fetal brain. *J. Neurocytol.*, **4**, 453–68.

Monnard, P.A., Oberholzer, T. and Luisi, P. (1997). Entrapment of nucleic acids in liposomes. *Biochim. Biophys. Acta*, **1329**, 39–50.

Montagnoli, A., Guardavaccaro, D., Starace, G. and Tirone, F. (1996). Overexpression of the nerve growth factor-inducible PC-3 immediate early gene is associated with growth inhibition. *Cell Growth Diff.*, **7**, 1327–36.

Moos, T., Oates, P.S. and Morgan, E.H. (1999). Iron-independent neuronal expression of transferrin receptor mRNA in the rat. *Mol. Brain Res.*, **72**, 231–4.

Morgan, M.E., Singhal, D. and Anderson, B.D. (1996). Quantitative assessment of blood–brain barrier damage during microdialysis. *J. Pharmacol. Exp. Ther.*, **277**, 1167–76.

Mori, A., Klibanov, A.L., Torchilin, V.P. and Huang, L. (1991). Influence of the steric barrier activity of amphipathic poly(ethyleneglycol) and ganglioside GM_1 on the circulation time of liposomes and on the target binding of immunoliposomes in vivo. *FEBS Lett.*, **284**, 263–6.

Moro, V., Kacem, K., Springhetti, V., Seylaz, J. and Lasbennes, F. (1995). Microvessels isolated from brain: localization of muscarinic sites by radioligand binding and immunofluorescent techniques. *J. Cereb. Blood Flow. Metab.*, **15**, 1082–92.

Moroni, M.C., Willingham, M.C. and Beguinot, L. (1992). EGF-R antisense RNA blocks expression of the epidermal growth factor receptor and suppresses the transforming phenotype of a human carcinoma cell line. *J. Biol. Chem.*, **267**, 2714–22.

Morris, C.M., Keith, A.B., Edwardson, J.A. and Pullen, R.G.L. (1992). Uptake and distribution of iron and transferrin in the adult rat brain. *J. Neurochem.*, **59**, 300–6.

Morrison, P.F., Laske, D.W., Bobo, H., Oldfield, E.H. and Dedrick, R.L. (1994). High-flow microinfusion: tissue penetration and pharmacodynamics. *Am. J. Physiol.*, **266**, R292–305.

Morrow, B.A., Starcevic, V.P., Keil, L.C. and Severs, W.B. (1990). Intracranial hypertension after cerebroventricular infusions in conscious rats. *Am. J. Physiol.*, **258**, R1170–6.

Mounkes, L.C., Zhong, W., Cipres-Palacin, G., Heath, T.D. and Debs, R.J. (1998). Proteoglycans mediate cationic lipsome-DNA complex-based gene delivery in vitro and in vivo. *J. Biol. Chem.*, **273**, 26164–70.

Mouritsen, O.G. and Jorgensen, K. (1997). Small-scale lipid-membrane structure: simulation versus experiment. *Curr. Opin. Struct. Biol.*, **7**, 518–27.

Muchardt, C. and Yaniv, M. (1993). A human homologue of *Saccharomyces cerevisiae* SNF32/SWI2 and *Drosophila* brm genes potentiates transcriptional activation by the glucocorticoid receptor. *EMBO J.*, **12**, 4279–90.

Muckerheide, A., Apple, R.J., Pesce, A.J. and Michael, J.G. (1987). Cationization of protein antigens. *J. Immunol.*, **138**, 833–7.

Mueckler, M., Caruso, C., Baldwin, S.A. et al. (1985). Sequence and structure of a human glucose transporter. *Science*, **229**, 941–5.

Mun-Bryce, S. and Rosenberg, G.A. (1998). Gelatinase B modulates selective opening of the blood–brain barrier during inflammation. *Am. J. Physiol.*, **274** (*Regulatory Integrative Comp. Physiol.*, **43**), R1203–11.

Murphy, L.J., Bell, G.I. and Friesen, H.G. (1987). Tissue distribution of insulin-like growth factor I and II messenger ribonucleic acid in the adult rat. *Endocrinol.*, **120**, 1279–82.

Nadal, A., Fuentes, E., Pastor, J. and McNaughton, P.A. (1995). Plasma albumin is a potent trigger of calcium signals and DNA synthesis in astrocytes. *Proc. Natl Acad. Sci. USA*, **92**, 1426–30.

Nadeau, S. and Rivest, S. (1999). Effects of circulating tumor necrosis factor on the neuronal activity and expression of the genes encoding the tumor necrosis factor receptors (p55 and p75) in the rat brain: a view from the blood–brain barrier. *Neurosci.*, **93**, 1449–64.

Nag, S. (1985). Ultrastructural localization of lectin receptors on cerebral endothelium. *Acta Neuropathol.*, **66**, 105–10.

Nag, S. (1995). Role of the endothelia cytoskeleton in blood–brain barrier permeability to protein. *Acta Neuropathol.*, **90**, 454–60.

Nagamatsu, S., Kornhauser, J.M., Burant, C.F. et al. (1992). Glucose transporter expression in brain. CDNA sequence of mouse GLUT3, the brain facilitative glucose transporter isoform, and identification of sites of expression by in situ hybridization. *J. Biol. Chem.*, **267**, 467–72.

Nagy, Z., Peters, H. and Huttner, I. (1983). Charge-related alterations of the cerebral endothelium. *Lab. Invest.*, **49**, 662–71.

Nakamura, E., Sato, M., Yang, H. et al. (1999). 4F2 (CD98) heavy chain is associated covalently with an amino acid transporter and controls intracellular trafficking and membrane topology of 4F2 heterodimer. *J. Biol. Chem.*, **274**, 3009–16.

Negri, L., Lattanzi, R., Tabacco, F., Scolaro, B. and Rocchi, R. (1998). Glycodermorphins: opioid peptides with potent and prolonged analgesic activity and enhanced blood–brain barrier penetration. *Br. J. Pharmacol.*, **124**, 1516–22.

Nestler, E.J., Walaas, S.I. and Greengard, P. (1984). Neuronal phosphoproteins: physiological and clinical implications. *Science*, **225**, 1357–64.

Neuwelt, E.A. and Rapoport, S.I. (1984). Modification of the blood–brain barrier in the chemotherapy of malignant brain tumors. *Fed. Proc.*, **43**, 214–19.

Neuwelt, E.A., Barnett, P.A., Bigner, D.D. and Frenkel, E.P. (1982). Effects of adrenal cortical steroids and osmotic blood–brain barrier opening on methotrexate delivery to gliomas in the rodent: the factor of the blood–brain barrier. *Proc. Natl Acad. Sci. USA*, **79**, 4420–3.

Nielsen, P.E., Egholm, M., Berg, R.H. and Buchardt, O. (1991). Sequence-selective recognition of DNA by strand displacement with a thymidine-substituted polyamide. *Science*, **254**, 1497–500.

Nielsen, P.E., Egholm, M., Berg, R.H. and Buchardt, O. (1993). Peptide nucleic acids (PNAs): potential anti-sense and anti-gene agents. *Anti-Cancer Drug Des.*, **8**, 53–63.

Nielsen, P.E., Egholm, M. and Buchardt, O. (1994). Peptide nucleic acid (PNA). A DNA mimic with a peptide backbone. *Bioconj. Chem.*, **5**, 3–7.

Niidome, T., Ohmori, N., Ichinose, A. et al. (1997). Binding of cationic α-helical peptides to plasmid DNA and their gene transfer abilities into cells. *J. Biol. Chem.*, **272**, 15307–12.

Nilaver, G., Muldoon, L.L., Kroll, R.A. et al. (1995). Delivery of herpesvirus and adenovirus to nude rat intracerebral tumors after osmotic blood–brain barrier disruption. *Proc. Natl Acad. Sci. USA*, **92**, 9829–33.

Nishikawa, R., Ji, X.-D., Harmon, R.C. et al. (1994). A mutant epidermal growth factor receptor common in human glioma confers enhanced tumorigenicity. *Proc. Natl Acad. Sci. USA*, **91**, 7727–31.

Nishino, H., Kumazaki, M., Fukuda, A. et al. (1997). Acute 3-nitropropionic acid intoxication induces striatal astrocytic cell death and dysfunction of the blood–brain barrier: involvement of dopamine toxicity. *Neurosci. Res.*, **27**, 343–55.

Noble, E.P., Wurtman, R.J. and Axelrod, J. (1967). A simple and rapid method for injecting H$_3$-norepinephrine into the lateral ventricle of the rat brain. *Life Sci.*, **6**, 281–91.

Noe, B., Hagenbuch, B., Stieger, B. and Meier, P.J. (1997). Isolation of a multispecific organic anion and cardiac glycoside transporter from rat brain. *Proc. Natl Acad. Sci. USA*, **94**, 10346–50.

Nordstedt, C., Naslund, J., Tjernberg, L.O. et al. (1994). The Alzheimer Aβ peptide develops protease resistance in association with its polymerization into fibrils. *J. Biol. Chem.*, **269**, 30773–6.

Nutt, J.G., Woodward, W.R., Hammerstad, J.P., Carter, J.H. and Anderson, J.L. (1984). The "on-off" phenomenon in Parkinson's disease: relation to levodopa absorption and transport. *N. Engl. J. Med.*, **310**, 483–8.

Ny, T., Leonardsson, G. and Hsueh, A.J.W. (1988). Cloning and characterization of a cDNA for rat tissue-type plasminogen activator. *DNA*, **7**, 671–7.

O'Donnell, M., Garippa, R.J., O'Neill, N.C., Bolin, D.R. and Cottrell, J.M. (1991). Structure-activity studies of vasoactive intestinal polypeptide. *J. Biol. Chem.*, **266**, 6389–92.

Ogawa, M., Hiraoka, Y., Taniguchi, K. and Aiso, S. (1998). Cloning and expression of a human/mouse Polycomb group gene, ENX-2/Enx-2. *Biochim. Biophys. Acta*, **1395**, 151–8.

Oldendorf, W.H. (1970). Measurement of brain uptake of radiolabeled substances using a tritiated water internal standard. *Brain Res.*, **24**, 372–6.

Oldendorf, W.H. (1971). Brain uptake of radiolabeled amino acids, amines, and hexoses after arterial injection. *Am. J. Physiol.*, **221**, 1629–39.

Oldendorf, W.H. (1973). Carrier-mediated blood–brain barrier transport of short-chain monocarboxylic organic acids. *Am. J. Physiol.*, **224**, 1450.

Oldendorf, W.H., Hyman, S., Braun, L. and Ordendorf, S.Z. (1972). Blood–brain barrier penetration of morphine, codeine, heroin, and methadone after carotid injection. *Science*, **178**, 984.

Oldendorf, W.H., Stoller, B.E. and Harris, F.L. (1993). Blood–brain barrier penetration abolished by N-methyl quaternization of nicotine. *Proc. Natl Acad. Sci. USA*, **90**, 307–11.

Oldendorf, W.H., Stoller, B.E., Tishler, T.A., Williams, J.L. and Oldendorf, S.Z. (1994). Transient blood–brain barrier passage of polar compounds at low pH. *Am. J. Physiol.*, **267**, H2229–36.

Olivier, J.C., Fenart, L., Chauvet, R. et al. (1999). Indirect evidence that drug brain targeting using polysorbate 80-coated polybutylcyanoacrylate nanoparticles is related to toxicity. *Pharm. Res.*, **16**, 1836–42.

Olney, R.C. and Mougey, E.B. (1999). Expression of the components of the insulin-like growth factor axis across the growth-plate. *Mol. Cell. Endocrinol.*, **156**, 63–71.

Osaka, G., Carey, K., Cuthbertson, A. et al. (1996). Pharmacokinetics, tissue distribution, and expression efficiency of plasmid [^{33}P]DNA following intravenous administration of DNA/cationic lipid complexes in mice: use of a novel radionuclide approach. *J. Pharm. Sci.*, **85**, 612–18.

Owens, H., Destaches, C.J. and Dash, A.K. (1999). Simple liquid chromatographic method for the analysis of the blood brain barrier permeability characteristics of ceftriaxone in an experimental rabbit meningitis model. *J. Chromatogr.*, **728**, 97–105.

Oztas, B. and Kucuk, M. (1995). Intracarotid hypothermic saline infusion: a new method for reversible blood–brain barrier disruption in anesthetized rats. *Neurosci. Lett.*, **190**, 203–6.

Paccaud, J.-P., Siddle, K. and Carpentier, J.-L. (1992). Internalization of the human insulin receptor. The insulin-independent pathway. *J. Biol. Chem.*, **267**, 13101–6.

Pahler, A., Hendrickson, W.A., Kolks, M.A.G., Argarana, C.E. and Cantor, C.R. (1987). Characterization and crystallization of core streptavidin. *J. Biol. Chem.*, **262**, 13933–7.

Pan, W., Banks, W.A. and Kastin, A.J. (1998). Permeability of the blood–brain barrier to neurotrophins. *Brain Res.*, **788**, 87–94.

Papahadjopoulos, D., Allen, T.M., Gabizon, A. et al. (1991). Sterically stabilized liposomes: improvements in pharmacokinetics and antitumor therapeutic efficacy. *Proc. Natl Acad. Sci. USA*, **88**, 11460–4.

Pardridge, W.M. (1976). Inorganic mercury: selective effects on blood–brain barrier transport systems. *J. Neurochem.*, **27**, 333–5.

Pardridge, W.M. (1977a). Kinetics of competitive inhibition of neutral amino acid transport across the blood–brain barrier. *J. Neurochem.*, **28**, 103–8.

Pardridge, W.M. (1977b). Regulation of amino acid availability to the brain. In *Nutrition and the Brain*, ed. R.J. Wurtman and J.J. Wurtman, vol. 1, pp. 141–204. New York: Raven Press.

Pardridge, W.M. (1979). Carrier-mediated transport of thyroid hormones through the blood–brain barrier. Primary role of albumin-bound hormone. *Endocrinol.*, **105**, 605–12.

Pardridge, W.M. (1983a). Brain metabolism: a perspective from the blood–brain barrier. *Physiol. Rev.*, **63**, 1481–535.

Pardridge, W.M. (1983b). Neuropeptides and the blood–brain barrier. *Annu. Rev. Physiol.*, **45**, 73–82.

Pardridge, W.M. (1986). Receptor-mediated peptide transport through the blood–brain barrier. *Endocr. Rev.*, **7**, 314–30.

Pardridge, W.M. (1991). *Peptide Drug Delivery to the Brain*, pp. 1–357. New York: Raven Press.

Pardridge, W.M. (1997). Drug delivery to the brain. *J. Cereb. Blood Flow Metab.*, **17**, 713–31.

Pardridge, W.M. (1998a). CNS drug design based on principles of blood–brain barrier transport. *J. Neurochem.*, **70**, 1781–92.

Pardridge, W.M. (1998b). Targeted delivery of hormones to tissues by plasma proteins. In *Handbook of Physiology*. Section 7: *The Endocrine System*, vol. 1: *Cellular Endocrinology*, ed. P.M. Conn, pp. 335–82. New York: Oxford University Press.

Pardridge, W.M. (1998c). Vector-mediated peptide drug targeting to the brain. In *Peptide and Protein Drug Research*, Alfred Benzon Symposium 43, ed. S. Frokjaer, L. Christrup and P. Krogsgaard-Larsen, pp. 381–96. Copenhagen: Munksgaard.

Pardridge, W.M. (1998d). Blood–brain barrier methodology and biology. In *Introduction to the Blood–Brain Barrier: Methodology, Biology, and Pathology*, ed. W.M. Pardridge, pp. 1–8. Cambridge, UK: Cambridge University Press.

Pardridge, W.M. (1999a). A morphological approach to the analysis of blood–brain barrier transport function. In *Brain Barrier Systems*, Alfred Benzon Symposium 45, ed. O. Paulson, G.M. Knudsen and T. Moos, pp. 19–42. Copenhagen: Munksgaard.

Pardridge, W.M. (1999b). Non-invasive drug delivery to the human brain using endogenous blood–brain barrier transport systems. *Pharm. Sci. Technol. Today*, **2**, 49–59.

Pardridge, W.M. and Connor, J.D. (1973). Saturable transport of amphetamine across the blood–brain barrier. *Experientia*, **29**, 302–4.

Pardridge, W.M. and Landaw, E.M. (1985). Testosterone transport in brain: primary role of plasma protein-bound hormone. *Am. J. Physiol.*, **249**, E534–42.

Pardridge, W.M. and Mietus, L.J. (1979). Transport of steroid hormones through the rat blood–brain barrier. Primary role of albumin-bound hormone. *J. Clin. Invest.*, **64**, 145–54.

Pardridge, W.M. and Mietus, L.J. (1980). Palmitate and cholesterol transport through the rat blood–brain barrier. *J. Neurochem.*, **34**, 463–6.

Pardridge, W.M. and Mietus, L.J. (1981). Enkephalin and blood–brain barrier: studies of binding and degradation in isolated brain microvessels. *Endocrinol.*, **109**, 1138–43.

Pardridge, W.M. and Oldendorf, W.H. (1975a). Kinetic analysis of blood–brain barrier transport of amino acids. *Biochim. Biophys. Acta*, **401**, 128–36.

Pardridge, W.M. and Oldendorf, W.H. (1975b). Kinetics of blood–brain barrier transport of hexoses. *Biochim. Biophys. Acta*, **382**, 377–92.

Pardridge, W.M. and Oldendorf, W.H. (1977). Transport of metabolic substrates through the blood–brain barrier. *J. Neurochem.*, **28**, 5–12.

Pardridge, W.M., Crawford, I.L. and Connor, J.D. (1973). Permeability changes in the blood–brain barrier induced by nortriptyline and chlorpromazine. *Toxicol. Appl. Parmacol.*, **26**, 49–57.

Pardridge, W.M., Connor, J.D. and Crawford, I.L. (1975). Permeability changes in the blood–brain barrier: causes and consequences. *CRC Crit. Rev. Toxicol.*, **3**, 159–99.

Pardridge, W.M., Cornford, E.M., Braun, L.D. and Oldendorf, W.H. (1979). Transport of choline and choline analogues through the blood–brain barrier. In *Nutrition and the Brain*, vol. 5, ed. A. Barbeau, J.H. Growdon and R.J. Wurtman, pp. 25–34. New York: Raven Press.

Pardridge, W.M., Van Herle, A.J., Naruse, R.T., Fierer, G. and Costin, A. (1983). In vivo quantification of receptor-mediated uptake of asialoglycoproteins by rat liver. *J. Biol. Chem.*, **258**, 990–4.

Pardridge, W.M., Sakiyama, R. and Fierer, G. (1984). Blood–brain barrier transport and brain sequestration of propranolol and lidocaine. *Am. J. Physiol.*, **247**, R582–8.

Pardridge, W.M., Eisenberg, J. and Yang, J. (1985a). Human blood–brain barrier insulin receptor. *J. Neurochem.*, **44**, 1771–8.

Pardridge, W.M., Yang, J. and Eisenberg, J. (1985b). Blood–brain barrier protein phosphorylation and dephosphorylation. *J. Neurochem.*, **45**, 1141–7.

Pardridge, W.M., Yang, J., Eisenberg, J. and Mietus, L.J. (1986). Antibodies to blood–brain barrier bind selectively to brain capillary endothelial lateral membranes and to a 46K protein. *J. Cereb. Blood Flow Metab.*, **6**, 203–11.

Pardridge, W.M., Eisenberg, J. and Yang, J. (1987a). Human blood–brain barrier transferrin receptor. *Metabolism*, **36**, 892–5.

Pardridge, W.M., Vinters, H.V., Yang, J. et al. (1987b). Amyloid angiopathy of Alzheimer's disease: amino acid composition and partial sequence of a 4200 Dalton peptide isolated from cortical microvessels. *J. Neurochem.*, **49**, 1394–401.

Pardridge, W.M., Triguero, D. and Buciak, J.B. (1989a). Transport of histone through the blood–brain barrier. *J. Pharmacol. Exp. Ther.*, **251**, 821–6.

Pardridge, W.M., Yang, J., Buciak, J. and Tourtellotte, W.W. (1989b). Human brain microvascular DR antigen. *J. Neurosci. Res.*, **23**, 337–41.

Pardridge, W.M., Boado, R.J. and Farrell, C.R. (1990a). Brain-type glucose transporter (GLUT-1) is selectively localized to the blood–brain barrier: studies with quantitative Western blotting and in situ hybridization. *J. Biol. Chem.*, **265**, 18035–40.

Pardridge, W.M., Triguero, D., Buciak, J.L. and Yang, J. (1990b). Evaluation of cationized rat albumin as a potential blood–brain barrier drug transport vector. *J. Pharmacol. Exp. Ther.*, **255**, 893–9.

Pardridge, W.M., Triguero, D., Yang, J. and Cancilla, P.A. (1990c). Comparison of in vitro and in vivo models of drug transcytosis through the blood–brain barrier. *J. Pharmacol. Exp. Ther.*, **253**, 884–91.

Pardridge, W.M., Yang, J., Buciak, J.L. and Boado, R.J. (1990d). Differential expression of 53 kDa and 45 kDa brain capillary-specific proteins by brain capillary endothelium and choroid plexus in vivo and by brain capillary endothelium in tissue culture. *Mol. Cell Neurosci.*, **1**, 20–8.

Pardridge, W.M., Buciak, J.L. and Friden, P.M. (1991). Selective transport of anti-transferrin receptor antibody through the blood–brain barrier in vivo. *J. Pharmacol. Exp. Ther.*, **259**, 66–70.

Pardridge, W.M., Buciak, J.L. and Yoshikawa, T. (1992). Transport of recombinant CD4 through the rat blood–brain barrier. *J. Pharmacol. Exp. Ther.*, **261**, 1175–80.

Pardridge, W.M., Buciak, J.L., Kang, Y.-S. and Boado, R.J. (1993). Protamine-mediated transport of albumin into brain and other organs in the rat. Binding and endocytosis of protamine–albumin complex by microvascular endothelium. *J. Clin. Invest.*, **92**, 2224–9.

Pardridge, W.M., Bickel, U., Buciak, J. et al. (1994a). Cationization of a monoclonal antibody to the human immunodeficiency virus rev protein enhances cellular uptake but does not impair antigen binding of the antibody. *Immunol. Lett.*, **42**, 191–5.

Pardridge, W.M., Kang, Y.-S. and Buciak, J.L. (1994b). Transport of human recombinant brain-derived neurotrophic factor (BDNF) through the rat blood–brain barrier in vivo using vector-mediated peptide drug delivery. *Pharm. Res.*, **11**, 738–46.

Pardridge, W.M., Yoshikawa, T., Kang, Y.-S. and Miller, L.P. (1994c). Blood–brain barrier transport and brain metabolism of adenosine and adenosine analogues. *J. Pharmacol. Exp. Ther.*, **268**, 14–18.

Pardridge, W.M., Boado, R.J. and Kang, Y.-S. (1995a). Vector-mediated delivery of a polyamide ("peptide") nucleic acid analogue through the blood–brain barrier in vivo. *Proc. Natl Acad. Sci. USA*, **92**, 5592–6.

Pardridge, W.M., Kang, Y.-S., Buciak, J.L. and Yang, J. (1995b). Human insulin receptor monoclonal antibody undergoes high affinity binding to human brain capillaries in vitro and rapid transcytosis through the blood–brain barrier in vivo in the primate. *Pharm. Res.*, **12**, 807–16.

Pardridge, W.M., Kang, Y.-S., Yang, J. and Buciak, J.L. (1995c). Enhanced cellular uptake and in vivo biodistribution of a monoclonal antibody following cationization. *J. Pharm. Sci.*, **84**, 943–8.

Pardridge, W.M., Golden, P.L., Kang, Y.-S. and Bickel, U. (1997). Brain microvascular and astrocyte localization of p-glycoprotein. *J. Neurochem.*, **68**, 1278–85.

Pardridge, W.M., Buciak, J., Yang, J. and Wu, D. (1998a). Enhanced endocytosis in cultured human breast carcinoma cells and in vivo biodistribution in rats of a humanized monoclonal antibody following cationization of the protein. *J. Pharmacol. Exp Ther.*, **286**, 548–54.

Pardridge, W.M., Wu. D. and Sakane, T. (1998b). Combined use of carboxyl-directed protein pegylation and vector-mediated blood–brain barrier drug delivery system optimizes brain uptake of brain-derived neurotrophic factor following intravenous administration. *Pharm. Res.*, 15, 576–82.

Paterson, P.Y., Koh, C.-S. and Kwaan, H.C. (1987). Role of the clotting system in the pathogenesis of neuroimmunologic disease. *Fed. Proc.*, 46, 91–6.

Paulson, O.B. and Newman, E.A. (1987). Does the release of potassium from astrocyte endfeet regulate cerebral blood flow? *Science*, 237, 896–8.

Pellerin, L., Pellegri, G., Martin, J.-L. and Magistretti, P.J. (1998). Expression of monocarboxylate transporter mRNAs in mouse brain: support for a distinct role of lactate as an energy substrate for the neonatal vs. adult brain. *Proc. Natl Acad. Sci. USA*, 95, 3990–5.

Peng, H., Wen, T.-C., Tanaka, J. et al. (1998). Epidermal growth factor protects neuronal cells in vivo and in vitro against transient forebrain ischemia- and free radical-induced injuries. *J. Cereb. Blood Flow Metab.*, 18, 349–60.

Penichet, M.L., Kang, Y.-S., Pardridge, W.M., Morrison, S.L. and Shin, S.-U. (1999). An anti-transferrin receptor antibody-avidin fusion protein serves as a delivery vehicle for effective brain targeting in an animal model. Initial applications in antisense drug delivery to the brain. *J. Immunol.*, 163, 4421–6.

Perales, J.C., Ferkol, T., Beegen, H., Ratnoff, O.D. and Hanson, R.W. (1994). Gene transfer in vivo: sustained expression and regulation of genes introduced into the liver by receptor-targeted uptake. *Proc. Natl Acad. Sci. USA*, 91, 4086–90.

Perales, J.C., Grossmann, G.A., Molas, M. et al. (1997). Biochemical and functional characterization of DNA complexes capable of targeting genes to haptocytes via the asialoglycoprotein receptor. *J. Biol. Chem.*, 272, 7398–407.

Pesonen, M., Bravo, R. and Simons, K. (1984). Transcytosis of the G protein of vesicular stomatitis virus after implantation into the apical membrane of Madin-Darby canine kidney cells. *J. Cell. Biol.*, 99, 803–9.

Peters, T. (1985). Serum albumin. *Adv. Protein Chem.*, 37, 161–245.

Petty, B.G., Cornblath, D.R., Adornato, B.T. et al. (1994). The effect of systematically administered recombinant human nerve growth factor in healthy human subjects. *Ann. Neurol.*, 36, 244–6.

Pineda, M., Fernandez, E., Torrents, D. et al. (1999). Identification of a membrane protein, LAT-2, that co-expresses with 4F2 heavy chain, an L-type amino acid transport activity with broad specificity for small and large zwitterionic amino acids. *J. Biol. Chem.*, 274, 19738–44.

Plank, C., Oberhauser, B., Mechtler, K., Koch, C. and Wagner, E. (1994). The influence of endosome-disruptive peptides on gene transfer using synthetic virus-like gene transfer systems. *J. Biol. Chem.*, 269, 12918–24.

Plank, C., Tang, M.X., Wolfe, A.R. and Szoka, F.C. (1999). Branched cationic peptides for gene delivery: role of type and number of cationic residues in formation and in vitro activity of DNA polyplexes. *Hum. Gene Ther.*, 10, 319–32.

Plate, K.H. and Risau, W. (1995). Angiogenesis in malignant gliomas. *Glia*, 15, 339–47.

Poduslo, J.F. and Curran, G.L. (1996). Permeability at the blood–brain and blood–nerve barriers of the neurotrophic factors: NGF, CNTF, NT-3, BDNF. *Mol. Brain. Res.*, 36, 280–6.

Poduslo, J.F., Curran, G.L., Sanyal, B. and Selkoe, D.J. (1999). Receptor-mediated transport of human amyloid β-protein 1–40 and 1–42 at the blood–brain barrier. *Neurobiol. Dis.*, 6, 190–9.

Pollack, I.F. and Lund, R.D. (1990). The blood–brain barrier protects foreign antigens in the brain from immune attack. *Exp. Neurol.*, 108, 114–21.

Polt, R., Porreca, F., Szabo, L.Z. et al. (1994). Glycopeptide enkephalin analogues produce analgesia in mice: evidence for penetration of the blood–brain barrier. *Proc. Natl Acad. Sci. USA*, 91, 7114–18.

Press, O.W., Shan, D., Howell-Clark, J. et al. (1996). Comparative metabolism and retention of iodine-125, yttrium-90, and indium-111 radioimmunoconjugates by cancer cells. *Cancer Res.*, 56, 2123–9.

Preston, E., Foster, D.O. and Mills, P.A. (1998). Effects of radiochemical impurities on measurements of transfer constants for [^{14}C]sucrose permeation of normal and injured blood–brain barrier of rats. *Brain Res.*, 45, 111–16.

Price, R.W., Brew, B., Sidtis, J. et al. (1988). The brain in AIDS: central nervous system HIV-1 infection and AIDS dementia complex. *Science*, 239, 586–92.

Prior, R., D'Urso, D., Frank, R. et al. (1996). Selective binding of soluble Aβ1–40 and Aβ1–42 to a subset of senile plaques. *Am. J. Pathol.*, 148, 1749–56.

Pullen, R.G.L., Candy, J.M., Morris, C.M. et al. (1990). Gallium-67 as a potential marker for aluminum transport in rat brain: implications for Alzheimer's disease. *J. Neurochem.*, 55, 251–9.

Puro, D.G. and Agardh, E. (1984). Insulin-mediated regulation of neuronal maturation. *Science*, 225, 1170–2.

Queen, C., Schneider, W.P., Selick, H.E. et al. (1989). A humanized antibody that binds to the interleukin 2 receptor. *Proc. Natl Acad. Sci. USA*, 86, 10029–33.

Quist, A.P., Rhee, S.K., Lin, H. and Lal, R. (2000). Physiological role of gap-junctional hemichannels extracellular calcium-dependent isoosmotic volume regulation. *J. Cell. Biol.*, 148, 1063–74.

Rabchevsky, A.G., Degos, J.-D. and Dreyfus, P.A. (1999). Peripheral injections of Freund's adjuvant in mice provoke leakage of serum proteins through the blood–brain barrier without inducing reactive gliosis. *Brain Res.*, 832, 84–96.

Radler, J.O., Kottover, I., Salditt, T. and Safinya, C.R. (1997). Structure of DNA-cationic liposome complexes: DNA intercalation in multilamellar membranes in distant interhelical packing regimes. *Science*, 275, 810–14.

Ram, Z., Culver, K.W., Oshiro, E.M. et al. (1997). Therapy of malignant brain tumors by intratumor implantation of retroviral vector-producing cells. *Nat. Med.*, 3, 1354–61.

Rapaka, R.S. and Porreca, F. (1991). Development of delta opioid peptides as nonaddicting analgesics. *Pharm. Res.*, 8, 1–8.

Rapoport, S.I., Fredericks, W.R., Ohno, K. and Pettigrew, K.D. (1980). Quantitative aspects of reversible osmotic opening of the blood–brain barrier. *Am. J. Physiol.*, 238, R421–31.

Raso, V. and Basala, M. (1984). A highly cytotoxic human transferrin-ricin A chain conjugate used to select receptor-modified cells. *J. Biol. Chem.*, 259, 1143–9.

Reed, R.G. and Burrington, C.M. (1989). The albumin receptor effect may be due to a surface-induced conformational change in albumin. *J. Biol. Chem.*, 264, 9867–72.

Regier, D.A., Boyd, J.H., Burke, J.D. Jr. et al. (1988). One-month prevalence of mental disorders in the United States. *Arch. Gen. Psychiatry*, **45**, 977–86.

Reinhardt, R.R. and Bondy, C.A. (1994). Insulin-like growth factors cross the blood–brain barrier. *Endocrinol.*, **135**, 1753–61.

Remen, E.C., Demel, R.A., De Grier, J. et al. (1969). Studies on the lysis of red cells and bimolecular lipids leaflets by synthetic lysolecithins, lecithins, and structural analogs. *Chem. Phys. Lipids*, **3**, 221–33.

Renkin, E.M. (1959). Transport of potassium-42 from blood to tissue in isolated mammalian skeletal muscles. *Am. J. Physiol.*, **197**, 1205–10.

Rennels, M.L., Gregory, T.F., Blaumanis, O.R., Fujimoto, K. and Grady, P.A. (1985). Evidence for a 'paravascular' fluid circulation in the mammalian central nervous system, provided by the rapid distribution of tracer protein throughout the brain from the subarachnoid space. *Brain Res.*, **326**, 47–63.

Reynolds, M.A., Arnold, L.J. Jr., Almazan, M.T. et al. (1994). Triple-strand-forming methylphosphonate oligodeoxynucleotides targeted to mRNA efficiently block protein synthesis. *Proc. Natl Acad. Sci. USA*, **91**, 12433–7.

Rigotti, A., Acton, S.L. and Krieger, M. (1995). The class B scavenger receptors SR-BI and CD36 are receptors for anionic phospholipids. *J. Biol. Chem.*, **270**, 16221–4.

Risau, W., Dingler, A., Albrecht, U., Dehouck, M.P. and Cecchelli, R. (1992). Blood–brain barrier pericytes are the main source of γ-glutamyltranspeptidase activity in brain capillaries. *J. Neurochem.*, **58**, 667–72.

Roach, A., Boylan, K.B., Horvath, S., Prusiner, S.B. and Hood, L.E. (1983). Characterization of cloned cDNA representing rat myelin basic protein: absence of expression in brain of shiverer mutant mice. *Cell*, **34**, 799–806.

Roberts, K.P. and Griswold, M.D. (1990). Characterization of rat transferrin receptor cDNA: the regulation of transferrin receptor mRNA in testes in Sertoli cells in culture. *Mol. Cell. Endocrinol.*, **14**, 531–42.

Roberts, R.L., Fine, R.E. and Sandra, A. (1993). Receptor-mediated endocytosis of transferrin at the blood–brain barrier. *J. Cell. Sci.*, **104**, 521–32.

Rockwel, P., O'Connor, W.J., King, K. et al. (1997). Cell-surface perturbations of the epidermal growth factor and vascular endothelial growth factor receptors by phosphorothioate oligodeoxynucleotides. *Proc. Natl Acad. Sci. USA*, **94**, 6523–8.

Rodriguez-Romero, A., Almog, O., Tordova, M., Randhawa, Z. and Gilliland, G.L. (1998). Primary and tertiary structures of the Fab fragment of a monoclonal anti-E-selectin 7A9 antibody that inhibits neutrophil attachment to endothelial cells. *J. Biol. Chem.*, **273**, 11770–5.

Roguska, M.A., Pedersen, J.T., Henry, A.H. et al. (1996). A comparison of two murine monoclonal antibodies humanized by CDR-grafting and variable domain resurfacing. *Prot. Engineering*, **9**, 895–904.

Romanic, A.M., White, R.F., Arleth, A.J., Ohlstein, E.H. and Barone, F.C. (1998). Matrix metalloproteinase expression increases after cerebral focal ischemia in rats: inhibition of matrix metalloproteinase-9 reduces infarct size. *Stroke*, **29**, 1020–30.

Rosebrough, S.F. (1993). Plasma stability and pharmacokinetics of radiolabeled desferroxamine-biotin derivatives. *J. Pharmacol. Exp. Ther.*, **265**, 408–15.

Rosenberg, G.A., Kyner, W.T. and Estrada, E. (1980). Bulk flow of brain interstitial fluid under normal and hyperosmolar conditions. *Am. J. Physiol.*, **238**, F42–9.

Rosenberg, M.B., Hawrot, E. and Breakefield, X.O. (1986). Receptor binding activities of biotinylated derivatives of β-nerve growth factor. *J. Neurochem.*, **46**, 641–8.

Roskams, A.J. and Connor, J.R. (1990). Aluminum access to the brain: a role for transferrin and its receptor. *Proc. Natl Acad. Sci. USA*, **87**, 9024–7.

Rothman, A.R., Freireich, E.J., Gaskins, J.R., Patlak, C.S. and Rall, D.P. (1961). Exchange of inulin and dextran between blood and cerebrospinal fluid. *Am. J. Physiol.*, **201**, 1145–8.

Rouselle, C., Clair, P., Lefauconnier, J.-M. et al. (2000). New advances in the transport of doxorubicin through the blood–brain barrier by a peptide vector-mediated strategy. *Mol. Pharmacol.*, **57**, 679–86.

Rusckowski, M., Paganelli, G., Hnatowich, D.J. et al. (1996). Imaging osteomyelitis with streptavidin and indium-111-labeled biotin. *J. Nucl. Med.*, **37**, 1655–62.

Ryser, H.J.-P., Levy, E.M., Mandel, R. and DiSciullo, G.J. (1994). Inhibition of human immunodeficiency virus infection by agents that interfere with thiol-disulfide interchange upon virus-receptor interaction. *Proc. Natl Acad. Sci. USA*, **91**, 4559–63.

Saija, A., Princi, P., Pisani, A. et al. (1992). Blood–brain barrier dysfunctions following systemic injection of kainic acid in the rat. *Life Sci.*, **51**, 467–77.

Saija, A., Princi, P., Trombetta, D., Lanza, M. and Pasquale, A.D. (1997). Changes in the permeability of the blood–brain barrier following sodium dodecyl sulphate administration in the rat. *Exp. Brain Res.*, **115**, 546–51.

Saito, Y., Buciak, J., Yang, J. and Pardridge, W.M. (1995). Vector-mediated delivery of [^{125}I]- labeled β-amyloid peptide Aβ$^{1-40}$ through the blood–brain barrier and binding to Alzheimer's disease amyloid of the Aβ$^{1-40}$/vector complex. *Proc. Natl Acad. Sci. USA*, **92**, 10227–31.

Sakamoto, A. and Ido, T. (1993). Liposome targeting to rat brain: effect of osmotic opening of the blood–brain barrier. *Brain Res.*, **629**, 171–5.

Sakanaka, M., Wen, T.-C., Matsuda, S. et al. (1998). In vivo evidence that erythropoietin protects neurons from ischemic damage. *Proc. Natl Acad. Sci. USA*, **95**, 4635–40.

Sakane, T. and Pardridge, W.M. (1997). Carboxyl-directed pegylation of brain-derived neutrophic factor markedly reduces systemic clearance with minimal loss of biologic activity. *Pharm. Res.*, **14**, 1085–91.

Sakane, T., Akizuki, M., Yamashita, S. et al. (1991). The transport of a drug to the cerebrospinal fluid directly from the nasal cavity: the relation to the lipophilicity of the drug. *Chem. Pharm. Bull.*, **39**, 2456–8.

Salahuddin, T.S., Johansson, B.B., Kalimo, H. and Olsson, Y. (1988). Structural changes in the rat brain after carotid infusions of hyperosmolar solutions. *Acta Neuropathol.*, **77**, 5–13.

Salgar, S.K., Kunz, H.W. and Gill, T.J. (1995). Nucleotide sequence and structural analysis of the rat RT1.Eu and RT1.Aw3l genes, and of genes related to RT1.O and RT1.C. *Immunogenetics*, **42**, 244–53.

Samii, A., Bickel, U., Stroth, U. and Pardridge, W.M. (1994). Blood–brain barrier transport of neuropeptides: analysis with a metabolically stable dermorphin analogue. *Am. J. Physiol.*, **267**, E124–31.

Samuel, A., Paganelli, G., Chiesa, R. et al. (1996). Detection of prosthetic vascular graft infection using avidin/indium-111-biotin scintigraphy. *J. Nucl. Med.*, **37**, 55–61.

Schabitz, W.-R., Schwab, S., Spranger, M. and Hacke, W. (1997). Intraventricular brain-derived neurotrophic factor reduces infarct size after focal cerebral ischemia in rats. *J. Cereb. Flow Metab.*, **17**, 500–6.

Schackert, G., Fan, D., Nayar, R. and Fidler, I.J. (1989). Arrest and retention of multilamellar liposomes in the brain of normal mice or mice bearing experimental brain metastases. *Selective Cancer Ther.*, **5**, 73–9.

Schechter, B., Silberman, R., Arnon, R. and Wilchek, M. (1990). Tissue distribution of avidin and streptavidin injected to mice. Effect of avidin carbohydrate, streptavidin truncation and exogenous biotin. *Eur. J. Biochem.*, **189**, 327–31.

Scheepens, A., Sirimanne, E., Beilharz, E. et al. (1999). Alterations in the neural growth hormone axis following hypoxic–ischemic brain injury. *Mol. Brain Res.*, **68**, 88–100.

Schena, M., Shalon, D., Davis, R.W. and Brown, P.O. (1995). Quantitative monitoring of gene expression patterns with a complementary DNA microarray. *Science*, **270**, 467–70.

Schenk, D., Barbour, R., Dunn, W. et al. (1999). Immunization with amyloid-β attenuates Alzheimer-disease-like pathology in the PDAPP mouse. *Nature*, **400**, 173–7.

Schinkel, A.H., Wagenaar, E., Deemter, L., Mol, C.A. and Borst, P. (1995). Absence of the mdr1a p-glycoprotein in mice affects tissue distribution and pharmacokinetics of dexamethasone, digoxin, and cyclosporin A. *J. Clin. Invest.*, **96**, 1698–705.

Schlageter, N.L., Carson, R.E. and Rapoport, S.I. (1987). Examination of blood–brain barrier permeability in dementia of the Alzheimer type with [^{68}Ga]EDTA and positron emission tomography. *J. Cereb. Blood Flow Metab.*, **7**, 1–8.

Schnitzer, J.E., Liu, J. and Oh, P. (1995). Endothelial caveolae have the molecular transport machinery for vesicle budding, docking, and fusion including VAMP, NSF, SNAP, annexins, and GPTases. *J. Biol. Chem.*, **270**, 14399–404.

Schröder, U. and Sabel, B.A. (1996). Nanoparticles, a drug carrier system to pass the blood–brain barrier, permit central analgesic effects of i.v. dalargin injections. *Brain Res.*, **710**, 121–4.

Schuberth, J. and Jenden, D.J. (1975). Transport of choline from plasma to cerebrospinal fluid in the rabbit with reference to the origin of choline and to acetylcholine metabolism in brain. *Brain Res.*, **84**, 245–56.

Schwartz, M.W., Seeley, R.J., Campfield, L.A., Burn, P. and Baskin, D.G. (1996). Identification of targets of leptin action in rat hypothalamus. *J. Clin. Invest.*, **98**, 1101–6.

Schwarze, S.R., Ho, A., Vocero-Akbani, A. and Dowdy, S.F. (1999). In vivo protein transduction: delivery of a biologically active protein into the mouse. *Science*, **285**, 1569–72.

Seeds, N.W., Basham, M.E. and Haffke, S.P. (1999). Neuronal migration is retarded in mice lacking the tissue plasminogen activator gene. *Proc. Natl Acad. Sci. USA*, **96**, 14118–23.

Seetharaman, S., Barrand, M.A., Maskell, L. and Scheper, R.J. (1998). Multidrug resistance-related transport proteins in isolated human brain microvessels and in cell cultured from these isolates. *J. Neurochem.*, **70**, 1151–9.

Segovia, J., Vergara, P. and Brenner, M. (1998). Astrocyte-specific expression of tyrosine hydroxylase after intracerebral gene transfer induces behavioral recovery in experimental Parkinsonism. *Gene Ther.*, **5**, 1650–5.

Service, R.F. (1995). Dendrimers: dream molecules approach real applications. *Science*, **267**, 458–9.

Shapiro, W.R., Voorhies, R.M., Hiesiger, E.M. et al. (1988). Pharmacokinetics of tumor cell exposure to [¹⁴C]methotrexate after intracarotid administration without and with hyperosmotic opening of the blood–brain barrier and blood–tumor barriers in rat brain tumors: a quantitative autoradiographic study. *Cancer Res.*, **48**, 694–701.

Shapiro, M.A., Fitzsimmons, S.P. and Clark, K.J. (1999). Characterization of a B cell surface antigen with homology to the S100 protein MRP8. *Biochem. Biophys. Res. Commun.*, **263**, 17–22.

Shashoua, V.E. and Hesse, G.W. (1996). N-Docosahexanoyl, 3 hydroxytyramine: a dopaminergic compound that penetrates the blood–brain barrier and suppresses appetite. *Life Sci.*, **58**, 1347–57.

Shechter, Y., Maron, R., Elias, D. and Cohen, I.R. (1982). Autoantibodies to insulin receptor spontaneously develop as anti-idiotypes in mice immunized with insulin. *Nature*, **216**, 542–5.

Shi, N. and Pardridge, W.M. (2000). Non-invasive gene targeting to the brain. *Proc. Natl Acad. Sci. USA*, **97**, 7567–72.

Shi, N., Boado, R.J. and Pardridge, W.M. (2000). Antisense imaging of gene expression in the brain in vivo. *Proc. Natl Acad. Sci. USA*, **97**, 14709–14.

Shih, L.B., Thorpe, S.R., Griffiths, G.L. et al. (1994). The processing and fate of antibodies and their radiolabels bound to the surface of tumor cells in vitro: a comparison of nine radiolabels. *J. Nucl. Med.*, **35**, 899–908.

Shimura, T., Tabata, S., Ohnishi, T., Terasaki, T. and Tsuji, A. (1991). Transport mechanism of a new behaviorally highly potent adrenocorticotropic hormone (ACTH) analog, ebiratide, through the blood–brain barrier. *J. Pharmacol. Exp. Ther.*, **258**, 459–65.

Shin, S.Y., Shimizu, M., Ohtaki, T. and Munekata, E. (1995). Synthesis and biological activity of N-terminal-truncated derivatives of human epidermal growth factor (h-EGF). *Peptides*, **16**, 205–10.

Shin, S.U., Wu, D., Ramanathan, R., Pardridge, W.M. and Morrison, S.L. (1997). Functional and pharmacokinetic properties of antibody/avidin fusion proteins. *J. Immunol.*, **158**, 4797–804.

Shoulson, I. (1998). Experimental therapeutics of neurodegenerative disorders: unmet needs. *Science*, **282**, 1072–4.

Siakotos, A.N., Rouser, G. and Fleischer, S. (1969). Isolation of highly purified human and bovine brain endothelial cells and nuclei and their phospholipid composition. *Lipids*, **4**, 234–9.

Sidtis, J.J., Gatsonis, C., Price, R.W. et al. (1993). Zidovudine treatment of the AIDS dementia complex: results of a placebo-controlled trial. *Ann. Neurol.*, **33**, 343–9.

Siminoski, K., Gonnella, P., Bernanke, J. et al. (1986). Uptake and transepithelial transport of nerve growth factor in suckling rat ileum. *J. Cell. Biol.*, **103**, 1979–90.

Simionescu, N. (1979). The microvascular endothelium segmental differentiations; transcytosis; selective distribution of anionic sites. In *Advances in Inflammation Research*, ed. G. Weissmann, B. Samuelsson and R. Paoletti, pp. 61–70. New York: Raven Press.

Skarlatos, S., Yoshikawa, T. and Pardridge, W.M. (1995). Transport of [¹²⁵I] transferrin through the blood–brain barrier in vivo. *Brain Res.*, **683**, 164–71.

Skorupa, A.F., Fisher, K.J., Wilson, J.M., Parente, M.K. and Wolfe, J.H. (1999). Sustained production of β-glucuronidase from localized sites after AAV vector gene transfer results in widespread distribution of enzyme and reversal of lysosomal storage lesions in a large volume of brain in mucopolysaccharidosis VII mice. *Exp. Neurol.*, **160**, 17–27.

Smith, M.-L., Bendek, G., Dahlgren, N. et al. (1984). Models for studying long-term recovery following forebrain ischemia in the rat. A 2-vessel occlusion model. *Acta Neurol. Scand.*, **69**, 385–401.

Smith, J.G., Raper, S.E., Wheeldon, E.B. et al. (1997). Intracranial administration of adenovirus expressing HSV-TK in combination with ganciclovir produces a dose-dependent, self-limiting inflammatory response. *Hum. Gene Ther.*, **8**, 943–54.

Sobolev, A.S., Rosenkranz, A.A., Smirnova, O.A. et al. (1998). Receptor-mediated transfection of murine and ovine mammary glands in vivo. *J. Biol. Chem.*, **273**, 7928–33.

Soderquist, A.M. and Carpenter, G. (1983). Developments in the mechanism of growth factor action: activation of protein kinase by epidermal growth factor. *Fed. Proc.*, **42**, 2615–20.

Song, Y.K., Liu, F., Chu, S. and Liu, D. (1997). Characterization of cationic liposome-mediated gene transfer in vivo by intravenous administration. *Hum. Gene Ther.*, **8**, 1585–94.

Soos, M.A., Siddle, K., Baron, M.D. et al. (1986). Monoclonal antibodies reacting with multiple epitopes on the human insulin receptor. *Biochem. J.*, **235**, 199–208.

Soos, M.A., O'Brien, R.M., Brindle, N.P.J. et al. (1989). Monoclonal antibodies to the insulin receptor mimic metabolic effects of insulin but do not stimulate receptor autophosphorylation in transfected NIH 3T3 fibroblasts. *Proc. Natl Acad. Sci. USA*, **86**, 5217–21.

Sparrow, L.G., McKern, N.M., Gorman, J.J. et al. (1997). The disulfide bonds in the C-terminal domains of the human insulin receptor ectodomain. *J. Biol. Chem.*, **272**, 29460–7.

Spector, R. (1981). Penetration of ascorbic acid from cerebrospinal fluid into brain. *Exp. Neurol.*, **72**, 645–53.

Spector, R. (1988). Transport of amantadine and rimantadine through the blood–brain barrier. *J. Pharmacol. Exp. Ther.*, **244**, 516–19.

Spector, R., Sivesind, C. and Kinzenbaw, D. (1986). Pantothenic acid transport through the blood–brain barrier. *J. Neurochem.*, **47**, 966–71.

Speth, R.C. and Harik, S.I. (1985). Angiotensin II receptor binding sites in brain microvessels. *Proc. Natl Acad. Sci. USA*, **82**, 6340–3.

Spigelman, M.K., Zappulla, R.A., Goldberg, J.D. et al. (1984). Effect of intracarotid etoposide on opening the blood–brain barrier. *Cancer Drug Del.*, **1**, 207–11.

Stacker, S.A., Stenvers, K., Caesar, C. et al. (1999). Biosynthesis of vascular endothelial growth factor-D involves proteolytic processing which generates non-covalent homodimers. *J. Biol. Chem.*, **274**, 32127–36.

Steele-Perkins, G., Turner, J., Edman, J.C. et al. (1988). Expression and characterization of a functional human insulin-like growth factor I receptor. *J. Biol. Chem.*, **263**, 11486–92.

Steil, G.M., Ader, M., Moore, D.M., Rebrin, K. and Bergman, R.N. (1996). Transendothelial insulin transport is not saturable in vivo. *J. Clin. Invest.*, **97**, 1497–503.

Stein, W.D. (1967). *The Movement of Molecules Across Cell Membranes*. New York: Academic Press.

Stein, C.A. and Cheng, Y.-C. (1993). Antisense oligonucleotides as therapeutic agents – is the bullet really magical? *Science*, **261**, 1004–12.

Steingold, K.A., Cefalu, W., Pardridge, W.M., Judd, H.L. and Chaudhuri, G. (1986). Enhanced hepatic extraction of estrogens used for replacement therapy. *J. Clin. Endocrinol. Metab.*, **62**, 761–6.

Stockinger, W., Hengstschlager-Ottnad, E., Novak, S. et al. (1998). The low density lipoprotein receptor gene family. *J. Biol. Chem.*, **273**, 32213–21.

Stott, K., Blackvurn, J.M., Butler, P.J.G. and Perutz, M. (1995). Incorporations of glutamine repeats makes protein oligomerize: implications for neurodegenerative diseases. *Proc. Natl Acad. Sci. USA*, **92**, 6509–13.

Stroemer, R.P. and Rothwell, N.J. (1997). Cortical protection by localized striatal injection of IL-1ra following cerebral ischemia in the rat. *J. Cereb. Blood Flow Metab.*, **17**, 597–604.

Sugawa, N., Uedo, S., Nakagawa, Y. et al. (1998). An antisense EGFR oligodeoxynucleotide enveloped in Lipofectin induces growth inhibition in human malignant gliomas in vitro. *J. Neuro-Oncol.*, **39**, 237–44.

Szentistvanyi, I., Patlak, C.S., Ellis, R.A. and Cserr, H.F. (1984). Drainage of interstitial fluid from different regions of rat brain. *Am. J. Physiol.*, **246**, F835–44.

Sztriha, L. and Betz, A.L. (1991). Oleic acid reversibly opens the blood–brain barrier. *Brain Res.*, **550**, 257–62.

Tafani, J.A.M., Lazorthes, Y., Danet, B. et al. (1989). Human brain and spinal cord scan after intracerebroventricular administration of iodine-123 morphine. *Int. J. Radiat. Appl. Instrum. Part B*, **16**, 505–9.

Takada, Y., Vistica, D.T., Greig, N.H. et al. (1992). Rapid high-affinity transport of a chemotherapeutic amino acid across the blood–brain barrier. *Cancer Res.*, **52**, 2191–6.

Takanaga, H., Tamai, I., Inaba, S. et al. (1995). cDNA cloning and functional characterization of rat intestinal monocarboxylate transporter. *Biochem. Biophys. Res. Commun.*, **217**, 370–7.

Takasawa, K., Terasaki, T., Suzuki, H. and Sugiyama, Y. (1997). In vivo evidence for carrier-mediated efflux transport of 3′-azido-3′-deoxythymidine and 2′,3′-dideoxyinosine across the blood–brain barrier via a probenecid-sensitive transport system. *J. Pharmacol. Exp. Ther.*, **281**, 369–35.

Tamaoka, A., Sawamura, N., Odaka, A. et al. (1995). Amyloid β protein 1–42/43 (Aβ 1–42/43) in cerebellar diffuse plaques: enzyme-linked immunosorbent assay and immunocytochemical study. *Brain Res.*, **679**, 151–6.

Tartaglia, L.A. (1997). The leptin receptor. *J. Biol. Chem.*, **272**, 6093–6.

Tavitan, B., Terrazzino, S., Kuhnast, B. et al. (1998). In vivo imaging of oligonucleotides with positron emission tomography. *Nat. Med.*, **4**, 467–71.

Terasaki, T. and Pardridge, W.M. (1987). Stereospecificity of triiodothyronine transport into brain, liver, and salivary gland: role of carrier- and plasma protein-mediated transport. *Endocrinol.*, **121**, 1185–91.

Terasaki, T. and Pardridge, W.M. (1988). Restricted transport of AZT and dideoxynucleosides through the blood–brain barrier. *J. Infect. Dis.*, **158**, 630–2.

Tewari, M., Mohn, K.L., Yue, F.E. and Taub, R. (1992). Sequence of rat RL/IF-1 encoding an IkappaB, and comparison with related proteins containing notch-like repeats. *Nucl. Acid Res.*, **20**, 607.

The BDNF Study Group (1999). A controlled trial of recombinant methionyl human BDNF in ALS (phase III). *Neurol.*, **52**, 1427–33.

Thomas, S.A. and Segal, M.B. (1997). The passage of azidodeoxythymidine into and within the central nervous system: does it follow the parent compound, thymidine? *J. Pharmacol. Exp. Ther.*, **281**, 1211–18.

Thorne, R.G., Emory, C.R., Ala, T.A. and Frey, W.H. (1995). Quantitative analysis of the olfactory pathway for drug delivery to the brain. *Brain Res.*, **692**, 278–82.

Tishler, D.M., Weinberg, K.I., Hinton, D.R. et al. (1995). MDR1 gene expression in brain of patients with medically intractable epilepsy. *Epilepsia*, **36**, 1–6.

Tjuvajev, J.G., Avril, N., Oku, T. et al. (1998). Imaging herpes virus thymidine kinase gene transfer and expression by positron emission tomography. *Cancer Res.*, **58**, 4333–41.

Tomatis, R., Marastoni, M., Balboni, G. et al. (1997). Synthesis and pharmacological activity of deltorphin and dermorphin-related glycopeptides. *J. Med. Chem.*, **40**, 2048–52.

Tomiyasu, K., Satoh, E., Oda, Y. et al. (1998). Gene transfer in vitro and in vivo with Epstein–Barr virus-based episomal vector results in markedly high transient expression in rodent cells. *Biochem. Biophys. Res. Commun.*, **253**, 733–8.

Torrence, P.F., Kinjo, J.-E., Khamnei, S. and Greig, N.H. (1993). Synthesis and pharmacokinetics of a dihydropyridine chemical delivery system for the antiimmunodeficiency virus agent dideoxycytidine. *J. Med. Chem.*, **36**, 529–37.

Träuble, H. (1971). The movement of molecules across lipid membranes: a molecular theory. *J. Membrane Biol.*, **4**, 193–208.

Triguero, D., Buciak, J.B., Yang, J. and Pardridge, W.M. (1989). Blood–brain barrier transport of cationized immunoglobulin G. Enhanced delivery compared to native protein. *Proc. Natl Acad. Sci. USA*, **86**, 4761–5.

Triguero, D., Buciak, J.B. and Pardridge, W.M. (1990). Capillary depletion method for quantification of blood–brain barrier transport of circulating peptides and plasma proteins. *J. Neurochem.*, **54**, 1882–8.

Triguero, D., Buciak, J.L. and Pardridge, W.M. (1991). Cationization of immunoglobulin G results in enhanced organ uptake of the protein following intravenous administration in rats and primate. *J. Pharmacol. Exp. Ther.*, **258**, 186–92.

Trouche, D., Chalony, C.L., Muchardt, C., Yaniv, M. and Kouzarides, T. (1997). RB and hbrm cooperate to repress the activation functions of E2F1. *Proc. Natl Acad. Sci. USA*, **94**, 11268–73.

Tseng, L.Y.-H., Brown, A.L., Yang, Y.W.-H. et al. (1989). The fetal rat binding protein for insulin-like growth factors is expressed in the choroid plexus and cerebrospinal fluid of adult rats. *Mol. Endocrinol.*, **3**, 1559–68.

Tsukamoto, H., Boado, R. and Pardridge, W.M. (1996). Differential expression in glioblastoma multiforme and cerebral hemangioblastoma of cytoplasmic proteins that bind to two different domains within the 3′-untranslated region of the human GLUT1 glucose transporter mRNA. *J. Clin. Invest.*, **97**, 2823–32.

Tsukamoto, H., Boado, R.J. and Pardridge, W.M. (1997). Site-directed deletion of a 10-nucleotide domain of the 3′-untranslated region of the GLUT1 glucose transporter mRNA eliminates cytosolic protein binding in human brain tumors and induction of reporter gene expression. *J. Neurochem.*, **68**, 1278–85.

Tsuzuki, N., Hama, T., Kawada, M. et al. (1994). Adamantane as a brain-directed drug carrier for poorly absorbed drug. AZT derivatives conjugated with the 1-adamantane moiety. *J. Pharm. Sci.*, **83**, 481–4.

Tyfield, L.A. and Holton, J.B. (1976). The effect of high concentrations of histidine on the level of other amino acids in plasma and brain of the mature rat. *J. Neurochem.*, **26**, 101–5.

Tyler, B.M., Jansen, K., McCormick, D.J. et al. (1999). Peptide nucleic acids targeted to the neurotensin receptor and administered i.p. cross the blood–brain barrier and specifically reduce gene expression. *Proc. Natl Acad. Sci. USA*, **96**, 7053–8.

Ueda, F., Raja, K.B., Simpson, R.J., Trowbridge, I.S. and Bradbury, M.W.B. (1993). Rate of ^{59}Fe uptake into brain and cerebrospinal fluid and the influence thereon of antibodies against the transferrin receptor. *J. Neurochem.*, **60**, 106–13.

Ueno, T., Takahashi, K., Matsuguchi, T., Endo, H. and Yamamoto, M. (1988). Transcriptional deviation of the rat insulin-like growth factor II gene initiated at three alternative leader exons between neonatal tissues and ascites hepatomas. *Biochim. Biophys. Acta*, **950**, 411–19.

Ueno, T., Takahashi, K., Matsuguchi, T. et al. (1989). Multiple polyadenylation sites in a large 3′-mast exon of the rat insulin-like growth factor II gene. *Biochim. Biophys. Acta*, **1009**, 27–34.

Unterberg, A., Wahl, M. and Baethmann, A. (1984). Effects of bradykinin on permeability and diameter of pial vessels in vivo. *J. Cereb. Blood Flow Metab.*, **4**, 574–85.

Urabe, T., Hattori, N., Nagamatsu, S., Sawa, H. and Mizuno, Y. (1996). Expression of glucose transporters in rat brain following transient focal ischemic injury. *J. Neurochem.*, **67**, 265–71.

Valentino, K.L., Pham, H., Ocrant, I. and Rosenfeld, R.G. (1988). Distribution of insulin-like growth factor II receptor immunoreactivity in rat tissues. *Endocrinol.*, **122**, 2753–63.

Van Houten, M. and Posner, B.I. (1979). Insulin binds to brain blood vessels in vivo. *Nature*, **282**, 623–5.

Vehaskari, V.M., Chang, C.T.C., Stevens, J.K. and Robson, A.M. (1984). The effects of polycations on vascular permeability in the rat. *J. Clin. Invest.*, **73**, 1053–61.

Vidovic, M., Sparacio, S.M., Elovitz, M. and Benveniste, E.N. (1990). Induction and regulation of class II major histocompatibility complex mRNA expression in astrocytes by interferon-γ and tumor necrosis factor-α. *J. Neuroimmunol.*, **30**, 189–200.

Vigne, P. and Frelin, C. (1992). C-type natriuretic peptide is a potent activator of guanylate cyclase in endothelial cells from brain microvessels. *Biochem. Biophys. Res. Commun.*, **183**, 640–4.

Vivés, E., Brodin, V. and Lebleu, B. (1997). A truncated HIV-1 tat protein basic domain rapidly translocates through the plasma membrane and accumulates in the cell nucleus. *J. Biol. Chem.*, **272**, 16010–17.

Vlassov, V.V. and Yakubov, L.A. (1991). Oligonucleotides in cells and in organisms: pharmacological considerations. In *Prospects for Antisense Nucleic Acid Therapy of Cancer and AIDS*, ed. E. Wickstrom, pp. 243–66. New York: Wiley-Liss.

Vogel, L.K., Noren, O. and Sjostrom, H. (1995). Transcytosis of aminopeptidase N in caco-2 cells is mediated by a non-cytoplasmic signal. *J. Biol. Chem.*, **270**, 22933–8.

Vogel, K., Wang, S., Lee, R.J., Chmielewski, J. and Low, P.S. (1996). Peptide-mediated release of folate-targeted liposome contents from endosomal compartments. *J. Am. Chem. Soc.*, **118**, 1581–6.

Vorbrodt, A.W. (1989). Ultracytochemical characterization of anionic sites in the wall of brain capillaries. *J. Neurocytol.*, **18**, 359–68.

Vorbrodt, A.W., Dobrogowska, D.H., Ueno, M. and Lossinsky, A.S. (1995). Immunocytochemical studies of protamine-induced blood–brain barrier opening to endogenous albumin. *Acta Neuropathol.*, **89**, 491–9.

Vorbrodt, A.W., Dobrogowska, D.H., Tarnawski, M., Meeker, H.C. and Carp, R.I. (1997). Immunocytochemical evaluation of blood–brain barrier to endogenous albumin in scrapie-infected mice. *Acta Neuropathol.*, **93**, 341–8.

Wade, L.A. and Katzman, R. (1975). Rat brain regional uptake and decarboxylation of ʟ-DOPA following carotid injection. *Am. J. Physiol.*, **228**, 352–9.

Wagner, H.-J., Pilgrim, Ch. and Brandl, J. (1974). Penetration and removal of horseradish peroxidase injected into the cerebrospinal fluid: role of cerebral perivascular spaces, endothelium and microglia. *Acta Neuropathol.*, **27**, 299–315.

Wagner, E., Zatloukal, K., Cotton, M. et al. (1992). Coupling of adenovirus to transferrin-polylysine/DNA complexes greatly enhances receptor-mediated gene delivery and expression of transfected genes. *Proc. Natl Acad. Sci. USA*, **89**, 6099–103.

Walker, L.C., Masters, C., Beyreuther, K. and Price, D.L. (1990). Amyloid in the brains of aged squirrel monkeys. *Acta Neuropathol.*, **80**, 381–7.

Walker, L.C., Price, D.L., Voytko, M.L. and Schenk, D.B. (1994). Labeling of cerebral amyloid in vivo with a monoclonal antibody. *J. Neuropathol. Exp. Neurol.*, **53**, 377–83.

Watanabe, K., Tachibana, O., Sato, K. et al. (1996). Overexpression of the EGF receptor and p53 mutations are mutually exclusive in the evolution of primary and secondary glioblastomas. *Brain Pathol.*, **6**, 217–24.

Watkins, L.R., Wiertelak, E.P. and Maier, S.F. (1992). Kappa opiate receptors mediate tail-shock induced antinociception at spinal levels. *Brain Res.*, **582**, 1–9.

Weber, M., Mehler, M. and Wollny, E. (1987). Isolation and partial characterization of a 56 000 Dalton phosphoprotein phosphatase from the blood–brain barrier. *J. Neurochem.*, **49**, 1050–6.

Weber, P.C., Ohlendorf, D.H., Wendoloski, J.J. and Salemme, F.R. (1989). Structural origin of high-affinity biotin binding to streptavidin. *Science*, **243**, 85–8.

Wecker, L. and Trommer, B.A. (1984). Effects of chronic (dietary) choline availability on the transport of choline across the blood–brain barrier. *J. Neurochem.*, **43**, 1762–5.

Weindl, A. (1973). Neuroendocrine aspects of circumventricular organs. In *Frontiers in Neuroendocrinology*, ed. W.F. Ganong and L. Martini, pp. 3–32. New York: Oxford University Press.

Weiner, H.L. (1994). Oral tolerance. *Proc. Natl Acad. Sci. USA*, **91**, 10762–5.

Weitman, S.D., Frazier, K.M. and Kamen, B.A. (1994). The folate receptor in central nervous system malignancies of childhood. *J. Neuro-oncol.*, **21**, 107–12.

Welford, S.M., Gregg, J., Chen, E. et al. (1998). Detection of differentially expressed genes in primary tumor tissues using representational differences analysis coupled to microarray hybridization. *Nucl. Acid Res.*, **26**, 3059–65.

Wen, D.Y., Hall, W.A., Conrad, J. et al. (1995). In vitro and in vivo variation in transferrin receptor expression on a human medulloblastoma cell line. *Neurosurg.*, **36**, 1158–64.

Werner, C.B.H., Roberts, C.T. and LeRoith, D. (1992). Cellular pattern of type-I insulin-like growth factor receptor gene expression during maturation of the rat brain: comparison with insulin-like growth factors I and II. *Neurosci.*, **46**, 909–23.

Westergren, I. and Johansson, B.B. (1993). Altering the blood–brain barrier in the rat by intra-carotid infusion of polycations: a comparison between protamine, poly-L-lysine and poly-L-arginine. *Acta Physiol. Scand.*, **149**, 99–104.

Westergren, I., Nystrom, B., Hamberger, A., Nordborg, C. and Johansson, B.B. (1994). Concentrations of amino acids in extracellular fluid after opening of the blood–brain barrier by intracarotid infusion of protamine sulfate. *J. Neurochem.*, **62**, 159–65.

Westergren, I., Nystrom, B., Hamberger, A. and Johansson, B.B. (1995). Intracerebral dialysis and the blood–brain barrier. *J. Neurochem.*, **64**, 229–34.

Westland, K.W., Pollard, J.D., Sander, S. et al. (1999). Activated non-neural specific T cells open the blood–brain barrier to circulating antibodies. *Brain*, **122**, 1283–91.

Weyerbrock, A. and Oldfield, E.H. (1999). Gene transfer technologies for malignant gliomas. *Curr. Opin. Oncol.*, **11**, 168–73.

Whelan, J.P., Eriksson, U.L.F. and Lampson, L.A. (1986). Expression of mouse β_2-microglobulin in frozen and formaldehyde-fixed central nervous tissues: comparison of tissue behind the blood–brain barrier and tissue I, a barrier-free region. *J. Immunol.*, **137**, 2561–6.

White, F.P., Dutton, G.R. and Norenberg, M.D. (1981). Microvessels isolated from rat brain: localization of astrocyte processes by immunohistochemical techniques. *J. Neurochem.*, **36**, 328–32.

Whitesell, L., Geselowitz, D., Chavany, C. et al. (1993). Stability, clearance, and disposition of intraventricularly administered oligodeoxynucleotides: implications for therapeutic application within the central nervous system. *Proc. Natl Acad. Sci. USA*, **90**, 4665–9.

Wilchek, M. and Bayar, E. (1993). Avidin-biotin immobilisation systems. In *Application of Immobilized Macromolecules*, ed. U.B. Sleytr, P. Messner, D. Pum and M. Sara, pp. 51–60. New York: Springer-Verlag.

Williams, S.A., Abbruscato, T.J., Hruby, V.J. and Davis, T.P. (1996). Passage of a δ-opioid receptor selective enkephalin, [D-penicillamine²,⁵] enkephalin, across the blood–brain and the blood–cerebrospinal fluid barriers. *J. Neurochem.*, **66**, 1289–99.

Williams, E.J., Dunican, D.J., Green, P.J. et al. (1997). Selective inhibition of growth factor-stimulated mitogenesis by a cell-permeable grb2-binding peptide. *J. Biol. Chem.*, **272**, 22349–54.

Wilson, D.A., O'Neill, J.T., Said, S.I. and Traystman, R.J. (1981). Vasoactive intestinal polypeptide and the canine cerebral circulation. *Circ. Res.*, **48**, 138–48.

Wilson, G.L., Dean, B.S., Wang, G. and Dean, D.A. (1999). Nuclear import of plasmid DNA in digitonin-permeabilized cells requires both cytoplasmic factors and specific DNA sequences. *J. Biol. Chem.*, **274**, 22025–32.

Winkler, T., Sharma, H.S., Stalberg, E., Olsson, Y. and Dey, P.K. (1995). Impairment of blood–brain barrier function by serotonin induces desynchronization of spontaneous cerebral cortical activity: experimental observations in the anaesthetized rat. *Neurosci.*, **68**, 1097–104.

Winkler, J., Ramirez, G.A., Kuhn, H.G. et al. (1997). Reversible schwann cell hyperplasia and sprouting of sensory and sympathetic neurites after intraventricular administration of nerve growth factor. *Ann. Neurol.*, **41**, 82–93.

Wizigmann-Voos, S., Breier, G., Risau, W. and Plate, K.H. (1995). Up-regulation of vascular endothelial growth factor and its receptors in von Hippel–Lindau disease-associated and sporadic hemangioblastomas. *Cancer Res.*, **55**, 1358–64.

Wojcik, W.J., Swoveland, P., Zhang, X. and Vanguri, P. (1996). Chronic intrathecal infusion of phosphorothioate or phosphodiester antisense oligonucleotides against cytokine responsive gene-2/IP-10 in experimental allergic encephalomyelitis of Lewis rat. *J. Pharmacol. Exp. Ther.*, **278**, 404–10.

Wong, A.J., Bigner, S.H., Bigner, D.D. et al. (1987). Increased expression of the epidermal growth factor receptor gene in malignant gliomas is invariably associated with gene amplification. *Proc. Natl Acad. Sci. USA*, **84**, 6899–903.

Wood, M.J.A., Charlton, H.M., Wood, K.J., Kajiwara, K. and Byrnes, A.P. (1996). Immune responses to adenovirus vectors in the nervous system. *Trends Neurosci.*, **19**, 497–501.

Wu, C. and Ghosh, S. (1999). β-TrCP mediates the signal induced ubiquitination of IκBβ. *J. Biol. Chem.*, **274**, 29591–4.

Wu, D. and Pardridge, W.M. (1996). CNS pharmacologic effect in conscious rats after intravenous injection of biotinylated vasoactive intestinal peptide analogue coupled to a blood–brain barrier drug delivery system. *J. Pharmacol. Exp. Ther.*, **279**, 77–83.

Wu, D. and Pardridge, W.M. (1998). Pharmacokinetics and blood–brain barrier transport of an anti-transferrin receptor monoclonal antibody (OX26) in rats after chronic treatment with the antibody. *Drug Metab. Disp.*, **26**, 937–9.

Wu, D. and Pardridge, W.M. (1999a). Blood–brain barrier transport of reduced folic acid. *Pharm. Res.*, **16**, 415–19.

Wu, D. and Pardridge, W.M. (1999b). Neuroprotection with noninvasive neurotrophin delivery to brain. *Proc. Natl Acad. Sci. USA*, **96**, 254–9.

Wu, G.Y., Wilson, J.M., Shalaby, F. et al. (1991). Receptor-mediated gene delivery in vitro. *J. Biol. Chem.*, **266**, 14338–42.

Wu, D., Boado, R.J. and Pardridge, W.M. (1996). Pharmacokinetics and blood–brain barrier transport of [^{3}H]-biotinylated phosphorothioate oligodeoxynucleotide conjugated to a vector-mediated drug delivery system. *J. Pharmacol. Exp. Ther.*, **276**, 206–11.

Wu, D., Kang, Y.-S., Bickel, U. and Pardridge, W.M. (1997a). Blood–brain barrier permeability to morphine-6-glucuronide is markedly reduced compared to morphine. *Drug Metab. Disp.*, **25**, 768–71.

Wu, D., Yang, J. and Pardridge, W.M. (1997b). Drug targeting of a peptide radiopharmaceutical through the primate blood–brain barrier in vivo with a monoclonal antibody to the human insulin receptor. *J. Clin. Invest.*, **100**, 1804–12.

Wu, D., Clement, J.G. and Pardridge, W.M. (1998). Low blood–brain barrier permeability to azidothymidine (AZT), 3TC^{TM} and thymidine and the rat. *Brain Res.*, **791**, 313–16.

Xiang, T.-X. and Anderson, B.D. (1994). The relationship between permeant size and permeability in lipid bilayer membranes. *J. Membr. Biol.*, **140**, 111–22.

Yakubov, L., Khaled, Z., Zhang, L.-M. et al. (1993). Oligonucleotides interact with recombinant CD4 at multiple sites. *J. Biol. Chem.*, **268**, 18818–23.

Yamada, K., Kinoshita, A., Kohmura, E. et al. (1991). Basic fibroblast growth factor prevents thalamic degeneration after cortical infarction. *J. Cereb. Blood Flow Metab.*, **11**, 472–8.

Yamamoto, T., Geiger, J.D., Daddona, P.E. and Nagy, J.I. (1987). Subcellular regional and immuno-histochemical localization of adenosine deaminase in various species. *Brain Res.*, 19, 473–84.

Yamane, A., Seetharam, L., Yamaguchi, S. et al. (1994). A new communication system between hepatocytes and sinusoidal endothelial cells in liver through vascular endothelial growth factor and FLT tyrosine kinase receptor family (FLT-1 and KDR/FLK-1). *Oncogene*, 9, 2683–90.

Yan, Q., Matheson, C., Sun, J. et al. (1994). Distribution of intracerebral ventricularly administered neurotrophins in rat brain and its correlation with Trk receptor expression. *Exp. Neurol.*, 127, 23–36.

Yarchoan, R. and Broder, S. (1987). Development of antiretroviral therapy for the acquired immunodeficiency syndrome and related disorders. *N. Engl. J. Med.*, 316, 557–64.

Yoshikawa, T. and Pardridge, W.M. (1992). Biotin delivery to brain with a covalent conjugate of avidin and a monoclonal antibody to the transferrin receptor. *J. Pharmacol. Exp. Ther.*, 263, 897–903.

Yuan, F., Salehi, H.A., Boucher, Y. et al. (1994). Vascular permeability and microcirculation of gliomas and mammary carcinomas transplanted in rat and mouse cranial windows. *Cancer Res.*, 54, 4564–8.

Zabner, J., Fasbender, A.J., Moninger, T., Poellinger, K.A. and Welsh, M.J. (1995). Cellular and molecular barriers to gene transfer by a cationic lipid. *J. Biol. Chem.*, 270, 18997–9007.

Zahniser, N.R., Goens, B., Hanaway, P.J. and Vinych, J.V. (1984). Characterization and regulation of insulin receptors in rat brain. *J. Neurochem.*, 42, 1354–62.

Zalipsky, S. (1995). Functionalized poly(ethylene glycol) for preparation of biologically relevant conjugates. *Bioconj. Chem.*, 6, 150–65.

Zendegui, J.G., Vasquez, K.M., Tinsley, J.H., Kessler, D.J. and Hogan, M.E. (1992). In vivo stability and kinetics of absorption and disposition of 3′ phosphopropyl amine oligonucleotides. *Nucl. Acids Res.*, 20, 307–14.

Zhang, Y. and Pardridge, W.M. (2001). Conjugation of brain-derived neurotrophic factor to a blood–brain barrier drug-targeting system enables neuroprotection in regional brain ischemia following intravenous injection of the neurotrophin. *Brain Res.*, 889, 49–56.

Zhang, B. and Roth, R.A. (1991). A region of the insulin receptor important for ligand binding (residues 450–601) is recognized by patients' autoimmune antibodies and inhibitory monoclonal antibodies. *Proc. Natl Acad. Sci. USA*, 88, 9858–62.

Zhang, E.T., Inman, C.B.E. and Weller, R.O. (1990). Interrelationships of the pia mater and the perivascular (Virchow–Robin) spaces in the human cerebrum. *J. Anat.*, 170, 111–23.

Zhang, R.-D., Price, J.E., Fujimaki, T., Bucana, C.D. and Fidler, I.J. (1992). Differential permeability of the blood–brain barrier in experimental brain metastases produced by human neoplasms implanted into nude mice. *Am. J. Pathol.*, 141, 1115–24.

Zhang, Y., Proenca, R., Maffei, M. et al. (1994). Positional cloning of the mouse obese gene and its human homologue. *Nature*, 372, 425–31.

Zhang, L., Ong, W.Y. and Lee, T. (1999a). Induction of p-glycoprotein expression in astrocytes following intracerebroventricular kainate injections. *Exp. Brain Res.*, 126, 509–16.

Zhang, W.R., Kitagawa, H, Hayashi, T. et al. (1999b). Topical application of neurotrophin-3 attenuates ischemic brain injury after transient middle cerebral artery occlusion in rats. *Brain Res.*, 842, 211–14.

Zhao, R., Seither, R., Brigle, K.E. et al. (1997). Impact of overexpression of the reduced folate carrier (RFC1), an anion exchanger, on concentrative transport in murine L1210 leukemia cells. *J. Biol. Chem.*, **272**, 21207–12.

Zhao, W., Chen, H., Xu, H. et al. (1999). Brain insulin receptors and spatial memory. *J. Biol. Chem.*, **274**, 34893–902.

Zhu, N., Liggitt, D., Liu, Y. and Debs, R. (1993). Systemic gene expression after intravenous DNA delivery into adult mice. *Science*, **261**, 209–11.

Zhu, J., Zhang, L., Hanisch, U.K., Felgner, P.L. and Reszka, R. (1996). A continuous intracerebral gene delivery system for in vivo liposome-mediated gene therapy. *Gene Ther.*, **3**, 472–6.

Zick, Y., Rees-Jones, R.W., Taylor, S.I., Gorden, P. and Roth, J. (1984). The role of antireceptor antibodies in stimulating phosphorylation of the insulin receptor. *J. Biol. Chem.*, **259**, 4396–400.

Zlokovic, B.V., Begley, D.J. and Chain-Eliash, D.G. (1985). Blood–brain barrier permeability to leucine-enkephalin, D-alanine^2-D-leucine^5-enkephalin and their N-terminal amino acid (tyrosine). *Brain Res.*, **336**, 125–32.

Zou, L.L., Huang, L., Hayes, R.L. et al. (1999). Liposome-mediated NGF gene transfection following neuronal injury: potential therapeutic applications. *Gene Ther.*, **6**, 994–1005.

Zünkeler, B., Carson, R.E., Olson, J. et al. (1996). Quantification and pharmacokinetics of blood–brain barrier disruption in humans. *J. Neurosurg.*, **85**, 1056–65.

Index